Type 2 Diabetes

Type 2 Diabetes

Prediction and Prevention

Edited by

GRAHAM A. HITMAN

St Bartholomew's and the
Royal London School of Medicine and Dentistry, London, UK

JOHN WILEY & SONS
Chichester • New York • Weinheim • Brisbane • Singapore • Toronto

National 01243 779777
International (+44) 1243 779777
e-mail (for orders and customer service enquiries): cs-books@wiley.co.uk
Visit our Home Page on http://www.wiley.co.uk
or http://www.wiley.com

Other Wiley Editorial Offices

John Wiley & Sons, Inc, 605 Third Avenue,
New York, NY 10158-0012, USA

WILEY-VCH Verlag GmbH, Pappelallee 3,
D-69469 Weinheim, Germany

Jacaranda Wiley Ltd, 33 Park Road, Milton
Queensland 4064, Australia

John Wiley & Sons (Asia) Pte Ltd, 2 Clementi Loop #02-01,
Jin Xing Distripark, Singapore 129809

John Wiley & Sons (Canada) Ltd, 22 Worcester Road,
Rexdale, Ontario M9W 1Ll, Canada

Library of Congress Cataloging-in-Publication Data

Type 2 diabetes : prediction and prevention / edited by Graham A. Hitman.
p. cm. — (Wiley practical diabetes series)
Includes bibliographical references and index.
ISBN 0-471-98595-3 (cased)
1. Non-insulin-dependent diabetes—Risk factors. 2. Non-insulin-dependent diabetes—Genetic aspects. 3. Non-insulin-dependent diabetes—Prevention. I. Hitman, Graham A. II. Title: Type two diabetes. III. Series.
[DNLM: 1. Diabetes Mellitus, Non-Insulin-Dependent—genetics.
2. Diabetes Mellitus, Non-Insulin-Dependent—prevention & control.
WK 810 T9913 1999]
RC662.18.T97 1999
616.4′62—dc21
DNLM/DLC
for Library of Congress 98–48819
CIP

British Library Cataloguing in Publication Data

A catalogue record for this book is available from the British Library

ISBN 0-471-98595-3

Typeset in 10/12pt Times from the author's disks by Keyword Typesetting Services Ltd, Wallington, Surrey.
Printed and bound in Great Britain by Biddles Ltd, Guildford and King's Lynn.
This book is printed on acid-free paper responsibly manufactured from sustainable forestry, in which at least two trees are planted for each one used for paper production.

Contents

Preface

It is currently estimated that there are 100 million people worldwide with diabetes and this figure is likely to increase two- to three-fold in the next 10 years, the predominant burden being felt in developing countries. Of the major forms of diabetes mellitus, cases of Type 2 diabetes outnumber Type 1 diabetes by ten to one. The challenge as we come into the next millennium must be how we might *predict* and *prevent* Type 2 diabetes mellitus, rather than just treat the consequences of the disease. The financial cost of diabetes accounts for four to five percent of the British health care budget, whereas in other countries it can be as much as ten percent. However, this does not take into account the indirect costs due to the person's reaction to their own illness.

Type 2 diabetes research has reached an extremely critical and exciting period where advances in its understanding have led to detection of some of the causes and important associated factors contributing to Type 2 diabetes. Thus, for the first time, we are in a real position to start planning how we might alleviate the future burden of Type 2 diabetes. Furthermore, many non-communicable diseases share antecedents with Type 2 diabetes mellitus and therefore any programme to prevent Type 2 diabetes mellitus will also impact on many other diseases such as ischaemic heart disease, hypertension, dyslipidaemia and obesity. The purpose of this book is to highlight the main areas of research whereby prediction and prevention of Type 2 diabetes will become a reality in the next millennium.

The book starts by setting the scene, providing the reader with an overview of Type 2 diabetes. It has been said that we are in the middle of an epidemic of diabetes. The evidence that there is an increasing prevalence of Type 2 diabetes is reviewed. Both Type 1 and Type 2 diabetes are multifactorial diseases with a strong genetic component. If a family member already has diabetes then other family members are likely to have markers of future susceptibility to disease and are a prime target group for testing prevention strategies. Indeed, in Type 1 diabetes, siblings at high risk of disease are currently being treated in large multicentre trials to assess strategies to prevent diabetes. Although for 10–15 years investigators have been trying to identify the precise genes involved in Type 2 diabetes susceptibility, it has only been comparatively recently that advances in technology have meant this is a real possibility. In 1999, we are likely to see the identification of at least 2 or 3 genes involved in Type 2 diabetes. The majority of the genetic causes of maturity onset diabetes of the young (MODY) and the insulin resistance syndromes have now been elucidated and this has been recognised in the new re-classification of diabetes adopted by the American Diabetes Association and proposed by the World Health Organisation. There are still many genes to be identified for the more common causes of diabetes and several chapters describe the exciting methods and progress in this area from the use of animal models to genome screening in man.

The elucidation of the environmental factors associated with Type 2 diabetes is another rapidly advancing research area. The realisation that environmental factors can affect intrauterine development and the subsequent risk of Type 2 diabetes has been an important advance in the field and remind us that environment affects disease predisposition throughout life, not just in adult life. The strategies that will be employed to prevent Type 2 diabetes will be manifold, some of which are already in progress, or indeed already applied to other non-communicable diseases. A large part of the book therefore deals with aspects of screening in the community and prevention strategies.

This book raises more questions than answers; the last section of the book therefore addresses future developments. The important impact of a rising prevalence of diabetes is discussed in detail. For instance, by the year 2010, it is predicted that India will have the largest number of subjects of diabetes in the world and by 2025 there will be the same number of subjects with diabetes in India as the total population of the UK. As the genes for Type 2 diabetes are identified, the medical community needs to consider the role of genetic counselling and ethical aspects of screening for monogenic and polygenic disease. Gene therapy may have a role in the future and the possible approaches to this are described. The last chapter considers the important aspect of costs and profits of prevention.

Graham A. Hitman

Contributors

L. Aerts *Laboratory of Obstetrics and Gynaecology, U.Z. Gasthuisberg, Herestraat 49, Leuven B-3000, Belgium*

P. Beales *Division of Medical and Molecular Genetics, 8th Floor, Guy's Tower, Guy's Hospital, London SE1 9RT, UK*

F. Beards *Division of Molecular Genetics, Diabetes Research, Postgraduate Medical School, University of Exeter, Barrack Road, Exeter, Devon EX2 5AX, UK*

K. Borch-Johnsen *Steno Diabetes Center, Niels Steensens Vej 2, 2820 Gentofte, Denmark*

B. J. Boucher *Medical Unit, St Bartholomew's and the Royal London School of Medicine and Dentistry, The Royal London Hospital, Whitechapel, London E1 1BB, UK*

M. de Courten *International Diabetes Institute, 260 Kooyong Road, Caulfield 3162, Victoria, Australia*

Professor K. Docherty *Department of Molecular and Cell Biology, University of Aberdeen, Institute of Medical Sciences, Foresterhill, Aberdeen AB25 2ZD, UK*

A. Dornhorst *Department of Metabolic Medicine, Imperial College School of Medicine, Hammersmith Hospital, London W12 0NN, UK*

M. R. Druce *Department of Metabolic Medicine, Imperial College School of Medicine, Hammersmith Hospital, London W12 0NN, UK*

T. Frayling *Division of Molecular Genetics, Diabetes Research, Postgraduate Medical School, University of Exeter, Barrack Road, Exeter, Devon EX2 5AX, UK*

Professor C. N. Hales *Department of Clinical Biochemistry, Box 232, Addenbrooke's Hospital, Hills Road, Cambridge CB2 2QR, UK*

A. Hattersley *Division of Molecular Genetics, Diabetes Research, Postgraduate Medical School, University of Exeter, Barrack Road, Exeter, Devon EX2 5AX, UK*

P. Havel *Department of Nutrition, University of California at Davis, Davis, California 95616, USA*

Professor R. J. Heine *Department of Endocrinology, Vrije Universiteit, University Hospital, PO Box 7057, 1007 MB Amsterdam, The Netherlands*

K. Holemans *Laboratory of Obstetrics and Gynaecology, U.Z. Gasthuisberg, Herestraat 49, Leuven B-3000, Belgium*

Professor P. G. Kopelman *Medical Unit, St Bartholomew's and the Royal London School of Medicine and Dentistry, Queen Mary and Westfield College, London E1 2AB, UK*

J. C. Levy *Diabetes Research Laboratories, The Radcliffe Infirmary, Oxford OX2 6HE, UK*

M. McCarthy *Unit of Metabolic Medicine, Imperial College School of Medicine at St. Mary's, Norfolk Place, London W2 1PG, UK*

D. McCarty *International Diabetes Institute, 260 Kooyong Road, Caulfield 3162, Victoria, Australia*

P. O'Connell *Department of Pathology, University of Texas Health Science Centre, 7703 Floyd Curl Drive, San Antonio, Texas 78284, USA*

Professor O. Pedersen *Steno Diabetes Center, Niels Steensens Vej 2, DK 2820 Gentofte, Denmark*

C.J. Petry *Department of Clinical Biochemistry, Box 232, Addenbrooke's Hospital, Hills Road, Cambridge CB2 2QR, UK*

A. Ramachandran *Diabetes Research Centre, 4 Main Road, Royapuram, Madras-600 013, India*

N. Schonfeld-Warden *Department of Paediatrics, University of California at Davis, Davis, California 95616, USA*

J. A. M. Shaw *Department of Molecular and Cell Biology, University of Aberdeen, Institute of Medical Sciences, Foresterhill, Aberdeen AB25 2ZD, UK*

D. Simmons *Department of Rural Health, University of Melbourne, c/o Gouldburn Valley Base Hospital, Graham Street, Shepparton, Victoria 3630, Australia*

C. Snehalatha *Diabetes Research Centre, 4 Main Road, Royapuram, Madras-600 013, India*

M. P. Stern *Department of Medicine, University of Texas Health Science Centre, 7703 Floyd Curl Drive, San Antonio, Texas 78284, USA*

Professor J. Tuomilehto *Diabetes and Genetic Epidemiology Unit, Department of Epidemiology and Health Promotion, National Public Health Institute, , Mannerheimintie 166, FIN-00300, Helsinki, Finland*

Dr F. A. van Assche *Laboratory of Obstetrics and Gynaecology, U.Z. Gasthuisberg, Herestraat 49, Leuven B-3000, Belgium*

M. Walker *Human Diabetes and Metabolism Research Centre, School of Clinical Medical Sciences, Floor 4, William Leech Building, The Medical School, Newcastle upon Tyne NE2 4HH, UK*

C. H. Warden *Rowe Genetics and Department of Paediatrics, University of California at Davis, Davis, California 95616, USA*

R. Wing *University of Pittsburgh Medical Center, Western Psychiatric Institute and Clinic, 3811 O'Hara Street, Pittsburgh, PA 15213-2593, USA*

Professor P. Zimmet *International Diabetes Institute, 260 Kooyong Road, Caulfield 3162, Victoria, Australia*

Part A

Introduction

1

Aetiology

J.C. LEVY

Diabetes Research Laboratories, The Radcliffe Infirmary, Oxford OX2 6HE, UK

The National Diabetes Data Group (NDDG)[1] and the World Heath Organization (WHO)[2] classifications of diabetes in the 1980s clarified research into the aetiology of diabetes by separating primary diabetes into insulin-dependent diabetes mellitus (or type 1 diabetes) and non-insulin-dependent diabetes mellitus (or type 2 diabetes). However, although the former was a relatively homogeneous pathophysiological entity, the latter was essentially a clinical entity and a diagnosis of exclusion, and over the subsequent two decades, its heterogeneity has become evident. The recent proposals by the American Diabetes Association (ADA)[3] and the World Health Organization (WHO)[4] have attempted to reclassify diabetes on aetiological grounds, though it was recognized by the committees that any such attempt at the present time must necessarily be provisional (Table 1.1). The committees adopted, with modifications, the terms type 1 and type 2 diabetes, which dated from the recognition in the late 1970s of the genetically distinct autoimmune aetiology of 'juvenile diabetes'[5]. It has recently been recognized that an appreciable minority of type 2 patients also share serological and genetic features, with autoimmune diabetes usually presenting in children[6–10]. Although it is possible that such serological markers are secondary to islet β-cell damage from some other cause, it seems likely that a primary autoimmune aetiology may account for about 10% of type 2 diabetes[6–10]. A further subset of type 2 diabetes has been splintered off in recent years by precise genetic characterization. Single gene defects have been identified for a substantial proportion of cases of maturity-onset diabetes of the young.[11–14], but, together with mitochondrial mutations[15,16], which are typically associated with maternally inherited diabetes and deafness, these account for only a small percentage of idiopathic type 2 diabetes. In common with autoimmune diabetes, these simple genetic forms of diabetes primarily affect the β cell, and the new classifications assume

Type 2 Diabetes: Prediction and Prevention. Edited by Graham A. Hitman

Table 1.1. WHO provisional aetiological classification of disorders of glycaemia

Type 1 (β-cell destruction, usually leading to absolute insulin deficiency)
Autoimmune
Idiopathic

Type 2 (may range from predominantly insulin resistance with relative deficiency to a predominantly secretory defect with or without insulin resistance)

Other specific types

Genetic defects of β-cell function
- Chromosome 20, HNF-4α (MODY1)
- Chromosome 7, glucokinase (MODY2)
- Chromosome 12, HNF-1α (MODY3)
- Mitochondrial DNA 3243 mutation
- Others

Genetic defects of insulin action
- Type A insulin resistance
- Leprechaunism
- Rabson–Mendenhall syndrome
- Lipoatrophic diabetes
- Others

Diseases of exocrine pancreas
- Fibrocalculous pancreatopathy
- Pancreatitis
- Trauma/pancreatectomy
- Neoplasia
- Cystic fibrosis
- Haemochromatosis
- Others

Endocrinopathies
- Cushing's syndrome
- Acromegaly
- Phaeochromocytoma
- Glucagonoma
- Hyperthyroidism
- Somatostatinoma
- Others

Drug or chemical induced
- Nicotinic acid
- Glucorticoids
- Thyroid hormone
- α-Adrenergic agonists
- β-Adrenergic agonists
- Thiazides
- Phenytoin
- Pentamidine
- Interferon-α therapy
- Others

Infections
- Congenital rubella
- Cytomegalovirus
- Others

Uncommon forms of immune-mediated diabetes
- Insulin autoimmune syndrome (antibodies to insulin)
- Anti-insulin receptor antibodies
- 'Stiff man' syndrome
- Others

Other genetic syndromes
- Down's syndrome
- Friedreich's ataxia
- Huntington's disease
- Klinefelter's syndrome
- Laurence–Moon–Biedel syndrome
- Myotonic dystrophy
- Porphyria
- Prader–Willi syndrome
- Turner's syndrome
- Wolfram's syndrome
- Others

Gestational diabetes (includes former categories of gestational impaired glucose tolerance and gestational diabetes)

HNF-4α, hepatic nuclear factor 4α.
From American Diabetes Association Export Committee[3].

that the aetiologyof diabetes is characterized by a major dichotomy between diabetes resulting from 'β-cell' defects and that caused by a combination of β-cell defect and insulin resistance (Table 1.1). Nevertheless, even after hiving off these specific genetically and serologically characterized subtypes, type 2 diabetes remains a heterogeneous disease.

For a complete understanding of the aetiology of the condition, it would be necessary to identify mechanisms at every level of biology: from genetics through biochemistry to molecular biology and physiology; it would also be necessary to describe the interaction between the organism and the environment. We are very far from this goal. Specific disciplines have shed some light in many of these areas, though in many instances this only illuminates further complexity.

GENES

Type 2 diabetes is a familial disease, and there are convincing arguments to support its partial genetic determination. The lifetime risk of a first-degree relative of a patient with type 2 diabetes has been estimated at about 35%, with the relative risk of diabetes compared with the general population, of between three- and fourfold. Twin studies have shown much higher concordance among homozygotic (50–90%) compared with dizygotic twins[17,18]. Different ethnic groups sharing the same environment have different rates of diabetes[19] and in ethnically mixed populations the prevalence of diabetes relates to the degree of genetic admixture[20]. The nature of the genetic contribution is unclear. Segregation analyses have pointed towards complex genetic models[21,22], and it is likely that several genes confer diabetes susceptibility. It is also possible that diabetes in different populations is the product of different patterns of these genes. Genome-wide scanning has identified loci linked to type 2 diabetes on chromosome 2q in a Mexican–American population[23], and on chromosome 12 in a subgroup of Finnish families[24]; as yet, no consistent genetic locus has been identified across different populations. Similarly, the screening of candidate genes has yielded little consistent association with diabetes itself, although a mutation in the gene for the insulin receptor substrate 1 has been associated with insulin resistance in subgroups of more than one population[25,26]. The methodological difficulties of genetic studies in type 2 diabetes are considerable. Not only is the genetic predisposition complex and the penetrance age related and highly dependent on environmental factors, but also its late onset and increased mortality make pedigree collections difficult[27,28] and identity-by-descent information hard to obtain. Nevertheless, the technology and science of genetic research in complex disease such as diabetes are developing rapidly, and promise significant advances in our understanding of their aetiology.

ENVIRONMENT

There is also ample evidence of an important environmental contribution to the aetiology of type 2 diabetes[29]. Secular changes in prevalence within populations, differing prevalence in urban and rural communities within the same ethnic groups, and migration studies showing increased prevalence in populations moving from relatively underdeveloped to 'Westernized' societies all support the hypothesis that changes in diet and physical activity have a marked influence on the development of the condition. Within populations, obesity, particularly if centrally distributed[30], and the habitual level of exercise and physical fitness[31,32], are strong determinants of risk. However, as mentioned above, the impact of the environment on these intermediate risk factors differs between different ethnic groups and between families within ethnic groups and undoubtedly interacts with genetic determinants.

BIRTHWEIGHT

A specific environmental effect that has received considerable attention recently is the relationship of intrauterine growth to the subsequent development of diabetes, obesity and several cardiovascular risk factors[33,34]. Babies who are small or thin at birth have a relative impairment of glucose tolerance and an increased prevalence of type 2 diabetes in later life, which has been attributed to defects in both pancreatic function[35,36] and to insulin sensitivity[37,38]. Although the effect of birthweight has been confirmed in several populations, it is unlikely to be the major contributor to the pathogenesis of diabetes, and intergenerational relationships of birthweight and cardiovascular risk make these observations intriguing but complex.

NATURAL HISTORY

Type 2 diabetes is a progressive disease, characterized by a steady increase in hyperglycaemia from the time of diagnosis. Underlying this is a concomitant deterioration in pancreatic β-cell function, with no significant change in insulin resistance[39]. The reasons for this have not been elucidated. Neither sulphonylureas, which stimulate insulin secretion, nor metformin, which potentiates insulin action, affects the rate of deterioration[40]. As both these agents significantly lower plasma glucose concentrations, it would appear unlikely that alterations in plasma glucose within the diabetic range significantly affect the rate of decline.

PHYSIOLOGY AND BIOCHEMISTRY

From the discovery of the insulin deficiency in juvenile diabetes and the recognition by Himsworth of the phenomenon of relative ineffectiveness of exogenous insulin in a large proportion of patients with diabetes of later onset[41], the principal causes of hyperglycaemia have been seen in terms of either pancreatic dysfunction or insulin resistance. Most researchers now recognize that both defects coexist in most people with type 2 diabetes.

CHARACTERISTICS OF TYPE 2 DIABETES AND SUBGROUPS PRONE TO TYPE 2 DIABETES

Hyperglycaemia can itself have deleterious effects on both β-cell function and insulin resistance[42,43] and, to avoid the confounding effects of this 'glucose toxicity', researchers have tried to identify its physiological antecedents in groups particularly at risk of developing diabetes. Cross-sectional studies of individuals with impaired control of either basal glycaemia or the response to administered glucose (impaired glucose tolerance or IGT) have identified defects of both insulin secretion and insulin sensitivity at the earliest stages of the disease. The same has been found in non-diabetic women who have had gestational diabetes[44], and in first-degree relatives of patients with diabetes[45,46]. Whether this early coexistance of the two disorders represents an underlying physiological link, or whether it is an artefact of the study of heterogeneous groups is not yet known.

β-CELL FUNCTION

Pancreatic β cells have an enormous capacity to adapt to sustained increases in demand, as demonstrated by the fact that extremes of insulin resistance produced by genetic insulin receptor abnormalities lead to greatly increased plasma insulin concentrations, but do not necessarily result in diabetes[47]. Although this may partly reflect impaired insulin clearance, reversible changes in insulin resistance, such as pregnancy, illness or obesity, also demonstrate significant degrees of adaptation. This adaptation is seen even in the presence of demonstrable β-cell impairment[48] and has two distinct implications. The first concerns experimental method: an obese subject with impaired glucose tolerance may have higher plasma insulin concentrations than a non-obese, non-diabetic control, and it is only by relating insulin secretion to the degree of insulin resistance that impairment in β-cell function can be demonstrated[49]. The second implication is that, in the presence of hyperglycaemia, insulin resistance is necessarily accompanied by a degree of β-cell failure, in the sense of a failure to adapt.

GLOBAL DEFICIT IN INSULIN SECRETION

In vitro studies of β-cell function have described two phases of insulin secretion in response to a step change in glucose concentration, the first phase consisting of a large, but transient, burst and the second a slow, steady increase in insulin release. This is seen in vivo in the plasma insulin response to an intravenous bolus of glucose. Marked diminution of the in vivo first phase has long been associated with mild type 2 diabetes[50]. The apparently maintained second phase response is, however, difficult to interpret because of the relative hyperglycaemia in the diabetic group and, after the development of the glucose clamp technique, there is evidence to suggest that the impairment of glucose-stimulated insulin secretion is applies to both phases[51].

DISPROPORTIONATE SECRETION OF PROINSULIN MOLECULES

The translation product of the insulin gene, pre-proinsulin, is processed by successive proteolytic cleavages through proinsulin, various species of split proinsulin, with the eventual removal of C-peptide to insulin. In non-diabetic individuals, small quantities of partially processed peptides are secreted alongside insulin. Secretion of these proinsulin species increases with β-cell stimulation, but the proportion of proinsulin to insulin remains fairly constant. Therefore, insulin-resistant subjects will have higher concentrations of plasma proinsulin molecules than normal controls. However, in people with type 2 diabetes, in pre-diabetic states, and in particular circumstances such as corticosteroid administration, the proportion of proinsulin to insulin is increased, possibly indicating an intrinsic β-cell defect[52]. However, it has not been established whether this is primary or secondary, for example, to a sustained, excessive increase in demand. An increased proinsulin to insulin ratio is seen in siblings of people with type 1 diabetes and in subtotal pancreatectomy in humans and animal models, where there would be no reason to expect a primary β-cell defect[53].

AMYLOID

The pancreatic islets of 95% of both humans with type 2 diabetes and diabetic rhesus monkeys, and some other species, are characterized by the deposition of a specific amyloid, the fibrils of which are primarily composed of islet amyloid polypeptide (IAPP; synonym amylin)[54], which is a peptide made up of 37 amino acids co-secreted with insulin from the granules of normal β cells[55]. Islet amyloid is rarely found in non-diabetic subjects. The striking specificity of this histological change for type 2 diabetes has not been explained and may represent either a primary or a secondary abnormality.

The cause of the deposition has not been determined, but IAPP in people with diabetes is structurally normal, and mutations related to the IAPP gene have not been described. In diabetic islets it is accompanied by some depletion of β-cell numbers[56]. In vitro evidence suggests that it may be toxic to the β cell.

MECHANISMS OF STIMULATION OF INSULIN SECRETION

The biochemical pathways of the stimulation of insulin secretion have been greatly clarified over the past decade. In the nutrient pathway, molecules that can be metabolized, such as glucose, cause an increase in the ATP:ADP ratio, altered binding to the 'sulphonylurea receptor', SUR-1, and the associated inwardly rectifying potassium channel, KIR 6.2. This closes the channel, with subsequent cell depolarization, voltage-dependent calcium channel activation and granule secretion. Mutations in glucokinase, the principal enzyme responsible for glucose phosphorylation in the β cell and the so-called 'glucose sensor' of the β cell, cause a dominantly inherited, stable form of mild diabetes[11]. Mutations in mitochondrial DNA also cause β-cell deficiency and maternally transmitted diabetes, in addition to a wide spectrum of other congenital abnormalities, including sensorineural deafness[57], presumably because of the central role of mitochondrial respiration in the generation of ATP. In most of the people with type 2 diabetes, however, no genetic abnormalities of this pathway have been described[58].

Physiological non-nutrient secretagogues are primarily hormonal and act by binding to cell surface receptors, not through substrate metabolism. These include circulating peptides such as gastrointestinal polypeptide (GIP) and glucagon-like peptide-1 (GLP-1), which work by stimulating intracellular cyclic AMP (cAMP), and other molecules such as acetylcholine, cholecystokinin and some neurotransmitters, which stimulate phospholipase C, generating inositol phosphates and diacylglycerol. This leads to the liberation of intracellular calcium stores and the activation of protein kinase C. Non-nutrient secretagogues generally potentiate nutrient-stimulated insulin secretion, but they cannot initiate it by themselves. Defects in this pathway have not been identified in type 2 diabetes, but GLP-1, in concentrations only two to three times the upper limit of the physiological range, has been shown to be able to stimulate insulin secretion into the normal range in diabetic patients who are poorly controlled on maximal sulphonylurea therapy. The degree to which this highlights intrinsic defects in the adenylyl cyclase–cAMP pathway has still to be elucidated.

INSULIN RESISTANCE

Insulin sensitivity is the measure of effectiveness of insulin action, at either the tissue or the whole body level. Decreased insulin sensitivity, or insulin resistance in the context of impaired insulin secretion, causes the hyperglycaemia in a substantial proportion of people with type 2 diabetes. A wide variety of different aetiological mechanisms will decrease the effectiveness of insulin action at the tissue or whole body level, and the aetiology of insulin resistance in type 2 diabetes is likely to be heterogeneous. Potential contributors include: obesity, particularly central obesity; inactivity; altered concentrations of metabolites, such as sustained high glucose or non-esterified fatty acids; possibly hormones, such as growth hormone, corticosteroids or catecholamines; acute phase reactants, such as tumour necrosis factor α; or interleukins 1 or 6. Insulin resistance has been shown to have a familial association, although the degree to which this is environmental or genetic has not been determined. Although insulin resistance refers to impairment in the glucose-lowering actions of insulin, it may be accompanied by impaired insulin action on metabolism of fatty acids, triglycerides or amino acids. In the context of glycaemic control, however, the principal defects in insulin action are at the level of the muscle or the liver.

PERIPHERY AND LIVER

In the postprandial state, plasma glucose is maintained by the balance of endogenous glucose production, primarily by the liver, and tissue glucose uptake, by either (1) insulin-insensitive tissues, such as the brain, intestine and blood cells, or (2) insulin-sensitive tissues, such as muscle and adipose tissue. As the latter account for only about 25% of glucose uptake in the fasting state, the control of fasting glucose is primarily the result of the rate of hepatic glucose output (HGO). This will depend on the balance of insulin in the portal blood, and 'counterregulatory' factors, including portal glucagon and fatty acids. Hepatic glucose output is progressively elevated with deterioration of control in type 2 diabetes.[59], and has been shown to be resistant to the suppressive effect of insulin, in parallel with insulin resistance in muscle[60]. Recently, insulin resistance in the hepatocyte has been postulated to be caused by an indirect pathway. By this hypothesis, insulin resistance at the level of adipocyte lipolysis would lead to increased fatty acid delivery to the liver, and consequent stimulation of hepatic glucose output[61].

After a glucose load, however, the clearance of glucose from the blood by muscle tissue becomes the dominant mechanism for controlling hyperglycaemia, with disposal of glucose in both oxidative and non-oxidative (glycogen synthesis and glycolysis with lactate release) pathways. In type 2 diabetes, the sensitivity of muscle tissue to insulin is decreased, and normal rates of glucose disposal can be maintained only with the additional mass action effect of the hyperglycaemia. Hypotheses to explain the insulin resistance of muscle in diabetes include abnormalities in capillary density, insulin transport across the capillary and abnormal distributions of muscle fibre types[62]. However, a great deal of attention has concentrated on the biochemical mechanisms mediating insulin action at the cellular level.

INSULIN RECEPTORS

Rare genetic defects of the insulin receptor give rise to marked insulin resistance and can lead to diabetes, but a genetic link with the insulin gene has not been confirmed in type 2 diabetes. Decreased numbers of insulin receptors have been described in insulin-resistance states, such as obesity, but consideration of the kinetic effects of this would account only for a right shift in the insulin dose–response curve, and not the decrease in maximum effect found in type 2 diabetes. The focus has thus shifted to the investigation of postreceptor defects.

POSTRECEPTOR ABNORMALITIES

Insulin has a multiplicity of cellular actions. Particularly important for the peripheral disposal of glucose are the translocation of glucose transporters (GLUT-4) to the cell surface, and the activation of glycogen synthesis and glycolysis. Physiological studies have identified that the defect in peripheral glucose utilization in diabetes is primarily the result of a decrease in non-oxidative metabolism, and impairment in the covalent activation of the glycogen synthesis has been identified in diabetes[63], in pre-diabetic states[64,65] and in cultured fibroblast lines derived from diabetic patients[66]. Markers associated with the glycogen synthase gene, or with its activator, protein phosphatase 1, have not been consistently found to be associated with type 2 diabetes, suggesting abnormalities in the postreceptor signalling cascade. This is, however, complex, incorporates multiple branching pathways and redundancies, and has not been fully characterized. Although the tyrosine kinase activity of the insulin receptor, the first component of the signalling cascade, is reduced in obese people with type 2 diabetes, this is reversible after weight loss, in contrast to the defect in whole body insulin sensitivity[67]. Mutations in insulin receptor substrate 1, one of the docking proteins proximal in the cascade, have been associated with alterations in insulin sensitivity in type 2 diabetes[26,68,69] and in obese non-diabetic subjects[70], but it is likely that it is only one of several potential genetic modulators of insulin action remaining to be identified.

ASSOCIATED FEATURES

Type 2 diabetes is associated with an increased cardiovascular risk and, at diagnosis, is characterized by hypertension and adverse biochemical risk factors[71]. These factors, comprising hypertriglyceridaemia, low plasma high-density lipoprotein and abnormalities of the coagulation and lipolytic systems, also characterize pre-diabetic hyperglycaemia[72,73] and the normoglycaemic siblings and children of people with type 2 diabetes[74], and the offspring of subjects with IGT[75]. Reaven has linked glucose intolerance and cardiovascular risk factors through insulin resistance[76], and the terms 'Reaven's syndrome', 'metabolic syndrome' or 'syndrome X' have been applied to this clustering of variables. Although Reaven hypothesized that insulin resistance was the fundamental link connecting the syndrome, this has not yet been clearly established, and the variables to be included in the syndrome may vary in different population groups[77]. Nevertheless, the combination of hyperglycaemia, obesity and cardiovascular risk factors appears to be a fundamental one in a large proportion of people with type 2 diabetes, and it is this association that explains much of the excess cardiovascular morbidity and mortality conferred by the disease.

CONCLUSION

In spite of intensive research over recent decades, and undoubted advances in the understanding of the pathogenesis of type 2 diabetes, the fundamental questions are still unanswered. The genes and gene products responsible, and the interactions between these and the environment, at the biochemical, cellular, tissue and whole body levels, remain to be discovered. The toll of the disease in human and economic terms is enormous and is to be contrasted with the limitations in our ability to prevent or treat it. Fundamental understanding of the pathogenesis of the condition will be essential for the development of new treatments, and it is only by continued collaboration of research at all levels that we will achieve the necessary advances.

REFERENCES

1. National Diabetes Data Group. Classification and diagnosis of diabetes mellitus and other categories of glucose intolerance. *Diabetes* 1979 **28**:1039–57.
2. World Health Organization. *Diabetes Mellitus, WHO Technical Report Series*, vol 727. Geneva: WHO, 1985.
3. American Diabetes Association Expert Committee. Report of the Expert Committee on the Diagnosis and Classification of Diabetes Mellitus. *Diabetes Care* 1997; **20**:1183–97.

4. Alberti, KGMM, Zinmet PZ, for the WHO Consultation. Definition, diagnoses and classification of diabetes mellitus and its complications. Part I: Diagnosis and classification of Diabetes Mellitus: Provisional Report of a WHO consultation. *Diabetic Med* 1998, **15**:539–553.
5. Cudworth AG. Type I diabetes mellitus. *Diabetologia* 1978; **14**:281–91.
6. Irvine WJ, Dimario U, Feek CM et al. Autoimmunity and HLA antigens in insulin-dependent (type 1) diabetes. *Clin Lab Immunol 1978;* **1**:107–10.
7. Gleichman H, Zorcher B, Greulich B et al. Correlation of islet cell antibodies and HLA-DR phenotypes with diabetes mellitus in adults. *Diabetologia* 1984; **27** (suppl): 90–2.
8. Groop LC, Bottazzo GF, Doniach D. Islet cell antibodies identify latent type I diabetes in patients aged 35–75 years at diagnosis. *Diabetes* 1986; **35**:237–41.
9. Tuomi T, Groop LC, Zimmet PZ, Rowley MJ, Knowles W, Mackay IR. Antibodies to glutamic acid decarboxylase reveal latent autoimmune diabetes mellitus in adults with a non-insulin-dependent onset of disease. *Diabetes* 1993; **42**:359–62.
10. Turner R, Stratton I, Horton V et al. UKPDS 25: autoantibodies to islet-cell cytoplasma and glutamic acid decarboxylase for prediction of insulin requirement in type 2 diabetes. *Lancet* 1997; **350**:1288–93.
11. Froguel P, Vaxillaire M, Sun F et al. Close linkage of glucokinase locus on chromosome 7p to early-onset non-insulin-dependent diabetes mellitus. *Nature* 1992; **356**:162–4.
12. Hattersley AT, Turner RC, Permutt MA et al. Linkage of type 2 diabetes to the glucokinase gene. *Lancet* 1992; **339**:1307–10.
13. Yamagata K, Furuta, H, Oda N et al. Mutations in the hepatocyte nuclear factor-4alpha gene in maturity-onset diabetes of the young (MODY1). *Nature* 1996; **384**:458–60.
14. Yamagata K, Oda N, Kaisaki PJ et al. Mutations in the hepatocyte nuclear factor-1alpha gene in maturity-onset diabetes of the young (MODY3). *Nature* 1996; **384**:455–8.
15. Alcolado JC, Thomas AW. Maternally inherited diabetes mellitus: the role of mitochondrial DNA defects. *Diabetic Med.* 1995; **12**:102–8.
16. Maassen JA, Kadowaki T. Maternally inherited diabetes and deafness: a new diabetes subtype. *Diabetological* 1996; **39**:375–82.
17. Barnett AH, Eff C, Leslie RD, Pyke DA. Diabetes in identical twins. A study of 200 pairs. *Diabetologia* 1981; **20**:87–93.
18. Newman B, Selby JV, King MC, Slemenda C, Fabsitz R, Friedman GD. Concordance for type 2 (non-insulin-dependent) diabetes mellitus in male twins. *Diabetologia* 1987; **30**:763–8.
19. Mather HM, Keen H The Southall Diabetes Survey: prevalence of known diabetes in Asians and Europeans. *BMJ* 1985; **291**:1081–4.
20. Knowler WC, Williams RC, Pettitt DJ, Steinberg AG. Gm3;5,13,14 and type 2 diabetes mellitus: an association in American Indians with genetic admixture. *Am J Hum Genet* 1988; **43**:520–6.
21. Cook JT, Shields DC, Page RC et al. Segregation analysis of NIDDM in Caucasian families. *Diabetologica* 1994; **37**:1231–40.
22. McCarthy MI, Hitman GA, Sheilds DC et al. Family studies of non-insulin-dependent diabetes mellitus in South Indians. *Diabetologia* 1994; **37**:1221–30.
23. Hanis CL, Boerwinkle E, Chakraborty R et al. A genome-wide search for human non-insulin-dependent (type 2) diabetes genes reveals a major susceptibility locus on chromosome 2. *Nat. Genet* 1996; **13**:161–6.

24. Mahtani MM, Widen E, Lehto M et al. Mapping of a gene for type 2 diabetes associated with an insulin secretion defect by a genome scan in Finnish families *Nat Genet* 1996; **14**:90–4.
25. Almind K, Inoue G, Pedersen O, Kahn CR. A common amino acid polymorphism in insulin receptor substrate-1 causes impaired insulin signalling. Evidence from transfection studies. *J Clin Invest* 1996; **97**:2569–75.
26. Zhang Y, Wat N, Stratton IM et al. UKPDS 19: heterogeneity in NIDDM: separate contributions of IRS-1 and beta 3-adrenergic-receptor mutations to insulin resistance and obesity respectively with no evidence for glycogen synthase gene mutations. UK Prospective Diabetes Study. *Diabetologia* 1996; **39**:1505–11.
27. O'Rahilly SP, Wainscoat JS, Turner RC. Type 2 (non-insulin-dependent) diabetes mellitus. New genetics for old nightmares. *Diabetologia* 1988; **31**:407–14.
28. Cook JTE, Page RCL, O'Rahilly S et al. Availability of type II diabetic families for detection of diabetes susceptibility genes. *Diabetes* 1993; **42**:1536–43.
29. Bennett PH, Bogardus C, Jaakko T, Zimmet P. Epidemiology and natural history of NIDDM: non-obese and obese. In: Alberti KGMM, Defronzo RA, Keen H, Zimmet P, eds. *International Textbook of Diabetes Mellitus*, Vol. 1. John Wiley & Sons Ltd, Chichester, 1992: 147–176.
30. Carey VJ, Walters EE, Colditz GA et al. Body fat distribution and risk of non-insulin-dependent diabetes mellitus in women. The Nurses' Health Study. *Am J Epidemiol* 1997; **145**:614–9.
31. Helmrich SP, Ragland DR, Leung RW, Paffenbarger RS Jr 1991; Physical activity and reduced occurrence of non-insulin-dependent diabetes mellitus. *N Engl J Med* 1991; **325**:147–52.
32. Eriksson KF, Lindgarde F. Poor physical fitness, and impaired early insulin response but late hyperinsulinaemia, as predictors of NIDDM in middle-aged Swedish men. *Diabetologia* 1996; **39**:573–9.
33. Hales CN, Barker DJ, Clark PM et al. Fetal and infant growth and impaired glucose tolerance at age 64. *BMJ* 1991; **303**:1019–22.
34. Barker DJ, Hales CN, Fall CH, Osmond C, Phipps K, Clark PM. Type 2 (non-insulin-dependent) diabetes mellitus, hypertension and hyperlipidaemia (syndrome X): relation to reduced fetal growth. *Diabetologia* 1993; **36**:62–7.
35. Cook JT, Levy JC, Page RC, Shaw JA, Hattersley AT, Turner RC. Association of low birth weight with beta cell function in the adult first degree relatives of non-insulin dependent diabetic subjects. *BMJ* 1993; **306**:302–6.
36. Phillips DI, Hirst S, Clark PM, Hales CN, Osmond C. Fetal growth and insulin secretion in adult life. *Diabetologia* 1994; **37**:592–6.
37. Phillips DI, Barker DJ, Hales CN, Hirst S, Osmond C. Thinness at birth and insulin resistance in adult life. *Diabetologia* 1994; **37**:150–4.
38. Lithel HO, McKeigue PM, Berglund L, Mohsen R, Lithell UB, Leon DA. Relation of size at birth to non-insulin dependent diabetes and insulin concentrations in men aged 50–60 years. *BMJ* 1996; **312**:406–10.
39. Rudenski AS, Hadden DR, Atkinson AB et al. Natural history of pancreatic islet B-cell function in type 2 diabetes mellitus studied over six years by homeostasis model assessment. *Diabetic Med* 1988; **5**:36–41.
40. UKPDS Group UK Prospective Diabetes Study 16: Overview of six years' therapy of type 2 diabetes – a progressive disease. *Diabetes* 1995; **44**:1249–58.
41. Himsworth HP. Diabetes mellitus: its differentiation into insulin-sensitive and insulin-resistant types. *Lancet* 1936; **i**:127–52.
42. Rossetti L. Glucose toxicity: the implications of hyperglycaemia in the pathophysiology of diabetes mellitus. *Clin Invest Med* 1995; **18**:255–60.

43. Yki Jarvinen H. Acute and chronic effects of hyperglycaemia on glucose metabolism: implications for the development of new therapies. *Diabetic Med* 1997; **14** (suppl 3). S32–7.
44. Ward WK, Johnstone CLW, Beard JC, Benedette TJ, Halter JB, Porte D. Insulin resistance and impaired insulin secretion in subjects with histories of gestational diabetes mellitus. *Diabetes* 1985; **34**:861–9.
45. O'Rahilly SP, Rudenski AS, Burnett MA et al. Beta-cell dysfunction, rather than insulin insensitivity is the primary defect in familial type 2 diabetes. *Lancet* 1986; 360–4.
46. Martin BC, Warram JH, Krolewski AS, Bergman RN, Soeldner JS, Kahn CR. Role of glucose and insulin resistance in development of Type 2 diabetes mellitus: results of a 25-year follow-up study. *Lancet* 1992; **340**:925–9.
47. Moller DE, O'Rahilly S. Syndromes of severe insulin resistance: clinical and pathophysiological features. In: Moller D, ed. *Insulin Resistance*. John Wiley & Sons, Chichester, 1997: 49–82.
48. Levy JC, Rudenski A, Burnett M, Knight R, Matthews DR, Turner RC. Simple empirical assessment of beta-cell function by a constant infusion of glucose test in normal and type 2 (non-insulin-dependent) diabetic subjects. *Diabetologia* 1991: **34**:488–99.
49. Kahn SE, Prigeon RL, McCulloch DK et al. Quantification of the relationship between insulin sensitivity and beta-cell function in human subjects. Evidence for a hyperbolic function. *Diabetes* 1993: **42**:1663–72.
50. Brunzel JD, Robertson RP, Lerner RL et al. Relationships between fasting plasma glucose levels and insulin secretion during intravenous glucose tolerance tests. *J Clin Endocrinol Metab* 1976; **42**:222–9.
51. Hosker JP, Rudenski AS, Burnett MA, Matthews DR, Turner RC. Similar reduction of first- and second-phase B-cell responses at three different glucose levels in type II diabetes and the effect of gliclazide therapy. *Metabolism* 1989; **8**:767–72.
52. Porte D Jr, Kahn SE. Hyperproinsulinemia and amyloid in NIDDM. Clues to etiology of islet beta-cell dysfunction? *Diabetes* 1989; **38**:1333–6.
53. Seaquist ER, Kahn SE, Clark PM, Hales CN, Porte D Jr, Robertson RP. Hyperproinsulinemia is associated with increased beta cell demand after hemipancreatectomy in humans. *J Clin Invest* 1996; **97**:455–60.
54. Cooper GJ, Willis AC, Clark A, Turner RC, Sim RB, Reid KB. Purification and characterization of a peptide from amyloid-rich pancreases of type 2 diabetic patients. *Proc Natl Acad Sci USA* 1987; **84**:8628–32.
55. Clark A, Edwards CA, Ostle LR et al. Localisation of islet amyloid peptide in lipofuscin bodies and secretory granules of human B-cells and in islets of type-2 diabetic subjects. *Cell Tissue Res* 1989; **257**:179–85.
56. Sanke T, Hanabusa T, Nakano Y et al. Plasma islet amyloid polypeptide (Amylin) levels and their responses to oral glucose in type 2 (non-insulin-dependent) diabetic patients. *Diabetologia* 1991; **34**:129–32.
57. Reardon W, Ross RJ, Sweeney MG et al. Diabetes mellitus associated with a pathogenic point mutation in mitochondrial DNA. *Lancet* 1992; **340**:1376–9.
58. McCarthy M, Cassell P, Tran T et al. Evaluation of the importance of maternal history of diabetes and of mitochondrial variation in the development of NIDDM. *Diabetic Med* 1996; **13**:420–8.
59. DeFronzo RA. Lilly lecture 1987. The triumvirate: beta-cell, muscle, liver. A collusion responsible for NIDDM. *Diabetes* 1988; **37**:667–87.
60. Firth R, Bell P, Rizza R. Insulin action in non-insulin-dependent diabetes mellitus: the relationship between hepatic and extrahepatic insulin resistance and obseity. *Metabolism* 1987; **36**:1091–5.

61. Rebrin K, Steil GM, Getty L, Bergman RN. Free fatty acid as a link in the regulation of hepatic glucose output by peripheral insulin. *Diabetes* 1995; **44**:1038–45.
62. Marin P, Andersson B, Krotkiewski M, Bjorntorp P. Muscle fiber composition and capillary density in women and men with NIDDM. *Diabetes Care* 1994; **17**:382–6.
63. Bogardus C, Lillioja S, Stone K, Mott D. Correlation between muscle glycogen synthase activity and in vivo insulin action in man. *J Clin Invest* 1984; **73**:1185–90.
64. Eriksson J, Franssila Kallunki A, Ekstrand A et al. Early metabolic defects in persons at increased risk for non-insulin-dependent diabetes mellitus. *N Engl J Med* 1989; **321**:337–43.
65. Vaag A, Henriksen JE, Beck Nielsen H. Decreased insulin activation of glycogen synthase in skeletal muscles in young nonobese Caucasian first-degree relatives of patients with non-insulin-dependent diabetes mellitus. *J Clin Invest* 1992; **89**:782–8.
66. Wells AM, Sutcliffe IC, Johnson AB, Taylor R. Abnormal activation of glycogen synthesis in fibroblasts from NIDDM subjects. Evidence for an abnormally specific to glucose metabolism. *Diabetes* 1993; **42**:583–9.
67. Freidenberg GR, Reichart D, Olefsky JM, Henry RR. Reversibility of defective adipocyte insulin receptor kinase activity in non-insulin-dependent mellitus. Effect of weight loss. *J Clin Invest* 1988; **82**:1398–406.
68. Almind K, Bjorbaek C, Vestergaard H, Hansen T, Echwald S, Pedersen O. Aminoacid polymorphisms of insulin receptor substrate-1 in non-insulin-dependent diabetes mellitus. *Lancet* 1993; **342**:828–32.
69. Hitman GA, Hawrami K, McCarthy MI et al. Insulin receptor substrate-1 gene mutations in NIDDM; implications for the study of polygenic disease. *Diabetologia* 1995; **38**:481–6.
70. Clausen JO, Hansen T, Bjorbaek C et al. Insulin resistance: interactions between obesity and a common variant of insulin receptor substrate-1. *Lancet* 1995; **346**:397–402.
71. UKPDS Group. UK Prospective Diabetes Study VI: Complications in newly diagnosed type 2 diabetic patients and their association with different clinical and biochemical risk factors. *Diabetes Res* 1990; **13**:1–11.
72. Nijpels G, Popp Snijders C, Kostense PJ, Bouter LM, Heine RJ. Cardiovascular risk factors prior to the development of non-sinulin-dependent diabetes mellitus in persons with impaired glucose tolerance: the Hoorn Study. *J Clin Epidemiol* 1997; **50**:1003–9.
73. Fujimoto WY, Bergstrom RW, Leonetti DL, Newell Morris LL, Shuman WP, Wahl PW. Metabolic and adipose risk factors for NIDDM and coronary disease in third-generation Japanese–American men and women with impaired glucose tolerance. *Diabetologia* 1994; **37**:524–32.
74. Walker M, Berrish TS, Stewart MW, Humphriss DB, Barriocanal L, Alberti KG. Metabolic heterogeneity in impaired glucose tolerance. *Metabolism* 1997; **46**: 914–17.
75. Leslie RD, Volkmann HP, Poncher M, Hanning I, Orskov H, Alberti KG. Metabolic abnormalities in children of non-insulin dependent diabetics. *Br Med J [Clin Res]* 1986; **293**:840–2.
76. Reaven GM. Role of insulin resistance in human disease. *Diabetes* 1988; **37**: 1595–1607.
77. Saad MF, Lilloja S, Nyomba BL et al. Racial differences in the relation between blood pressure and insulin resistance. *N Engl J Med* 1991; **324**:733–9.

2

Diagnosis: The Scale of the Problem and Future Risks

M. DE COURTEN, D. McCARTY AND P. ZIMMET

International Diabetes Institute, 260 Kooyong Road, Caulfield 3162, Victoria, Australia

Diabetes mellitus is a major global health problem[1] and causes substantial morbidity and mortality primarily in the form of cardiovascular, eye and kidney diseases, and limb amputations. There is overwhelming evidence that diabetes is increasing rapidly in many developing and newly industrialized nations. Estimates suggest a doubling of the prevalence over the next 15 years[1]. Although there seems to be general agreement about the principles in the prevention and control of diabetes and its complications, the most appropriate strategies to achieve the desired outcome still need to be found. This chapter highlights general aspects of risk, prevention and control of type 2 diabetes mellitus, by far the most prevalent form of diabetes.

Primary prevention (i.e. prevention before any evidence of disease is present) of type 2 diabetes is the ideal method for controlling the increasing rates of diabetes. Primary prevention involves addressing the major risk determinants, particularly obesity and low physical activity levels. It can be targeted at individuals who are at high risk for diabetes (e.g. obese persons, those aged >40 years, certain high-susceptibility ethnic groups and those with a family history of diabetes) or a community-wide approach can be used to try to reduce risk factor levels overall[2]. In type 2 diabetes there is likely to be a role for both strategies.

WORLDWIDE PREVALENCE OF DIABETES MELLITUS

To assist in raising the profile of diabetes and to encourage governments to initiate or improve local diabetes monitoring and prevention strategies, we

Type 2 Diabetes: Prediction and Prevention. Edited by Graham A. Hitman

recently published global diabetes estimates for 1997 and projections for the years 2000 and 2010[3]. Estimates for 1995 and the age-specific rates employed for the estimates were also shown to allow comparisons with a recent World Health Organization (WHO) report[4].

In 1997 we estimated that 123 million people probably had diabetes globally (Table 2.1), or about 2.1% of the world population. Of these, approximately 3.5 million people have type 1 diabetes mellitus and 120 million have type 2.

By the year 2010 (Table 2.2), the total number of people with diabetes is projected to reach 220 million worldwide: 5 million with type 1 diabetes and 215 million with type 2. The regions with greatest potential increase are Asia and Africa where diabetes could become two to three times more common than it is today. Asia will probably be home to 61% of the total globally projected number of people with diabetes by 2010.

The greatest increase in diabetes for the period 1995–2010 will probably be seen in western Asia (3.6–11.4 million), south-central Asia (28.8–57.5 million), south-east Asia (8.6–9.5 million) and east Asia (21.7–44 million).

Paradoxically, for many countries, type 2 diabetes has evolved as a major health problem because of increasing life expectancy. Over the past century, improved nutrition, better hygiene and the control of many communicable (infectious) diseases have resulted in dramatically improved longevity, but these benefits have unmasked many age-related non-communicable diseases (NCDs) such as type 2 diabetes, cardiovascular disease (CVD), hypertension, strokes and some cancers. These formerly uncommon NCDs have replaced many communicable diseases and are now major contributors to ill-health and death. The term 'epidemiological transition'[5] has been used to describe the shift in disease patterns that has occurred in developed countries over the past 50 years, but are currently affecting many developing countries today. This transition has catapulted type 2 diabetes from a rare disease at the

Table 2.1. Global estimates of diabetes in 1997 (in thousands)

Region	Population[a]	Type 1 diabetes < 15	Type 1 diabetes ≥ 15	Type 2 diabetes All ages	Total Diabetes
World	5846130	408	3135	119994	123537
Africa	758101	21	64	7644	7729
Asia	3538451	220	820	65008	66048
North America	301591	53	832	12463	13348
Latin America	490971	35	274	12847	13156
Europe	728498	74	1068	21157	22299
Oceania	28518	5	77	875	957

Adapted from Amos et al.[3]
[a] In thousands.

Table 2.2. Global estimates of diabetes – 1995 to 2010 (in thousands)

Region	1995				2000			2010		
	Population[a]	Type 1 diabetes	Type 2 diabetes	Total	Type 1 diabetes	Type 2 diabetes	Total	Type 1 diabetes	Type 2 diabetes	Total
World	5697038	3539	114878	118417	4423	146804	151227	5446	215272	220718
Africa	731470	85	7209	72984	142	9270	9412	219	13933	14152
Asia	3437786	1030	61752	62782	1608	82902	84510	2241	130056	132297
North America	296517	879	12098	12977	1019	13174	14193	1175	16360	17535
Latin America	475704	309	12094	12403	389	15177	15566	479	22062	22541
Europe	727787	1155	20885	22040	1182	25325	26507	1245	31620	32865
Oceania	27774	81	840	921	83	956	1039	87	1241	1328

Adapted from Amos et al.[3]
[a] In thousands.

beginning of this century to its current position as a major global contributor to disability and death.

In addition to shifting disease patterns, lifestyle changes are also greatly contributing to the problem of type 2 diabetes. This phenomenon has been well illustrated in Pacific and Indian Ocean island populations[6], and also in Australian Aboriginal communities[7]. Rapid socioeconomic development over the last 40–50 years has resulted in a change of way of life from traditional to modern, often referred to as 'Coca-colonisation[8]. In virtually all populations, diets high in saturated fat and decreased physical activity have accompanied the benefits of modernisation. These dietary and physical activity changes, combined with increasing longevity, form the basis of the dynamic type 2 diabetes epidemic that we are witnessing today. Hales and Barker[9] have suggested that intrauterine malnutrition may be the cause of the epidemic but this remains unproven. In any case, type 2 diabetes will continue to affect every region of the world, although its greatest impact will probably be felt in newly industrialized and developing nations. The corresponding burden of complications and premature mortality resulting from diabetes will constitute a major public health and socioeconomic problem for most countries.

RISK FACTORS AND DETERMINANTS OF DIABETES

Type 2 diabetes is a multi-factorial disease and shows heterogeneity in numerous respects[10]. The understanding of type 2 diabetes has undergone a radical change in recent years, particularly with the new discoveries from molecular biology and immunology[11]. Previously, it was regarded as a relatively distinct disease entity, but, in reality, type 2 diabetes (and its associated hyperglycaemia) is a descriptive term and a manifestation of a much broader underlying disorder[12]. This probably also includes the metabolic syndrome[10,13] – a cluster of CVD risk factors which, apart from hyperglycaemia (manifesting as type 2 diabetes or impaired glucose tolerance (IGT)), includes hyperinsulinaemia, dyslipidaemia, hypertension, central obesity and hyperleptinaemia.

Social, behavioural and environmental risk determinants[14] appear to unmask the effects of genetic susceptibility, with the result that type 2 diabetes now occurs in epidemic proportions in many populations. This has occurred too quickly to be the result of altered gene frequencies[15] and the significance of this is reflected in preventive approaches. Oversecretion of insulin (hyperinsulinaemia) and insulin resistance characterize type 2 diabetes in many populations, although pancreatic β-cell failure also occurs as the disease progresses[10], and it may also play an adjunctive role to insulin resistance in the initial stages of the development of IGT and type 2 diabetes.

Risk factors are characteristics that are associated with or predict disease. Although they are not necessarily causal, risk factors can be modified through intervention. In contrast, demographic characteristics of a disease, such as age, sex and ethnicity, are determinants of disease occurrence and cannot be modified (Table 2.3). However, lack of knowledge about the status of several factors (e.g. insulin, resistance, genetic susceptibility, etc.), and the interaction of the different factors, limits division into modifiable and non-modifiable factors. In addition, not only the causes but also the means to prevent the disease may differ according to the ethnic group studied.

NEW DIAGNOSTIC CRITERIA FOR GLUCOSE INTOLERANCE

The contemporary classification of diabetes and other categories of glucose intolerance was developed by the international workgroups, the National Diabetes Data Group (NDDG) of the National Institutes of Health, USA in 1979[16], and the World Health Organization (WHO) Expert Committee on Diabetes in 1980[17]. The NDDG/WHO classification system incorporated data from research conducted during the previous decades, which clearly established that diabetes was an aetiologically and clinically heterogeneous group of disorders sharing hyperglycaemia in common. A new risk category, IGT, was introduced at that time. The inclusion of IGT followed recognition

Table 2.3. Aetiological determinants and risk factors of type 2 diabetes

Genetic factors
Genetic markers
Family history
'Thrifty gene(s)', etc.
Demographic characteristics
Sex
Age
Ethnicity
Behavioural and lifestyle-risk factors
Obesity (including distribution of obesity and duration)
Physical inactivity
Diet
Stress
'Westernization, urbanization, modernization'
Metabolic determinants and intermediate risk categories of type 2 diabetes
Impaired glucose tolerance
Insulin resistance
Pregnancy-related determinants (parity, gestational diabetes, diabetes in offspring of women with diabetes during pregnancy, intrauterine malnutrition or overnutrition)

that a zone of diagnostic uncertainty existed in the oral glucose tolerance test (OGTT) between what was clearly normal glucose tolerance and diabetes. Many subjects with IGT subsequently develop overt diabetes. The introduction of the IGT category had other important implications for people with glucose intolerance. Until 1980, people with 2-hour post-glucose load plasma glucose (2h-PG) between 7.8 mmol/l (140 mg/dl) and 11 mmol/l (199 mg/dl) were diagnosed with diabetes. The new categorization rescued them from a disease that could restrict life insurance and certain jobs, and have other social penalties in some countries.

In 1985, he WHO Study Group on Diabetes Mellitus proposed a slightly revised classification which, although not ideal, has been adopted internationally[18]. There were two major types – type 1 diabetes and type 2 diabetes – plus several from a numerical perspective less important forms. Types 1 and 2 diabetes were recognized to be quite heterogeneous, particularly type 2. Regarding the 1985 WHO classification, at the time that it was proposed, the WHO committee recognized that this would require review in the light of ongoing research.

The diagnostic cutpoint of 11.1 mmol/l for the 2h-PG concentration was originally adopted for two reasons. First, the bimodality of glucose distributions in populations with high prevalence of diabetes suggested that 11.1 mmol/l represented the cut-off point separating the two components of the frequency distribution. Second, when the prevalence of microvascular complications was plotted against the 2h-PG value, it became obvious that the former sharply increased at about 11.1 mmol/l. However, the choice of a distinct cut-off point will always be somewhat arbitrary because blood glucose levels are continuously distributed in a population.

Using the WHO cut-off point values to define type 2 diabetes, it became apparent that fasting plasma glucose (FPG) and 2h-PG detect different sectors of the hyperglycaemic state. The WHO FPG criterion for diabetes (7.8 mmol/l or 140 mg/dl) represents a greater degree of hyperglycaemia than the 2h-PG criterion for diabetes (11.1 mmol/l or 199 mg/dl).

The 1985 WHO classification was widely accepted and has been used internationally, although it is a compromise between a clinical and an aetiological classification. However, calls continued for revisiting the NDDG and WHO recommendations and, in a rather impassioned editorial in 1990, Abourizk and Dunn[19] stated that 'a revised classification is needed to further fulfil the aims declared by the NDDG in 1979. For clinicians, teachers and researchers, the revision should go beyond the narrow type $1^{1/2}$ distinction. It should also take into account the dynamic phasic nature of diabetes. We see a need to revisit the landmark NDDG classification. We are ready for NDDG II'.

Their wish may have been fulfilled in part by the recently published American Diabetes Association's (ADA) report[20]. Here, it is recommended that the classification of diabetes mellitus be based on staging of glucose tolerance status with a complementary subclassification according to aetiological type (Table 2.4). The concepts for the new staging/aetiological classification were proposed by Kuzuya and Matsuda in an excellent and thought-provoking article[21]. Their proposals sought to separate clearly the criteria related to aetiology and those related to the degree of deficiency of insulin action, and to define each patient on the basis of these two criteria.

The change in diagnostic criteria is discussed in detail in the ADA report. The most substantive change is that the FPG concentration for the diagnosis of diabetes has been lowered from 7.8 mmol/l (140 mg/dl) to 7 mmol/l (126 mg/dl). A new category of impaired FPG of 6.1–7.0 mmol/l (111–126 mg/dl) has been created because the ADA recommended abolition of the OGTT for routine clinical use. It is unlikely that the WHO, in their future revision of diabetes classification will go so far as to agree with this last recommendation and more likely that they will recommend its use for when blood sugar is in an uncertain range for the diagnosis of diabetes. Furthermore, as there are a number of major IGT intervention studies now in progress, it would seem pointless to continue these studies aimed at showing the best way to interrupt the progression of IGT to type 2 diabetes, and then renounce the very test, i.e. OGTT that is used to diagnose IGT.

The OGTT is not used very often to diagnose diabetes in a clinical setting and has been used mainly for clinical research and epidemiological studies. Although the OGTT may appear to be unpopular for diagnosis of type 2 diabetes among general physicians, fewer than 20% of diabetic patients being diagnosed by OGTT[22–24], it is also true that many cases of type 2

Table 2.4. Aetiological classification of diabetes mellitus

I	Type 1 diabetes (β-cell destruction, usually leading to absolute insulin deficiency)
	A Immune-mediated diabetes
	B Idiopathic
II	Type 2 diabetes (ranging from predominantly insulin resistance with relative insulin deficiency to predominantly insulin secretory defect with insulin resistance)
III	Other specific types of diabetes
	A Genetic defects of the β-cell
	B Genetic defects in insulin action
	C Diseases of the exocrine pancreas
	D Endocrinopathies
	E Drug- or chemically-induced diabetes
	F Infections
	G Uncommon forms of immune-mediated diabetes
	H Other genetic syndromes sometimes associated with diabetes
IV	Gestational diabetes mellitus (GDM)

Adapted from American Diabetic Association[20].

diabetes can be diagnosed without an OGTT[18]. However, this is not the case for IGT. Only recently, the logistics and costs of measuring glycated haemoglobin (HbA1c) have become less than those of obtaining fasting blood or performing an OGTT. Yet the current disadvantage of glycated haemoglobin is the lack of standardization of methodology, as well as the fact that there is no universal reference standard for interlaboratory calibration[25]. In addition, there are fewer outcome data available than for the OGTT. However, these limitations may be overcome in the near future, so further evaluation of the properties of HbA1c measurements for screening and diagnosis could justify postponing a change in screening recommendations.

There are several arguments for abolishing the OGTT as a routine screening test for type 2 diabetes. First the complexity of the current diagnostic criteria reflects both the difficulty in distinguishing diabetic from non-diabetic patients on the basis of a single measurement, and the considerable test/retest variability of the OGTT[26].

However, a major argument for continuing the OGTT relates to the identification of high-risk subjects, i.e. those with IGT for clinical trials of type 2 diabetes prevention as alluded to above. In addition, the 2h-PG value from the OGTT was in particular recommended by WHO for epidemiological studies, to overcome uncertainties about whether or not study subjects were fasting sufficiently.

GESTATIONAL DIABETES MELLITUS

Gestational diabetes mellitus (GDM) is defined as carbohydrate intolerance of variable severity with onset or first recognition during pregnancy. The definition applies irrespective of whether or not insulin is used for treatment or the condition persists after pregnancy. It does not exclude the possibility that unrecognized glucose intolerance may have antedated or begun together with the pregnancy. After pregnancy ends, the woman has to be reclassified, either into diabetes mellitus (type 2 or 1), IGT or normal glucose tolerance. In most cases of GDM, glucose tolerance will return to normal after delivery.

Those with GDM represent a very important group as far as potential for prevention of type 2 diabetes is concerned, so the question of diagnostic criteria assumes great importance. Unfortunately, this is the major area where international groups, particularly the ADA and WHO, have not been able to come anywhere near consensus. It is highly likely that the WHO recommendations for the diagnosis of GDM are different from those of the ADA. Ideally all pregnant women should be screened between 24 and 28 weeks of gestation in order to detect the appearance of GDM.

It may be appropriate to screen pregnant women belonging to high-prevalence populations or high-risk individuals, during first trimester of pregnancy, in order to detect diabetes that might have been present even before the pregnancy but was not known about.

It is likely that the WHO will stay with its 1985 recommendation that an OGTT should be performed after overnight fasting (8–14 hours) by giving 75 g glucose. Plasma glucose is measured after 2 hours. Pregnant women who meet WHO criteria for diabetes for IGT should be classified as having GDM. After the pregnancy ends, the woman should be reclassified based on the results of 75-g load OGTT, 6 weeks or more after delivery.

SCREENING TO DETECT DIABETES

The purpose of screening is to discriminate, by the use of a rapid and simple test or examination, between people who are and those who are not likely to have a disease. By implication, a definite diagnostic procedure has to be used to confirm the presence or absence of the disease. Screening for diabetes is somewhat unusual because, depending on the test(s) chosen, the same test may be used for screening and diagnosis[27].

The current WHO criteria for type 2 diabetes[18] define the disease in terms of blood glucose levels during a 2-hour 75-g OGTT. Studies show that there are a proportion of asymptomatic people with normal fasting glucose levels who will be diagnosed only on the basis of abnormal 2-hour glucose levels during an OGTT[18,26]. These individuals will be detected during screening surveys, but would not be detected during normal clinical practice relying on fasting glucose testing alone[18,26].

Earlier detection of diabetes through screening might provide an important opportunity to reduce the progression of microvascular or macrovascular disease caused by asymptomatic hyperglycaemia. Numerous epidemiological studies and some animal models suggest that the degree of hyperglycaemia and the duration of disease are closely associated with microvascular (retinopathy and nephropathy) and neuropathic complications of diabetes[28,29], and many newly identified cases of type 2 diabetes have several other CVD risk factors in evidence[30]. In cases of GDM, the evidence that infants born to diabetic women are at increased risk of fetal malformation, prematurity, spontaneous abortion, macrosomia and metabolic abnormalities[31,32] adds further support to early detection and control of diabetes.

However, detection of type 2 diabetes in asymptomatic adults is unlikely to provide optimal benefit unless it is accompanied by a comprehensive health assessment, during which other lifestyle-related conditions requiring treatment may also be detected[27]. Screening asymptomatic people may also have some harmful effects, including false-positive diagnoses.

Today, there is no definitive evidence that detection of type 2 diabetes in the asymptomatic period can significantly improve long-term health outcomes or that it is cost-beneficial[26,33,34]. Even if improving blood glucose control can reduce long-term complications of type 2 diabetes, many other factors[25] must be considered in determining the likely benefits and risks of screening in asymptomatic people, e.g. efficacy of diet or medications in reducing glucose levels; compliance of asymptomatic people with lifestyle advice; inconvenience and costs of screening, follow-up and treatment; potential adverse effects of screening; and possible risks of drug or insulin therapy.

Targeting screening to high-risk groups, so-called opportunistic screening, such as certain ethnic groups, older and overweight subjects or people with previous gestational diabetes or other CVD risk factors, and emphasizing interventions that are inexpensive and safe (exercise, prudent diet and weight loss) are likely to minimize potential adverse effects of screening[26]. However, most of these interventions are already recommended for all adults, and the additional benefit of screening to promote lifestyle interventions remains uncertain.

The risk factor profile of age, ethnicity and body mass index (BMI) or other factors at which opportunistic screening will be recommended may vary across populations.

GENES AND PREVALENCE OF TYPE 2 DIABETES

Although the rise of diabetes and other NCDs in developing populations seems to be an accompaniment of modern lifestyle (reflected by high fat/low fibre diets and lower levels of physical activity), differences in the rates of diabetes and its complications among different populations point towards underlying genetic differences. The incidence rates of diabetes are now in fact higher in some developing countries than in some developed nations where lifestyle-related factors associated with diabetes can be assumed to be similar.

The thrifty genotype hypothesis[35] is one attempt to explain the high prevalence of obesity and type 2 diabetes in the American Pima Indians, Australian Aborigines and Pacific Islanders. The basis for the susceptibility to obesity and type 2 diabetes in such populations is unclear. A 'thrifty' genotype that promoted fat deposition[36,37] and conferred a survival advantage when food supplies were irregular may account for some of the observed differences in rates of type 2 diabetes. Such a metabolism would result in type 2 diabetes once populations adopted a more sedentary lifestyle and a diet with an excess of energy. However, the thrifty gene(s) has evaded genetic researchers so far.

Nevertheless, rapid progress is being made in the study of the genetics of diabetes mellitus, in terms of both methods applied to the problem and recent findings[38,39].

Several lines of evidence point to the important contribution of genes to diabetes. Type 2 diabetes is familial, but in most families the pattern is not consistent with inheritance by a single gene, unless other factors are postulated to account for a major part of susceptibility to the diseases. The familial occurrence of diabetes has been studied extensively in the Pima Indians, where diabetes below the age of 25 years is strongly familial, occurring only in those with at least one diabetic parent[40]. Data from many other populations also support genetic causes of diabetes. Concordance rates for type 2 diabetes in identical twins in reported series range from about 34% to 100%[41–43]. This frequency is at least twofold greater than that reported among non-identical twins, siblings or other first-degree relatives. There are markedly different prevalence rates of type 2 diabetes in different ethnic groups, even among those living in similar environments[14]. Genetic admixture of populations is of great importance to explain disease-marker associations because the admixture can give specific clues to the genes involved or account for confounding factors. Finally, maternal excess of type 2 diabetes has been shown in many different ethnic groups[44].

Identification of disease susceptibility loci is an important step towards understanding the genetic and environmental causes of that disease. The rapid application of molecular biology to public health will depend in large part on how many such genetic defects are ultimately discovered, and whether any single gene or multiple genes will account for most of the people with diabetes.

After a disease susceptibility locus has been successfully mapped on the genome, there are in general two major implications/outcomes. First, almost paradoxically, the discovery of susceptibility genes can be extremely useful in longitudinal investigations of environmental risk factors for diabetes. A typical investigation of environmental risk factors as causes of diabetes follows a cohort of people and retrospectively tries to detect the difference between the environments of those who did and those who did not develop the disease. However, the people who did not develop the disease may be a mixture of those who avoided the environmental trigger and those who encountered the trigger but did not develop the disease, because they were not genetically susceptible. Analysis of the impact of the environment on disease aetiology would be far more sensitive if a cohort of susceptible people could be identified (prospectively or retrospectively). Genetic markers of susceptibility to diabetes make this possible.

The second benefit of mapping diabetes susceptibility genes is in the development of novel therapies. Even if a diabetes gene were identified, population screening for the susceptibility locus would not be socially useful and ethically acceptable, unless an effective treatment would be available. The most important issue in identifying individuals at risk for diabetes should be to reduce that risk. However, if one cannot change one's genes, knowing that one has a high-risk genotype is not particularly helpful. This issue might be considered differently in the future if it concerns susceptibility loci for diabetes or obesity-related complications, such as renal disease or ischaemic heart disease and novel therapies were deduced from the genetic findings.

Once the relevant genetic factors are identified, in the case of diabetes it might still be easier to alter the environment. By that stage, population screening might conceivably be useful to identify the minority of people whose environment must be changed, while allowing the genetically non-susceptible majority to lead their lives as before. This scenario in the context of diabetes might apply in the future to interventions in women with gestational diabetes.

THE ROLE OF DIET IN TYPE 2 DIABETES AETIOLOGY

Diet has long been suspected to play a major role in the development of diabetes[14]. As early as the sixth century Hindu physicians attributed diabetes to an overindulgence in rich foods. By 1875 Bouchardat had already described what we now call type 2 diabetes as being associated with obesity, and observed that the rates of diabetes declined during the siege of Paris and this was attributed to food shortage[45]. Subsequently, declining diabetes mortality has been observed during war situations with severe food shortages, in contrast to areas where there was no food shortage and mortality from diabetes remained constant or even increased[46,47]. These findings were recently confirmed by observations of improved glycaemic control and blood pressure of type 2 diabetes patients during the war in Sarajevo[48] but can only provide indirect evidence for a role of diet, because the effects are confounded by rapid weight loss, increased physical activity and other changes during those times.

THE ROLE OF PHYSICAL ACTIVITY AND OBESITY IN TYPE 2 DIABETES AETIOLOGY

Obesity and physical inactivity have been found to be independently associated with both prevalence[49,50] and incidence[51–55] of type 2 diabetes in men and women. From epidemiological data, it can be estimated that risk of type 2 diabetes could be reduced 50–75% by control of obesity and 30–50% by increasing physical activity levels[56]. Physical activity may lower risk of type 2 diabetes via reducing total body fat[50,51,53–55,57,58] and abdominally distributed fat[50,53,57,58], and/or through its action in improving insulin sensitivity[57,58]. These mechanisms are closely linked, but the independent effects of physical activity and obesity suggest that the former can modify the risk of type 2 diabetes even within a given level of obesity. The best evidence yet that type 2 diabetes can be prevented in people with IGT comes from a large-scale, randomized intervention study published recently from the Da Qing Study in China[59]. Over a period of 6 years, there were significant and similar reductions in the incidence of diabetes in people randomized to diet, exercise or combined diet/exercise treatment groups.

It is likely that average physical activity levels have decreased over recent years in many populations, and this has to be considered as a major contributor to the current global rise of obesity[60], which is one of the major risk factors for type 2 diabetes.

THE ROLE OF LOW BIRTHWEIGHT IN TYPE 2 DIABETES AETIOLOGY

Birthweight is an important health measure, influenced by factors such as maternal health and nutrition. Not only does birthweight directly impact on neonatal and infant survival, it is also statistically associated with increased risk of type 2 diabetes, hypertension and CVD in some populations[61–65].

Hales and colleagues have proposed that poor intrauterine nutrition, and perhaps poor nutrition in early infancy, reflected in low birthweights and decreased rates of postnatal growth, can increase the risk of type 2 diabetes and CVD in later life, through either reducing pancreatic β-cell function or increasing insulin resistance[61–63,66]. The effects of low birthweight appear to be enhanced by adult obesity[63,64,67]. Data in support of the so-called 'thrifty phenotype' hypothesis have been reported in Europeans[61–65,68], Indians[69], Mexican–Americans[67] and Native Americans[70], although at least two studies in Europeans have failed to show the expected associations[71,72].

In many available data sets it is not known whether low birthweights reflect poor intrauterine growth or pre-term delivery, but this could affect the type of interventions recommended and the relevance of the thrifty phenotype hypothesis in the aetiology of type 2 diabetes. Gestational age if often not well documented, and a large number of pre-term births could be misclassified as intrauterine growth retardation and make a contribution to low-birthweight statistics. Low weight at 1 year of age was also associated with increased risk of developing type 2 diabetes in adulthood in British men[62].

However, McCance et al.[70] have challenged the validity of the 'thrifty phenotype' hypothesis. Among the Pima Indians of Arizona, they described a U-shaped relationship between birthweight and type 2 diabetes prevalence. Risk of type 2 diabetes in infants weighing <2500 g at birth was 3.8 times that of infants weighing 2500–4500 g, whereas those with birthweights ≥ 4500 g had a 1.8-fold increased risk relative to the normal weight group. The authors interpret the increased risk of type 2 diabetes in low-birthweight infants as being compatible with more accepted hypothesis of susceptibility to type 2 diabetes, which are a result of interaction between genetic and postnatal environmental factors. In their view, the increased prevalence of type 2 diabetes among adults with low birthweights reflects selective survival of low-birthweight infants who carry 'diabetogenic' genes, i.e., the survival advantage suggested by proponents of the 'thrifty genotype' hypothesis. Joseph and Kramer[73] have criticized the 'thrifty phenotype' on a number of grounds, suggesting that the reported associations between low birthweight and adult health may be the result of bias rather than being causal. Specifically, they point out the inadequacy of control for the confounding health consequences of social deprivation (low socioeconomic status). Conversely, the finding, in both monozygotic and dizygotic twin pairs discordant for type 2 diabetes, that the twins with diabetes have lower birthweights is supportive of the 'thrifty phenotyoe' hypothesis[68].

TYPE 2 DIABETES AND CHANGE IN LIFESTYLE

Change in the behavioural aspects of our lifestyle is thought to be at the centre of the diabetes epidemic and management if we accept that lifestyle has a major influence on incidence and progression of the disease. Interventions aiming at lifestyle change recognize the causal involvement in the aetiology of type 2 diabetes and other NCDs, such as CVD. What also cannot be ignored are the recent socioeconomic and cultural factors, associated with globalization, which have a direct impact on people's behaviour and lifestyle[74].

The concept of population health transition[5] has led to the dichotomy in thinking about 'traditional' lifestyle, which as been equated to physical activity and 'good' diet, and 'modern' or 'Western' or 'urban' lifestyle, which has been associated with stress, high-fat/low-fibre diet and sedentary behaviour. However, historical information about traditional lifestyle and diet of indigenous people and documentation about the presumed very low rates of diabetes are insufficient. In addition, the successful early spread of indigenous populations worldwide into vastly different living conditions leads to the conclusion that, for millennia, there have been very different lifestyles and diets between the groups. The term 'traditional lifestyle' has at least two dimensions that should be clearly delineated. 'Traditional', in the context of the history of indigenous people, can mean the time before contact with the European settlers (pre-contact), i.e. historical dimension, or it can denote a lifestyle according to (what we now assume to be) behavioural traditions, which have an impact on patterns of physical activity, composition of the diet and amount of food and other factors of daily living – the behavioural dimension. Terms such as 'Westernized', 'modernized' or 'industrialized' are generalizations of many lifestyle-related behaviours. More useful conclusions may be drawn regarding causality and prevention strategies or comparisons between populations if the specific components of the lifestyle were identified[75,76].

The recognition of the marked heterogeneity of indigenous populations regarding genetic background, lifestyle and diet implies that uniform programmes across populations are of limited assistance in reducing type 2 diabetes or other lifestyle-related diseases.

THE IMPACT OF TYPE 2 DIABETES COMPLICATIONS

In the UK, diabetic complications account for over 80% of health service costs for care[77]. These complications are thought to be largely preventable through early detection and good diabetes care. Compared with people who do not have diabetes, those with diabetes are two to four times at greater risk of heart disease, two to six times more at risk of strokes and 12 times at greater risk of amputations[78]. In the USA, diabetes is the leading cause of legal blindness[79] and the most common cause of kidney failure[80]. Fetal and maternal pregnancy complications are also seen two to six times more often in patients with diabetes[81]. In newly diagnosed patients with diabetes there is also a high frequency of treatable cardiovascular risk factors, which calls not only for earlier detection, but also for integrated diabetes management that addresses all modifiable risk factors immediately after diagnosis.

SOCIOCULTURAL AND PSYCHOLOGICAL ASPECTS ASSOCIATED WITH TYPE 2 DIABETES

Issues to be considered in planning preventive strategies include cultural differences and the special socioeconomic circumstances under which the specific population is living. These issues can enhance success and sustainability or undermine preventive campaigns. They operate not only on the level of the individual or the community at risk, but also among the health service providers and policy-makers involved in decisions that determine health. These issues are:

- psychological factors, such as illusion of immortality, which can impact on the commitment for prevention
- insufficient knowledge about prevention, which can result in apathy of participants and decision makers alike
- low priority among academics and institutions for research and funding of prevention
- socioeconomic and cultural factors which can inhibit changes in diet and lifestyle

- vested commercial interest in certain aspects of lifestyle and nutrition
- economic benefits of curative medicine, which de-emphasizes prevention
- late benefits of prevention, which are often initially intangible, but require upfront financial investment. Support for prevention is therefore difficult to obtain in politics governed by the quest for short-term results.

CONCLUSION

Diabetes affects an increasing number of people worldwide and is responsible for considerable personal and health care costs. Unless effective action is taken, diabetes and its complications will continue to increase with continued ageing and urbanization of populations, more sedentary lifestyles and an increase in people being overweight. Despite the evidence for the type 2 diabetes epidemic, the knowledge has still not been translated into effective public health action in most countries.

Although the WHO has called for global and country action, few nations have taken up the challenge. The future remains gloomy with over 123 million people today suffering from diabetes and with the predictions of well over 220 million people by 2010. Most of the new cases will be type 2 diabetes and these will be in China, the Indian subcontinent and Africa.

The major molecular biological, behavioural, environmental and social determinants are defined for type 2 diabetes; they provide the basis for intervention programmes emphasizing healthy lifestyle practices such as physical activity, good nutrition, maintenance of ideal bodyweight, smoking cessation and reduced alcohol consumption. The prevention and control of diabetes needs to receive highest priority and should be integrated with prevention and control of other NCDs. Effective, culturally appropriate intervention strategies also addressing the social environment of the community at risk need to be implemented and evaluated.

REFERENCES

1. McCarty D, Zimmet P. Diabetes 1994 to 2010: *Global Estimates and Projections*. Melbourne: International Diabetes Institute; 1994.
2. World Health Organization. Prevention of diabetes mellitus. Geneva: WHO; 1994.
3. Amos A, McCarty D, Zimmet P. The rising global burden of diabetes and its complications: Estimates and projections to the year 2010. *Diabetic Med* 1997; **14**:S1–S85.
4. World Health Organization. *The World Health Report 1997*. Geneva: WHO; 1997.
5. Omran A. The epidemiologic transition: A theory of the epidemiology of population change. *Milbank Q 1971;* **49**:509–38.

6. Zimmet P. Kelly West Lecture 1991, Challenges in diabetes epidemiology – from West to the Rest. *Diabetes Care* 1992; **15**:232–52.
7. O'Dea K. Westernisation, insulin resistance and diabetes in Australian Aborigines. *Med J Austr* 1995; **155**:258–64.
8. Koestler A. The Call Girls. London: Pan Books; 1976.
9. Hales CN, Barker DJP. Type 2 (non-insulin-dependent) diabetes mellitus: The thrifty phenotype hypothesis. *Diabetologia* 1992; **35**:595–601.
10. Zimmet P. The pathogenesis and prevention of diabetes in adults. *Diabetes Care* 1995; **18**:1050–64.
11. Zimmet P. Non-insulin-dependent (Type 2) diabetes mellitus – does it really exist? *Diabetic Med* 1989; **6**:728–35.
12. Zimmet P. Hyperinsulinaemia – how innocent a bystander. *Diabetes Care* 1993; **16**:56–70.
13. Reaven G. Role of insulin resistance in human disease. *Diabetes* 1988; **37**: 1595–1607.
14. de Courten M, Bennett P, Tuomilehto, J. Zimmet P. Epidemiology of NIDDM in non-Europids, In: Alberti KGMM ZP, DeFronzo RA, Keen H, eds. *International Textbook of Diabetes Mellitus* 2nd edn. Chichester: John Wiley & Sons; 1997.
15. Diamond J. Diabetes running wild. *Nature* 1992; **357**:362–3.
16. National Diabetes Data Group. Classification and diagnosis of diabetes mellitus and other categories of glucose intolerance. *Diabetes* 1979; **28**:1039–57.
17. World Health Organization. *Expert Committee on Diabetes Mellitus, Second Report*. Geneva: WHO; 1980.
18. World Health Organization. *Diabetes Mellitus: Report of a WHO Study Group*. Geneva: WHO; 1985.,
19. Abourizk N, Dunn J. Types of diabetes according to National Diabetes Data Group Classification. Limited applicability and need to revisit. *Diabetes Care* 1990; 13:1120–3.
20. American Diabetes Association. Report of the expert committee on the diagnosis and classification of diabetes mellitus. *Diabetes Care* 1997; **20**:1183–97.
21. Kuzuya T, Matsuda A. Classification of diabetes on the basis of etiologies versus degree of insulin deficiency. Diabetes Care 1997; **20**:219–20.
22. Davidson M, Peters A, Schriger D. An alternative approach to the diagnosis of diabetes with a review of the literature. *Diabetes Care* 1995; **18**:1065–71.
23. Orchard T, Wagener D. The Pittsburgh insulin-dependent diabetes mellitus (IDDM) registry. The incidence of insulin-dependent diabetes mellitus in Allegheny Country, PA (1965–1976). *Diabetes* 1981; **30**:279–84.
24. Melton L. Ochi J, Pasquale B, Palumbo P, Chu C. Referral bias in diabetes research. *Diabetes Care* 1984; **7**:12–18.
25. de Courten M, Zimmet P. Screening for non-insulin-dependent diabetes mellitus: where to draw the line. *Diabetic Med* 1997; **14**:95–8.
26. Dowse G, Zimmet P, Alberti K. Screening for diabetes and glucose intolerance. In: Alberti K, Zimmet P, DeFronzo R, Keen HH, eds. *International Textbook of Diabetes Mellitus* 2nd edn. London: John Wiley & Sons; 1996; 1687–707.
27. Knowler W. Screening for NIDDM. Opportunities for detection, treatment, and prevention. *Diabetes Care* 1994; **17**:445–50.
28. Brownlee M. Glycation and diabetic complications. *Diabetes* 1994; **43**:836–41.
29. Bennett P, Bogardus C, Zimmet P, Tuomilehto J. The epidemiology of non-insulin dependent diabetes–non-obese and obese. In: Alberti K, DeFronzo R, Keen H, Zimmet P, eds. *International Textbook of Diabetes Mellitus*. London: John Wiley & Sons; 1992; 147–76.

30. Harris M, Couric C, Reiber G, Boyko E, Stern M, Bennett P, eds. *Diabetes in America*, 2nd edn. Washington DC: US Government Printing Office; 1995.
31. Garner P. Type 1 diabetes mellitus and pregnancy. *Lancet* 1995; **346**:157–61.
32. Miodovnik M, Mimouni F, Dignan P, et al. Major malformations in infants of IDDM women: vasculopathy and early-trimester poor glycemic control. *Diabetes Care* 1988; **11**:713–18.
33. Eastman R, Javitt J, Herman W, Dasbach E, Harris M. Prevention strategies for non-insulin-dependent diabetes mellitus: an economic perspective. In: Le-Roith D, Taylor S, Olefsky J, eds. *Diabetes mellitus: A Fundamental and Clinical Text*. New York: Lippincott-Raven Publishers; 1996: 621–30.
34. Carrington-Reid M, Sox H, Comi R, Atkins D. Screening for diabetes mellitus. In: US Preventive Services Task Force, ed. *Guide to Clinical Preventive Services*, 2nd ed. Baltimore, MA: Williams & Wilkins; 1996: 193–208.
35. Neel J. Diabetes mellitus: a thrifty genotype rendered detrimental by 'progress'? *Am J Hum Genet* 1962; **14**:353–62.
36. Dowse G, Zimmet P. The thrifty genotype in non-insulin-dependent diabetes. The hypothesis survives, *BMJ* 1993; **306**:532–3.
37. Neel J. The thrifty genotype revisited. In: Kobberling J, Tattersall R, eds. The genetics of diabetes mellitus. *Proceedings of the Serono Symposium*. London: Academic Press; 1982: 283–93.
38. Moller D, Bjorbaek, C. Vidal-Pluig A. Candidate genes for insulin resistance. *Diabetes Care* 1996; **19**:396–400.
39. Turner R, Hattersley A, Shaw J, Levy J. Type II diabetes: clinical aspects of molecular biologic studies. *Diabetes* 1995; 44:1–10.
40. Knowler W, Pettitt D, Saad M, Bennett P. Diabetes mellitus in the Pima Indians: incidence, risk factors and pathogenesis. *Diab Metabol Rev* 1990; **6**:1–27.
41. Newman B, Selby JV, Slemenda C, Fabsitz R, Friedman GD. Concordance for type 2 (non-insulin-dependent) diabetes mellitus in male twins. *Diabetologia* 1987; **30**:763–8.
42. Barnett A, Eff C, Leslie R, Pyke D. Diabetes in identical twins. A study of 200 pairs. *Diabetologia* 1981; **20**:87–93.
43. Lo S, Tun R, Hawa M, Leslie R. Studies of diabetic twins. *Diabetes Metab Rev* 1881; **7**:223–28.
44. Riley M, Blizzard C, McCarty D, Senator G, Dwyer T, Zimmet P. Parental history of diabetes in an insulin-treated diabetes registry. *Diabetic Med* 1997; **14**:35–41.
45. Bouchardat A. *De la glycosurie ou diabete sucre*, vol. 2. Paris: Germer-Baillière; 1875.
46. Himsworth H. Diet and the incidence of diabetes mellitus. *Clin Sci Mol Med* 1935–6; **2**:117–48.
47. Westlund K. Incidence of diabetes mellitus in Oslo, Norway, 1925 to 1954. *Br J Prev Soc Med* 1966; **20**:105.
48. Kulenovic I, Robertson A, Grujic M, Suljevic E, Smajkic A. The impact of war on Sarajevans with non-insulin-dependent diabetes mellitus. *Eur J Public Health* 1996; **6**:252–6.
49. Dowse G, Zimmet P, Gareeboo H, et al. Abdominal obesity and physical inactivity as risk factors for NIDDM and impaired glucose tolerance in Indian, Creole and Chinese Mauritians. *Diabetes Care* 1991; **14**:271–82.
50. Kriska A, LaPorte R, Pettit D, et al. The association of physical activity with obesity, fat distribution and glucose intolerance in Pima Indians. *Diabetologia* 1993; **36**:863–9.
51. Manson J, Rimm E, Stampfer M, et al. Physical activity and incidence of non-insulin-dependent diabetes mellitus in women. *Lancet* 1991; **338**:774–8.

52. Helmrich SP, Ragland DR, Leung RW, Paffenbarger RS. Physical activity and reduced occurrence of non-insulin-dependent diabetes mellitus. *N. Engl J Med* 1991; **325**:147–52.
53. Burchfiel C, Sharp D, Curb J, et al. Physical activity and incidence of diabetes: The Honolulu Heart Program. *Am J Epidemiol* 1995; **141**:360–8.
54. Manson J, Nathan D, Krolewski A, Stampfer M, Willett W. Hennekens C. A prospective study of exercise and incidence of diabetes among US male physicians. *JAMA* 1992; **268**:63–7.
55. Schranz A, Tuomilehto J, Marti B, Jarrett R, Grabaukas V, Vassallo A. Low physical activity and worsening of glucose tolerance: results from a 2-year follow-up of a population sample in Malta. *Diabetes Res Clin Practice* 1991; **11**:127–36.
56. Manson J, Spelsberg A. Primary prevention of non-insulin-dependent diabetes mellitus. *Am J Prev Med* 1994; **10**:172–84.
57. Bouchard C, Després J-P, Tremblay A. Exercise and obesity. *Obes Res* 1993; 1:133–47.
58. Houmard J, McCulley C, Roy L, Bruner R, McCammon M, RG Isreal. Effects of exercise training on absolute and relative measurements of regional adiposity. *Int J Obes* 1994; **18**:243–8.
59. Pan X, Li G, Hu Y, et al. Effects of diet and exercise in preventing NIDDM in people with impaired glucose tolerance: The Da Qing IGT and Diabetes Study. *Diabetes Care* 1997; **204**:537–44.
60. Prentice A, Jebb S. Obesity in Britain: gluttony or sloth? *BMJ* 1995; **311**:437–9.
61. Barker D, Hales C, Fall C, Osmond C, Phipps K, Clark P. Type 2 (non-insulin-dependent) diabetes mellitus, hypertension and hyperlipidaemia (syndrome X): relation to reduced fetal growth. *Diabetologia* 1993; **36**:62–7.
62. Hales CN, Barker DJP, Clark PMS, et al. Fetal and infant growth and impaired glucose tolerance at age 64. *BMJ* 1991; **303**:1019–22.
63. Phillips D, Barker D, Hales C, Hirst S, Osmond C. Thinness at birth and insulin resistance in adult life. *Diabetologia* 1994; **37**:150–4.
64. Fall C, Osmond C, Barker D, Clark P, Hales C. Fetal and infant growth and cardiovascular risk factors in women. *BMJ* 1995; **310**:428–32.
65. Leon DA, Kuopiliva I, Lithell HO, et al. Failure to realise growth potential in utero and adult obesity in relation to blood pressure in 50 year old Swedish men. *BMJ* 1996; **312**:401–6.
66. Phillips D. Insulin resistance as a programmed response to fetal undernutrition. *Diabetologia* 1996; **39**:1119–22.
67. Valdez R, Athens M, Thompson G, Bradshaw B, Stern M. Birthweight and adult health outcomes in a biethnic population in the USA. *Diabetologia* 1994; **37**:64–31.
68. Poulsen P, Vaag A, Kyvik K, Møller Jensen D, Beck-Nielsen H. Low birth weight is associated with NIDDM in discordant monozygotic and dizygotic twin pairs. *Diabetologia* 1997; **40**:439–46.
69. Yajnik C, Fall C, Vaidya U, et al. Fetal growth and glucose and insulin metabolism in four-year-old Indian children. *Diabetic Med* 1995; **12**:330–6.
70. McCance D, Pettitt D, Hanson R, Jacobsson L, Knowler, W, Bennett P. Birth weight and non-insulin dependent diabetes: thrifty genotype, thrifty phenotype, or surviving small baby genotype? *BMJ* 1994; **308**:942–5.
71. Alvarsson M, Efendic S, Grill V. Insulin responses to glucose in healthy males are associated with adult height but not with birth weight. *J Intern Med* 1994; **236**:275–9.
72. Cook JT, Levy JC, Page RC, Shaw AG, Hattersley AT, Turner RC. Association of low birth weight with β cell function in the adult first degree relatives of non-insulin dependent diabetic subjects. *BMJ* 1993; **306**:302–6.

73. Joseph K, Kramer M. Review of the evidence on fetal and early childhood antecedents of adult chronic disease. *Epidemiol Rev* 1996; **18**:158–74.
74. Zimmet P, Lefebre P. The global NIDDM epidemic. Treating the disease and ignoring the symptom. *Diabetologia* 1996; **39**:1247–8.
75. Hodge AM, Dowse GK, Koki G, Mavo B, Alpers MP, Zimmet P. Modernity and obesity in coastal and Highland Papua New Guinea. *Int J Obesity* 1995; **19**: 154–61.
76. Muhilal. Transitions in diet and health: implication of modern lifestyles in Indonesia. *Asia Pacific J Clin Nutr* 1996; **5**:132–4.
77. Home P. Diagnosing the undiagnosed with diabetes. *BMJ* 1994; **308**:611–12.
78. Nathan D. Long term complications of diabetes mellitus. *N. Engl J Med* 1993; **328**:1676–85.
79. Klein R, Klein B. Vision disorders in diabetes. In: Harris M, ed. *Diabetes in America*, 2nd edn. Bethesda, MA: National Institutes of Health; 1995: 293–338.
80. Selby J, Fitzsimmons S, Newman J, Fatz P, Sepe S, Showstack J, The natural history and epidemiology of diabetes nephropathy: implications for prevention and control. *JAMA* 1990; **263**:1954–1960.
81. Buchanan T. Pregnancy in preexisting diabetes. In: Harris M, ed. *Diabetes in America*. 2nd ed. Bethesda, MA: National Institutes of Health; 1995: 719–33.

Part B

Genetics

3

An Introduction to the Genetics of Type 2 Diabetes

M.P. STERN AND P. O'CONNELL

Departments of Medicine and Pathology, University of Texas Health Science Center at San Antonio, 7703 Floyd Curl Drive, San Antonio, TX 78284, USA

In this chapter we review some of the basic principles of genetics as they relate to type 2 diabetes. As Chapters 4, 5 and 6 deal with the genetics of diabetes in Caucasian populations, in this chapter we draw examples primarily from US Hispanic and Native American populations to illustrate the principles that are presented. Moreover, we focus on the 'common' form of type 2 diabetes. Thus, although the genetics of many rare types of diabetes have been worked out in considerable detail – for example, diabetes in association with mutations of the insulin receptor gene[1] – and although much is known about the genetics of maturity – onset diabetes of the young (MODY) (see Chapter 8) – we do not address these types of diabetes in this chapter.

The topics covered include a discussion of possible heterogeneity of type 2 diabetes. This is followed by a summary of the evidence that type 2 diabetes has major genetic determinants; then we discuss the possible modes of inheritance of type 2 diabetes, namely, polygenic, oligogenic, or predominantly single gene inheritance. Segregation analysis is then discussed as a way of evaluating predominantly single gene inheritance, after which we discuss the principles that underlie molecular genetic approaches for the identification of diabetes susceptibility genes, followed by a discussion of the various analytic techniques that are commonly used to establish either association or linkage between a genetic marker and a trait. These techniques include analyses of associations, in both related and unrelated individuals, and linkage analysis using either segregation models or allele-sharing methods. The latter analyses include sib-pair or relative pair methods (which may or may not be limited to affected individuals) and methods using variance components.

Type 2 Diabetes: Prediction and Prevention. Edited by Graham A. Hitman

HETEROGENEITY OF TYPE 2 DIABETES

It is commonly asserted that type 2 diabetes is a heterogeneous disorder. The impression given is that, as more and more is learned about the etiology and pathogenesis of this disorder, and more distinct types of diabetes will be discovered, none of which will account for more than a small percentage of the total prevalence; no predominant type will therefore emerge. Another possibility is that, notwithstanding the gradual discovery of numerous subtypes of what is presently referred to as type 2 diabetes, one predominant type will, in fact, emerge. At the present time there is little evidence available that would enable us to distinguish between these two types of heterogeneity. Also, it is possible that the extent of heterogeneity varies between populations. For example, it is possible that in low-risk populations such as Caucasians, type 2 diabetes will some day disaggregate into multiple specific types without any predominant type, whereas in high-risk populations such as Mexican–Americans or Native Americans, a single predominant type will emerge.

The type of heterogeneity that underlies what we presently call type 2 diabetes has important implications for genetic studies of this disease. If one studies a single large pedigree, heterogeneity is not likely to be a problem. Such large, multiplex pedigrees, however, are often not representative of the common form of type 2 diabetes. If, on the other hand, one combines linkage data from multiple pedigrees, one must hope that a single type predominates in most of the pedigrees under study. Of course, one can always examine individual pedigrees within the pooled material, but, in the absence of strong prior hypotheses, this approach often tends to take on an aspect of 'data dredging'. Also, individual families in pooled pedigree studies tend to be small. Far and away the great majority of currently ongoing studies of the genetics of type 2 diabetes rely on combined linkage data from multiple pedigrees.

EVIDENCE THAT TYPE 2 DIABETES HAS GENETIC DETERMINANTS

Until such time as susceptibility genes for type 2 diabetes have been identified and the mechanisms by which they enhance diabetes risk have been elucidated, a genetic basis for this disorder cannot be regarded as having been absolutely proven. Nevertheless, there is extensive circumstantial evidence in favor of genetic determinants for type 2 diabetes. This evidence includes the familial nature of the disease and data derived from studies of hybrid populations descended from high- and low-risk ancestral populations. The familial nature of the disease has been established from epidemiologic studies in which family history has been confirmed as a diabetes risk factor, from family studies that show clustering of type 2 diabetes, and from twin studies.

Figure 3.1 shows the age- and sex-adjusted incidence type 2 diabetes in Pima Indians according to body mass index (BMI) and parental history of diabetes[2]. The data indicate that, although increasing obesity as judged by BMI is clearly associated with increasing diabetes risk, parental history is independently associated with a further increase in risk. Those who had at least one parent with 'late-onset' (>45 years) diabetes had an increased incidence of diabetes compared with those with similar BMI, but a negative family history. If either parent had 'early-onset' diabetes, the risk was enhanced still further. There is some evidence to suggest that a maternal family history of diabetes confers greater risk than a paternal history. (This is in contrast to type 1 diabetes where a maternal history is protective relative to a paternal history.) One has to be careful about interpreting these data, however, as respondent reports of parental history may be biased. Specifically, as women are more likely to receive health care than men, the respondent's mother, if diabetic, is more likely to have been diagnosed than the father, even if the latter also had the disease. Moreover, often the mother's health status is better known to the respondent than that of the father. In the San Antonio Family Diabetes Study, excess transmission

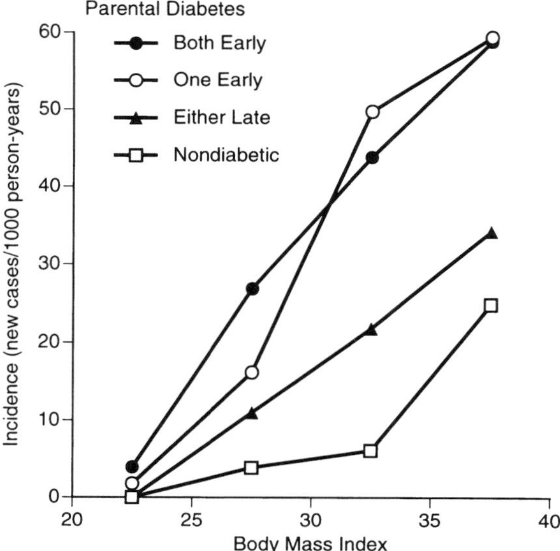

Figure 3.1. Age- and sex-adjusted incidence of type 2 diabetes in Pima Indians according to body mass index and parental history of diabetes. The incidence measures the new cases of diabetes per 1000 person-years. (Reproduced from Knowler et al.[2] with permission.)

through the mother compared with the father was observed when respondent reports were relied upon, whereas this effect was abolished when only parents who had been examined in the clinic and whose diabetic status had thereby been confirmed were relied upon[3]. Data from the Pima Indian study indicate that offspring of women who are already diabetic at the time of their pregnancy are up to nine times more likely to develop diabetes than offspring of women who develop diabetes later, i.e., who were prediabetic at the time of the pregnancy in question[4]. Although at lower risk compared with the offspring of diabetic women, the offspring of prediabetic women are nevertheless at greater risk of developing diabetes than the offspring of women who remain non-diabetic. These findings implicate some feature of the intrauterine environment of pregnant diabetic women that increases the risk to their offspring over and above the enhanced risk as a result of genetic factors. What this intrauterine environmental factor might be is, however, unclear, although it could involve the delivery of excess fuel and nutrients to the fetus, because the offspring of diabetic mothers are also larger for gestational age at birth and develop more obesity later in life than the offspring of pre-diabetic mothers[4]. A possible explanation for the failure to observe excess maternal transmission of type 2 diabetes in Mexican–Americans is that Pima Indians develop diabetes at a substantially younger age than do Mexican–Americans. Thus, fewer Mexican–Americans will have been subjected to a diabetic environment *in utero*, even if their mothers subsequently develop diabetes.

Apart from epidemiologic studies in which family history has emerged as a strong diabetes risk factor, numerous family studies have reported family clustering of diabetes directly. Table 3.1 presents data from the San Antonio Family Diabetes Study showing the risk to individuals who are related to a diabetic proband according to their degree of relatedness[5]. The background risk for each individual is estimated, based on his or her age and sex, from previously obtained epidemiologic data. These risks are then summed for each category of relatedness (i.e., for first-, second-, and third-degree relatives) to obtain the expected number of cases for each category of relative. This number is then compared to the number of cases actually observed in the family data for that category of relative, and the observed to expected ratios calculated. This ratio, which is referred to as the 'recurrent risk' to a certain class of relatives (first, second, etc.), was introduced by Risch and is referred to as Risch's λ[6]. As seen in Table 3.1, the recurrent risk to first-degree relatives of a diabetic proband is almost double the population risk, i.e., the risk to an individual from the same population and of the same age and sex, but without a first-degree relative with diabetes. The recurrent risks to second- and third-degree relatives are 33% and 13% higher than the corresponding age- and sex-adjusted population risks. These last two increases were not however statistically significant.

Table 3.1. Observed vs expected cases of type 2 diabetes according to degree of relatedness to the proband

	No. examined	Type 2 diabetes No. observed O (%)	Type 2 diabetes No. expected (E)	O/E
First-degree relatives				
Parents	18	13 (72.2)	6.5	2.00
Sibs	76	28 (36.8)	14.9	1.88
Children	81	9 (11.1)	3.9	2.31
Total	175	50 (28.6)	25.3	1.98[a]
Second-degree relatives				
Aunts/Uncles	18	8 (44.4)	6.5	1.23
Nieces/Nephews	93	7 (7.5)	5.3	1.32
Grandchildren	14	0 (0)	0.2	0
Other	3	2 (66.7)	0.8	2.50
Total	128	17 (13.3)	12.8	1.33
Third-degree relatives				
Cousins	46	6 (13.0)	6.2	0.97
Child of niece/nephew	14	0 (0)	0.2	0
Other	12	2 (16.7)	0.7	2.86
Total	72	8 (11.1)	7.1	1.13

[a] $p < 0.001$.

Twin studies have also provided evidence for a genetic basis for type 2 diabetes. Concordance for type 2 diabetes for monozygotic twins has ranged from 60% to 90%[7,8]. For type 1 diabetes, by contrast, the concordance rates for monozygotic twins are only in the range of 30–40%, indicating a substantially greater environmental contribution for this type of diabetes. For type 2 diabetes, however, the highest concordance rates may be inflated as a result of ascertainment bias. This can arise in a number of ways. If the cases are ascertained because they are diabetic, and not because they are twins, concordant twins have double the chance of being ascertained. Moreover, if cases are ascertained through clinical facilities, concordant twins, because they may be thought to be of greater interest, may be selectively referred. One study that avoided these biases by using a twin registry and examining all cases, rather than relying on a history given by the co-twin, reported a concordance rate of almost 60%[8]. Even this lower estimate is strikingly high and suggests that genes play an important role in the etiology of type 2 diabetes. Of course, it is still possible to assert that monozygotic twins share environments to a high degree and that this sharing is what produces their high diabetes concordance rates. This explanation is rendered less likely by the fact that type 2 diabetes develops late in life after the environments of twins have typically diverged, and by the fact that dizygotic or fraternal twins have much lower concordance rates.

Further evidence that type 2 diabetes has genetic determinants comes from studies of hybrids of high- and low-risk populations. A number of studies of this type have been performed, and several of them have relied on official records or the respondent's report of his or her ancestry. For example, in a study of the Three Affiliated Tribes of North Dakota, Indian Health Service records were used to classify tribe members into Indians with less than half inheritance, those with between half and full, and those with full inheritance[9]. Diabetes prevalence increased in parallel with increasing Native American admixture. Similar results have been reported for Pima Indians[2]. As Native Americans typically have exceedingly high rates of type 2 diabetes and Caucasians have much lower rates, these results are compatible with the hypothesis that Native American populations have a high frequency of diabetes susceptibility genes and that the rate of this disease in hybrid populations is proportional to the percent of their gene pool that is derived from the Native American source. Biochemical and anthropometric measurements have also been used to assess genetic admixture. For example, a reduced prevalence of type 2 diabetes has been associated with Caucasian admixture as judged by HLA typing in Micronesians from the South Pacific island of Nauru[10] and by a specific haplotype of the Gm system of human immunoglobulin G in Pima Indians[11]. Caucasian admixture has also been assessed in Mexican–Americans using skin color[12] and a combination of red cell antigens and polymorphic serum proteins[13]. Both approaches indicated that there was a stepwise increase in diabetes prevalence associated with increasing Native American admixture. A synthesis of the results of a number of studies in which diabetes prevalence has been correlated with genetic admixture, as assessed using red cell antigens and polymorphic serum proteins, is presented in Figure 3.2. It is apparent that there is a close correspondence between the degree of Native American admixture and the prevalence of type 2 diabetes[14]. Conceivably, this correspondence could be produced by environmental differences between the populations represented in Figure 3.2 but, for this to be the explanation, the environmental factor would have to track genetic admixture with extraordinary fidelity. This seems unlikely, and therefore a genetic explanation for these findings seems more plausible.

WHAT IS THE MODE OF INHERITANCE OF TYPE 2 DIABETES?

The mode of inheritance of type 2 diabetes is unknown. A number of theoretical possibilities may be considered. Polygenic inheritance refers to the situation in which many genes, possibly hundreds, contribute to diabetes

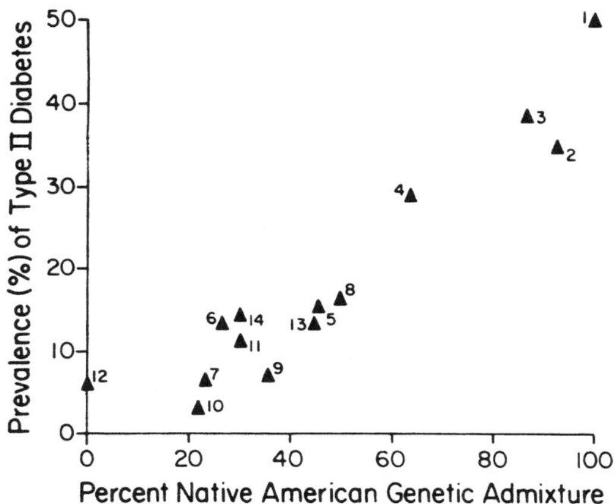

Figure 3.2. Correlation between percent Native American genetic admixture and prevalence of type 2 diabetes. The populations are as follows: (1) Pima Indians in Arizona; (2) Seminole Indians in Florida; (3) Seminole Indians in Oklahoma; (4) Cherokee Indians in North Carolina; (5) Barrio Mexican–American men; (6) transitional Mexican–American men; (7) suburban Mexican–American men; (8) Barrio Mexican–American women; (9) transitional Mexican–American women; (10) suburban Mexican–American women (groups 5–10 are from the San Antonio Heart Study[14]; (11) Mexican–Americans in Starr County, Texas; (12) non-Hispanic Whites from the San Antonio Heart Study; (13) Hispanics in Colorado; and (14) Puerto Ricans in Peurto Rico. (Reproduced from Stern and Haffner[14] with permission.)

susceptibility. These genes could have epistatic effects, either additive or multiplicative. In a worst case scenario, no single gene would explain more than a few percent of the overall variability in diabetes susceptibility between individuals. If this is the true situation, it will be exceedingly difficult to identify and characterize diabetes susceptibility genes. A more favorable scenario would be 'oligogenic' inheritance in which a few, say two to four 'major' genes, explain perhaps 15–30% each of the variability in diabetes susceptibility. In aggregate these oligogenes might explain perhaps 50–75% of the overall variability in disease occurrence. There could still be a polygenic 'background' in which many, possibly hundreds, of polygenes contribute to the residual variability in susceptibility, but these polygenes in aggregate would explain only a modest amount of the overall susceptibility. Lastly, one can imagine a scenario in which a single major gene accounts for, say, 70% or 80% of the variability in susceptibility, again with a polygenic background. If this last situation is the true one, it might be possible to develop segregation models to describe the mode of inheritance. These segregation models could then be used to study possible linkage to various genetic markers spanning the entire genome to locate the chromosomal regions that harbor diabetes susceptibility genes. This approach is discussed in a later section of this chapter.

SEGREGATION ANALYSES OF TYPE 2 DIABETES

With segregation analyses one attempts to infer the presence of major susceptibility genes from the distribution of phenotypes in pedigrees. For a fully penetrant, autosomal dominant trait it is usually relatively easy to recognize vertical transmission through two or more generations with the trait appearing in approximately half of the offspring of matings between affected and unaffected individuals. When penetrance is delayed until middle age, however, or when it is markedly influenced or even overriden by environmental factors, it is much more difficult to discern the mode of inheritance. In such instances the mode of inheritance that fits the observed distribution of the trait in families can be assessed best using complex segregation analysis in which maximum likelihood techniques are used to estimate the parameters and possibilities of various transmission models. These models are then compared using the likelihood ratio test. (The difference in two times the natural logarithm of the likelihoods is asymptotically distributed as a chi-squared statistic, thereby providing a basis for statistical inference.) A putative major susceptibility gene is posited, and the probability of having each of the three possible genotypes (AA, Aa, aa) is estimated for each individual in the pedigree, as are the probabilities of transmitting the hypothetical susceptibility allele (A) from parent to offspring. For mendelian traits, these transmission probabilities are, of course, 1.0 for the AA homozygote, 0.5 for the Aa heterozygote, and 0 for the aa homozygote.

If the data-derived estimates of the transmission probabilities are close to their mendelian expectations, one can suspect the presence of a major gene. One then constrains the transmission probabilities to be equal to their mendelian expectations, and compares the likelihood of the resulting 'mendelian' model to that of the 'general' model, i.e., the model in which the transmission probabilities were estimated. If the likelihoods are not significantly different, one may conclude that the mendelian model fits the data as well as the general model, i.e., it is not 'rejected.' These models also typically allow for residual family resemblance (reflecting polygenic 'background' and/or shared environment), after having accounted for the family resemblance attributable to the major gene. One may also construct models in which there is no parent-to-offspring transmission, i.e., a purely environmental model in which the phenotype of the offspring is independent of that of either parent. Finally, one may construct models in which pure polygenic inheritance is simulated. One then computes the likelihoods of these 'non-mendelian' models and compares them with the likelihood of the general model. If the latter is significantly better, one may conclude that the non-mendelian models, unlike the mendelian model, have been rejected.

A number of segregation analyses have suggested the presence of major genes for quantitative traits related to diabetes. For example, an analysis of 16 Caucasian pedigrees from Utah ascertained through two or more type 2 diabetic siblings found evidence for an autosomal recessive gene, which accounted for approximately 33% of the variance in fasting plasma insulin concentration[15]. Later, Mitchell et al.[16] reported evidence for a major gene which accounted for approximately 31% of the variance in 2-hour post-oral glucose load insulin levels in 27 Mexican–American pedigrees from San Antonio, Texas. This gene appeared to affect serum insulin levels in an autosomal dominant fashion. As hyperinsulinemia usually reflects a compensatory response to underlying insulin resistance, which is thought to play a critical role in the development of type 2 diabetes, these data suggest the presence of major gene(s) which influence insulin resistance.

Elston et al.[17] performed complex segregation analysis on 30 Seminole Indian families from Oklahoma and 27 families from Florida. The results in Oklahoma suggested a major gene for serum glucose concentration measured 1 hour after an oral glucose load. The data were fitted equally well by an autosomal dominant model with an allele frequency of 9% or an autosomal recessive model with an allele frequency of 41%. Evidence for a major gene affecting serum glucose levels in the Florida families was not, however, observed. Segregation analyses have also been performed on Micronesian families from the South Pacific island of Nauru[18]. These analyses provided evidence for an autosomal dominant susceptibility gene for type 2 diabetes with an allele frequency of 0.31, although recessive inheritance could not be ruled out[18]. More recent studies have provided evidence for a major gene for early onset of type 2 diabetes in Pima Indians[19] and Mexican–Americans from San Antonio, Texas[20]. In the Pima Indian study, non-mendelian transmission of the early onset trait was rejected, and the best fitting models tended to be codominant, with the estimated frequency of the early onset allele ranging from 0.37 to 0.42. Similar results were found in Mexican–Americans except that the best-fitting model in this study was autosomal dominant[20]. For Mexican–Americans the mean age of diabetes onset was 51 years for individuals who were either homozygous for the early onset allele or heterozygous, and 85 years for individuals who were homozygous for the late-onset allele. It was of interest that the estimated frequency of the early onset allele in Mexican–Americans ranged from 0.17 to 0.25, i.e., roughly half the frequency estimated for Pima Indians. This lower allele frequency fits well with admixture estimates, which suggests that about 40% of the gene pool of low-income San Antonio Mexican–Americans is derived from Native American ancestral sources[12,13]. A surprising feature of the segregation model for Mexican–Americans was the impressively high percentage of variability in age of diabetes onset which was accounted for by the putative major gene, namely, 70%. This gene appeared to account for all of the family resemblance in age of diabetes onset, because the parameter estimates for residual family resemblance in age of onset were not statistically significant once the major gene was taken into account.

GENETIC LINKAGE

Aside from adequate family material, accurate phenotyping and appropriate models of the mode of inheritance of a genetic disorder, a mechanism for examining the segregation of a disease trait with respect to specific genome segments is required to assess genetic linkage. Gregor Mendel's second law governing heredity, the principle of independent assortment, states that genes transmit from one generation to the next independently of one another. Although this is true for most genes, Mendel was unaware that genes are arranged in a linear fashion on chromosomes. Genes located close to one another on the same chromosome disobey Mendel's second law in that they do not assort independently; they are thus described as being 'linked.' This linkage is not perfect as a result of genetic 'crossing over' during gamete formation (meiosis) (Figure 3.3). As a consequence of meiotic crossing over from generation to generation, markers on the same chromosome will be separated with a frequency proportional to the distance between them. This genetic distance between loci is estimated by the recombination frequency. If markers A and B recombine in 5 out of 100 meioses, i.e., a 5% recombination frequency, they are considered to be close together,

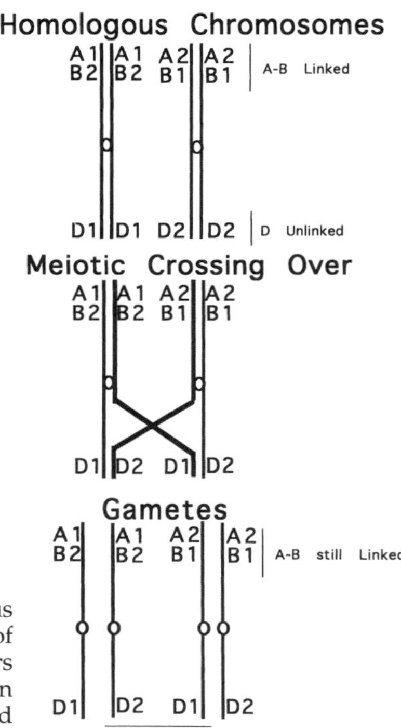

Figure 3.3. Meiotic crossing over. Homologous chromosomes pair during meiosis. The chance of a cross over separating tightly linked markers (A, B) is proportional to the distance between them. Distant markers (D), are unlinked and recombine at 50% frequency.

or tightly linked. If markers A and C undergo recombination 20 times out of 100 meioses, i.e., a 20% recombination frequency, they are linked, but much farther apart. Markers showing 50% recombination are not genetically linked even if they are on the same chromosome, because 50% recombination is indistinguishable from independent assortment. The phenomenon of genetic recombination permits the mapping and ordering of genetic markers; in the above example, if the recombination frequency between markers B and C is 15% then the gene map would be: A–5%–B–15%–C. Given an accurate model for the mode of transmission (e.g., autosomal dominant, autosomal recessive, etc.), a genetic phenotype can likewise be ordered with respect to markers on a genetic map.

The significance of a genetic linkage signal is assessed using the logarithm (base 10) of the odds (LOD) score method (reviewed in reference[21]). This method calculates iteratively a likelihood function for the pattern of segregation observed in a family for every possible linkage distance (θ) between two loci (e.g., between two markers or between a marker and a putative disease gene). The values of these likelihoods are compared with those calculated using a model of independent assortment ($\theta = 50\%$, or non-linkage). A ratio of likelihoods is plotted for all values of θ, and a LOD curve is generated. The best estimate of θ is the point on the LOD curve at which the LOD score is highest. A LOD score of 3.0 (i.e., the support for linkage is 1000 times greater than the support for non-linkage) has become accepted as the minimum criterion for establishing linkage. Conversely, LOD scores of less than -2.0 (i.e., the support for non-linkage is 100 times greater than the support for linkage) indicate that the loci are not linked.

Genetic distance is measured in centimorgans (cM) in honor of T.H. Morgan who, in his pioneering studies of fruit fly genetics, first described meiotic crossing over in 1910. The relationship between recombination frequency and centimorgans is approximate; measures of recombination frequency underestimate genetic disease, because double crossovers between markers are not scored as recombinants. At close distances, however, 1 cM approximates a 1% recombination frequency. The human genome spans approximately 3000 cM and has approximately 3.0×10^9 basepairs. Thus, 1 cM averages about 1 million basepairs. As a result of differences in the frequency of crossing over in different regions of the chromosome, however, 1 cM can range from well under a million basepairs at the tip of a chromosome, where crossing over is relatively common, to several million basepairs near the centromere, where crossing over is rare.

GENETIC MARKERS

To track the segregation of genomic segments, genetic markers are required. For maximum utility in linkage studies, these markers should be numerous, codominant, and demonstrate a high degree of heterozygosity. Codominance means that both classes of homozygotes are distinguishable from heterozygotes, insuring that the allele designation is unambiguous. Heterozygosity is defined as the proportion of individuals in a population who are heterozygous at a given locus. If, for example, a marker has five alleles, each of which occurs with a population frequency of 0.2, then 4% of the population (0.2×0.2) will be homozygous for each of the five alleles. The total percentage of homozygotes in the population will then be 20%, and the heterozygosity of the marker will be $1 - 0.20$ or 0.80. High heterozygosity is important because the efficiency of linkage studies is proportional to the number of informative matings, i.e., matings in which parent(s) are heterozygous for the marker (Figure 3.4).

Abundant, codominant, and highly polymorphic genetic markers for use in carrying out comprehensive genetic linkage studies have emerged only

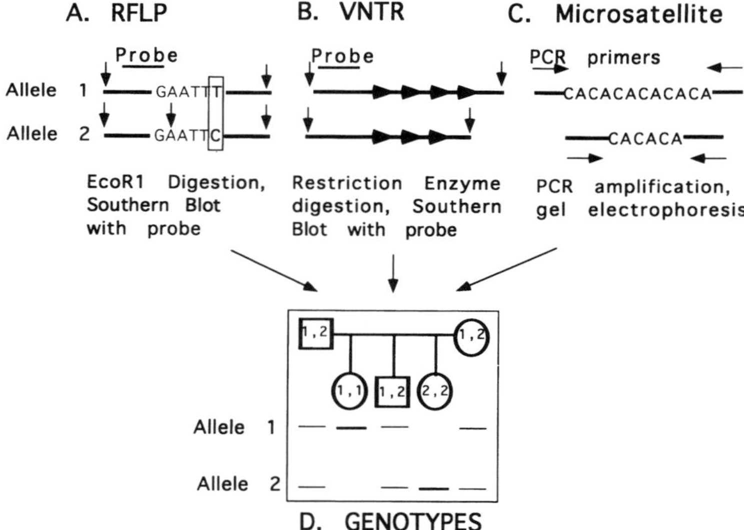

Figure 3.4. DNA-based polymorphic markers. (a) Restriction fragment length polymorphism markers result from DNA sequence changes. In this case, a T $\rightarrow$ C transition creates an EcoR1 site (GAATTC). The polymorphic base is boxed. Genotyping is by digestion with EcoR1, gel electrophoresis, and Southern blotting with a locus-specific probe (bar). (b) Variable number of tandem repeat (VNTR) markers are formed by differing numbers of tandem repeats (triangles). Genotyping is by restriction enzyme digestion, followed by gel electrophoresis and Southern blotting, with a locus-specific probe (bar). (c) Microsatellite markers are formed by very short tandem repeats (CA in this example). Genotyping is by polymerase chain reaction (PCR) with locus-specific primers (horizontal arrows). (d) Genotypes for a mating between two heterozygous (1, 2) parents, resulting in offspring who are either heterozygous (1, 2) or homozygous (1,1; 2,2).

within the last 15 years. Before that, only a few genetic markers, mainly protein polymorphisms, blood group antigens, or human lymphocyte antigen gene polymorphisms, were available. This situation changed dramatically with the advent of recombinant DNA technology. The resulting DNA-based markers exploit two common types of polymorphism in the human population (Figure 3.4). The first type of polymorphism results from single nucleotide sequence variants. These single base polymorphisms are very abundant, estimated to occur at a frequency of one every 400 basepairs[22]. They are easily genotyped because they frequently alter the recognition sites of site-specific restriction endonucleases. Thus, when genomic DNA is cleaved with a restriction enzyme, the fragmentation pattern of the locus varies depending on the presence or absence of the polymorphic base. As shown in Figure 3.4a, these alterations result in restriction fragments of differing lengths which can be detected by Southern blotting with locus-specific DNA probes or amplification by the polymerase chain reaction (PCR) and visualization after gel electrophoresis. These genetic markers are thus called 'restriction fragment length polymorphisms' or RFLPs[23]. Although numerous, the biallelic nature of these polymorphisms limits their heterozygosity to a maximum of 50%.

The second type of genetic polymorphism results from population variations in the number of copies of several categories of tandemly repeating genomic elements. These polymorphisms include variable numbers of tandem repeat (VNTR or minisatellite, see references[24,25]) and microsatellite[26] polymorphisms. As shown in Figure 3.4b, VNTR polymorphisms are detected by fragmenting genomic DNA with restriction endonucleases that flank the repeating unit, followed by Southern blot analysis with locus-specific probes. As shown in Figure 3.4c, microsatellite polymorphisms can be detected by PCR amplification using locus-specific oligonucleotide primers, followed by gel electrophoresis of the PCR products. Although tandem repeat polymorphisms are less abundant in the genome than RFLPs, they are still numerous and their high number of alleles typically raises the heterozygosity levels to more than 75%. The high heterozygosity and ease and efficiency of PCR amplification have made PCR-based microsatellite markers the mainstay of present-day genetic mapping exercises, although emerging technology to automate reading of single basepair polymorphisms may eclipse this technology in the future.

GENETIC MAPPING STRATEGIES

Before the development of high-resolution genetic maps, two basic approaches to linkage mapping emerged. One approach emphasized polymorphisms of genes which on theoretical grounds were possibly thought to play a causative role in the disorder under study (the candidate gene approach). The other approach utilized anonymous genetic markers spanning the entire genome (the general linkage approach). Initially, both methods were hampered. The candidate gene approach suffered from the fact that very few of the estimated 50 000–100 000 human genes had been cloned, so that the probability that the gene under study was in fact a susceptibility gene was remote. The general linkage approach was initially hampered by a lack of knowledge of the locations of the genetic markers with respect to one another. Often, even after many hundreds of markers had been typed, significant fractions of the genome remained untested. As the genetic maps matured, however, large numbers of markers and genes spanning the entire genome have been localized. By testing a series of markers known to be more or less equally spaced across the genome, a complete genome scan for linkage can be accomplished with 250–300 markers[27–29]. Once a signal has been detected in a genome scan, candidate genes known to map to the region in question can be tested.

LINKAGE DISEQUILIBRIUM

By the definition of genetic linkage, marker alleles near a disease gene locus will co-segregate with the disease gene in a pedigree containing affected individuals. This phenomenon leads to a family specific 'haplotype' (haploid genotype) for the chromosome bearing the disease gene. If the haplotypes associated with the disease susceptibility gene vary from family to family such that their frequency distribution reflects the distribution of haplotype frequencies in the general population, then the disease gene and the linked genetic markers are considered to be in linkage equilibrium. In some cases, there is non-random association between a particular haplotype and a disease gene locus *across* families, such that the frequency with which a particular haplotype is found on chromosomes bearing disease genes is much higher than the frequency of that haplotype in the general population. This phenomenon, referred to as 'linkage disequilibrium,' results when a new disease gene mutation occurs within a particular haplotype. Population dynamic events, such as founder effects, can also result in genetic disequilibrium. The resulting tight linkage between the disease gene and the surrounding markers is only slowly eroded by crossing-over events over many generations. The presence of linkage disequilibrium implies very tight genetic linkage between the markers and the disease gene; if detected, it is a useful tool for gene cloning studies (reviewed in reference[29]). Not uncommonly, linkage disequilibrium is intragenic, i.e., the marker in disequilibrium with the disease susceptibility gene is a polymorphism *within* the same gene that bears the functional mutation.

LINKAGE VERSUS ASSOCIATION

Linkage and association are commonly confused in discusssions of genetic analysis of human disease. Linkage implies that specific marker–phenotype combinations will segregate as haplotypes *within a family* because the markers and the disease gene are very near one another on the same chromosome. Association refers to non-random statistical associations (which may or may not be genetic in origin) between a marker allele and a phenotype in the *general population*, i.e., the two traits occur in the same individual more often than predicted by chance. The association may result from linkage disequilibrium and, if so, it should be possible to confirm it by linkage studies. In some cases, the association may indicate the presence of a nearby susceptibility gene as in the case of the association between the HLA-DR3 and DR4 alleles and type 1 diabetes[30]. On the other hand, statistical associations can be misleading, because they are highly sensitive to ethnic stratification within a population. For example, as noted earlier, an association between a particular IgG haplotype and reduced prevalence of type 2 diabetes was found in the Pima–Papago population. This association was explained, however, when it was found that the IgG haplotype in question specifically reflected European ancestry (a population at considerably lower risk of type 2 diabetes), and that it did not even occur in *full-blooded* Native Americans[11]!

TESTING FOR LINKAGE USING SEGREGATION MODELS

Although segregation models can be used to test for linkage, relative few attempts have been made to do this. Using the model described for the San Antonio population, we found weak evidence for linkage between the gene for insulin receptor substrate 1 and age of diabetes onset in Mexican–Americans[20]. We also found evidence for linkage to two regions on chromosome 11: one near the insulin gene and one near the sulfonylurea receptor gene[31]. The latter linkage was strongly confirmed by the variance components method (see below). It is important to emphasize that segregation models represent merely a parsimonious description of the data. The statistical approach allows the claim that the model describes the data better than those specific alternative models that have been examined and rejected. But, obviously, one cannot explicitly examine all possible alternatives. Thus, even when the model fits the data reasonably well, one cannot exclude the possibility that some other, perhaps more complex, model would fit the data even better. Although segregation analysis is a powerful method for identifying linkage, it is dependent on the accuracy of the model. If the model is seriously misspecified with respect to the true mode of inheritance, biased estimates of linkage are likely to result. Since there is no a priori way to be certain that the model is sufficiently accurate to be useful, other methods of detecting linkage have been developed that are relatively independent of models that specify the mode of inheritance. These 'model-independent' methods are less powerful, but also less vulnerable to misspecification. They are discussed in the next section.

TESTING FOR LINKAGE USING ALLELE-SHARING METHODS

ANALYSIS OF RELATIVE PAIRS

Testing for linkage using segregation models depends on co-segregation of the trait with the putatively linked marker. In contrast, allele-sharing methods are based on the idea that relatives who are concordant for a trait will share markers more often than would be predicted by their kinship relationships if the markers are linked, but not if they are not linked. For example, for sibs the probability of sharing an allele at a given locus is 0.5, and for first cousins the probability is 0.125. But, if the sibs or first cousins are concordant for a trait, and if the locus in question is linked to a susceptibility gene for that trait, then the likelihood of their sharing the marker in question will be higher than predicted by their kinship relationship. Allele sharing may be of two types: identical by state (IBS) or identical by descent (IBD). Two relatives may share an allele, but have inherited it either from different ancestors or from the same ancestor, but from different homologous chromosomes in the event that the common ancestor happened to be homozygous for the allele in question. This type of sharing is referred to as IBS. Only if two relatives have inherited copies of the same allele, i.e., from the same homologous chromosome of a common ancestor, are they said to share IBD. Only sharing that is IBD informs us about linkage, because, in the event that the common ancestor carried a disease susceptibility gene linked to the marker allele in question, only if the two relatives are IBD for this marker allele, and in the absence of recombination, will they both have inherited the haplotype bearing the disease susceptibility gene.

In some cases it is possible to infer unambiguously that an allele shared by two relatives is IBD. For example, if four alleles are identified in a sibship, it is obvious, barring non-parentage, that only one copy of each allele can be represented in the parental generation. Thus, any sharing of alleles within the sibship must be IBD. Also, when both or in some cases when only one parent has been genotyped, sharing IBD can sometimes be inferred unambiguously. In many situations, however, it is possible only to estimate the probability that the sharing is IBD. Clearly, when two relatives share a rare allele, the sharing is more likely to be IBD than when they share a common allele, because, in the former case, it is more likely that the allele in question entered the pedigree just once, and that all family members who share it do so IBD.

Linkage analyses based on allele-sharing methods may be restricted to affected individuals only, or they may include both affected and unaffected individuals. For diseases in which penetrance is delayed until middle age, restricting the analyses to affected individuals circumvents the problem of misclassifying as unaffected young individuals who may some day express the trait as they age. But, as it is often desirable to genotype unaffected, in addition to affected, family members to improve inferences about whether or not allele sharing is IBD, it seems wasteful to discard whatever linkage information is contained in the discordant and concordant unaffected relative pairs. In the former case, *lack* of sharing IBD constitutes evidence for linkage and, in the latter, sharing IBD still constitutes evidence for linkage just as in the case of affected relative pairs. If phenotypic information from unaffected individuals is to be used, it is desirable to weight the information from older unaffected individuals more heavily than that from younger unaffected individuals, i.e., a 20-year-old unaffected individual contains relatively weak information about linkage because he or she may well express the trait at an older age; a 70-year-old unaffected individual, however, contains nearly as much linkage information as an affected individual, because his or her affection status is unlikely to change with continued aging. As we shall see, an analytic technique known as the variance component method has the capability of appropriately weighting the information contained in unaffected individuals based on their age.

One popular study design that has been used to search for linkage to diabetes susceptibility genes is the affected sib-pair method. As the name implies, this method is restricted to affected individuals and considers only sibs. An example of this method is the study of 408 Mexican–Americans with type 2 diabetes living in Starr County, Texas[32]. These individuals were derived from 170 sibships that generated 330 affected sib-pairs. A genome-wide scan involving 490 markers with an average distance of 8.6 cM between adjacent markers was performed. A LOD score of 3.2 in favor of linkage between type 2 diabetes and a region near the q-terminal end of chromosome 2 was observed. No linkage between this region and type 2 diabetes was found in non-Hispanic white or Japanese populations. Later, possible evidence of linkage was confirmed with a LOD score of 0.86 (corresponding to a nominal p value of less than 0.05) in an independent set of sib-pairs from Starr County, but so far it has not been confirmed in other studies. Unfortunately, there are no candidate genes in this region. The affected sib-pair method was also used to demonstrate linkage between diabetes and a region on chromosome 7 (7q21–22) in Pima Indians[33].

Sib-pair linkage analyses need not be limited to affected pairs. For quantitative trait loci (QTLs), the Haseman–Elston method is commonly used[34].

This method is based on the expectation that, when a marker is linked to a quantitative trait, the mean squared difference between siblings for that trait will be inversely related to the number of marker alleles that the siblings share IBD. For an unlinked marker there should be no relationship between the mean squared difference in a quantitative trait and the number of alleles shared. The Haseman–Elston method can also be used with discrete traits such as diabetes. Using this method linkages between early onset diabetes (age of onset <45 years) and a region on chromosome 1 (1q21–23), and between diabetes adjusted for age and a region on chromosome 11 (11q23–25), were demonstrated in Pima Indians[33].

VARIANCE COMPONENTS METHOD

It is possible to partition the variance in a quantitative trait into its various components, namely, a component resulting from linkage with a marker locus, one resulting from residual additive genetic effects, and a random or environmental one. The first component depends on the IBD relationships between all relative pairs in a pedigree, the second on the kinship relationships between all relative pairs, and the last on the residual error variance. This method can be used on sibships, but is also suitable for extended pedigrees. In the latter case it is necessary to estimate the IBD relationships for all relative pairs, including whatever distant relatives are represented in the pedigree. The necessary computations for these estimates are more formidable and computer intensive than in the case of estimating the IBD relationships between sib pairs. Recently, however, techniques for performing these computations in a reasonable amount of time have become available. A LOD score for linkage can be calculated from the difference in likelihoods of a model in which the marker variance is constrained to be 0 and a model in which this component of variance is estimated. The former model simulates polygenic inheritance, because the only family resemblance that is allowed for depends exclusively on kinship relationships and not on any allele sharing at potentially linked loci.

A significantly higher likelihood of the unconstrained model compared to the constrained model constitutes evidence of linkage between the trait and the marker in question. Although initially developed for QTLs, the variance component approach has been adapted for discrete traits by using a continuous liability function and defining affectation status in terms of having crossed a threshold on the liability scale. The variance components method has been used in San Antonio Mexican–Americans to study linkage with glucose concentrations 2 hours after the ingestion of a standard oral glucose load. Figure 3.5 presents a multipoint LOD score curve summarizing the evidence for linkage between 2-hour glucose and points along chromosome 11[31]. As can be seen, strong evidence for linkage exists in a region approximately 60 cM from the p-terminal end of the chromosome. An interesting

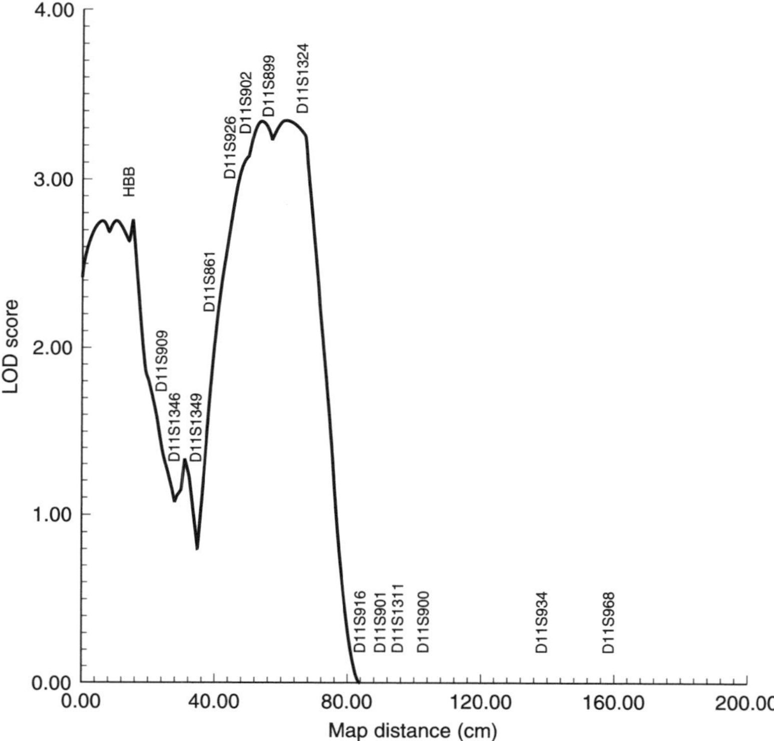

Figure 3.5. Linkage between 2-hour glucose concentration and points along chromosome 11. (Reproduced from Stern et al.[31] with permission.)

candidate gene – the high affinity sulfonylurea receptor (SUR1)/inward rectifier gene – is located in this region. SUR1 is one of the subunits that, along with the inward rectifier, forms the ATP-sensitive potassium channel that is expressed on the β-cell membrane and that is involved in regulating insulin secretion. Sulfonylureas stimulate insulin secretion by binding to this receptor. A number of mutations of the SUR1 gene have been described that produce a syndrome known as persistent hyperinsulinemic hypoglycemia of infancy (PHHI), a severe form of neonatal hypoglycemia[35]. Whether or not more subtle alterations of the SUR1 gene play a role in ordinary type 2 diabetes, as suggested by the above linkage results, remains to be demonstrated.

CONCLUSION

Although the genetic bases for a number of rare type of diabetes, such as insulin receptor mutations and maturity-onset diabetes of the young, have now been defined, susceptibility genes for ordinary type 2 diabetes remain to be discovered. Nevertheless, there is persuasive evidence that this type of diabetes has strong genetic determinants. This evidence includes the familial nature of type 2 diabetes, as shown by epidemiologic studies that have documented family history of diabetes as being a strong diabetes risk factor, by studies showing increased diabetes risk in relatives of diabetic patients, and by twin studies. Studies of hybrids of high- and low-risk diabetes populations have also provided evidence for a genetic basis for type 2 diabetes. Although the mode of inheritance of diabetes is unknown, there are several theoretical possibilities, including: polygenic inheritance in which diabetes risk is determined by the additive or multiplicative effects of many, possibly hundreds, of polygenes; oligogenic inheritance, in which diabetes risk is primarily determined by the action of a few, perhaps two or three, genes; and single gene inheritance, in which diabetes risk is determined primarily by the action of a single gene. Segregation analyses from a number of populations with a high prevalence of diabetes have supported single gene inheritance, although this is probably superimposed on a polygenic background, with the single gene accounting for up to 70% of the variance in phenotype expression in certain populations.

Two approaches have been used to locate and identify type 2 diabetes susceptibility genes: the candidate gene approach and the whole genome scan approach. Candidate genes are genes that, on theoretical grounds, are thought to play a causative role in the development of diabetes; they are therefore examined for variants to see if these are associated with increased diabetes risk. The whole genome scan approach involves searching for linkage between the disease and a series of anonymous genetic markers that span the entire genome. A number of statistical analytic approaches have been developed to establish linkage between these markers and diabetes itself and/or various diabetes-related phenotypes. Although thus far these molecular and statistical techniques have not led to the identification of susceptibility genes for type 2 diabetes, the remarkable pace of progress in DNA and computer technology holds out the promise that such genes will be discovered in the near future.

ACKNOWLEDGEMENTS

The authors would like to thank Jean MacCluer and John Blangero of the Southwest Foundation for Biomedical Research, San Antonio, TX for critically reading the manuscript and offering many helpful suggestions.

REFERENCES

1. Taylor S. Lilly lecture: molecular mechanisms of insulin resistance. Lessons from patients with mutations in the insulin-receptor gene. *Diabetes* 1992; **41**:1473–90.
2. Knowler WC, Pettitt DJ, Saad MF, Bennett PH. Diabetes mellitus in the Pima Indians: incidence, risk factors and pathogenesis. *Diabetes Metab Rev* 1990; **6**:1–27.
3. Mitchell BD, Kammerer CM, Reinhard LJ, Stern MP, MacCluer JW. Is there an excess in maternal transmission of NIDDM? *Diabetologia* 1995; **38**:314–7.
4. Pettitt DJ, Nelson RG, Saad MF, Bennett PH, Knowler WC. Diabetes and obesity in the offspring of Pima Indian women with diabetes during pregnancy. *Diabetes Care* 1993; **16** (suppl 1): 310–14.
5. Mitchell BD, Kammerer CM, Reinhart LJ, Stern MP. NIDDM in Mexican–American families. Heterogeneity by age of onset. *Diabetes Care* 1994; **17**:567–73.
6. Risch N. Linkage strategies for genetically complex traits. I. Multilocus models. *Am J Hum Genet* 1990; **46**:222–8.
7. Barnett AH, Eff C, Leslie RDG, Pyke DA. Diabetes in identical twins. A study of 200 pairs. *Diabetologia* 1981; **20**:87–93.
8. Newman B, Selby JV, King M-C, Slemenda C, Fabsitz R, Friedman GD. Concordance for type 2 (non-insulin-dependent) diabetes mellitus in male twins. *Diabetologia* 1987; **30**:763–8.
9. Brosseau JD, Eelkema RC, Crawford AC, Abe TA. Diabetes among the Three Affiliated Tribes: correlation with degree of Indian inheritance. *Am J Public Health* 1979; **69**:1277–8.
10. Serjeantson SW, Owerbach D, Zimmet P, Nerup J, Thoma K. Genetics of diabetes in Nauru: effects of foreign admixture, HLA antigens and the insulin-gene-linked polymorphism. *Diabetologia* 1983; **25**:13–17.
11. Knowler WC, Williams RC, Pettitt DJ, Steinberg AG. $Gm^{3;5,13,14}$ and type 2 diabetes mellitus: an association in American Indians with genetic admixture. *Am J Hum Gene* 1988; **43**:520–6.
12. Gardner LI, Stern MP, Haffner SM et al. Prevalence of diabetes in Mexican Americans: relationship to percent of gene pool derived from American Indian sources. *Diabetes* 1984; **33**:86–92.
13. Chakraborty R, Ferrell RE, Stern MP, Haffner SM, Hazuda HP, Rosenthal M. Relationship of prevalence of non-insulin dependent diabetes mellitus to Amerindian admixture in the Mexican Americans of San Antonio, Texas. *Gene Epidemiol* 1986; **3**:35–54.
14. Stern MP, Haffner SM. Type II diabetes and its complications in Mexican Americans. *Diabetes/Metab Rev* 1990; **6**:29–45.
15. Schumacher MC, Hasstedt SJ, Hunt SC, Williams RR, Elbein SC. Major gene effect for insulin levels in familial NIDDM pedigrees. *Diabetes* 1992; **41**:416–23.
16. Mitchell BD, Kammerer CM, Hixson JE et al. Evidence for a major gene affecting postchallenge insulin levels in Mexican-Americans. *Diabetes* 1995; **44**:284–9.
17. Elston RC, Namboodiri KK, Nino HV, Pollitzer WS. Studies on blood and urine glucose in Seminole Indians: indications for segregation of a major gene. *Am J Hum Genet* 1974; **26**:13–34.
18. Serjeantson S, Zimmet P. Diabetes in the Pacific: evidence for a major gene. In Baba S, Gould MK, Zimmet P, eds. *Diabetes Mellitus, Recent Knowledge on Etiology, Complications and Treatment*. Sydney: Academic Press Australia, 1984; pp. 23–30.
19. Hanson RL, Elston RC, Pettit DJ, Bennett PH, Knowler WC. Segregation analysis of non-insulin-dependent diabetes mellitus in Pima Indians: evidence for a major gene effect. *Am J Hum Genet* 1995; **57**:160–70.

20. Stern MP, Mitchell BD, Blangero et al. Evidence for a major gene for type II diabetes and linkage analyses with selected candidate genes in Mexican–Americans. *Diabetes* 1996; **45**:563–8.
21. Morton NE. LODs past and present. *Genetics* 1995; **140**:7–12.
22. Jeffreys AJ. DNA sequence variants in the Gγ-, Aγ-, δ- and β-globin genes in man. *Cell* 1979; **18**:1–10.
23. Botstein D, White RL, Skolnick M, Davis RW. Construction of a genetic map in man using restriction fragment length polymorphisms. *Am J Hum Genet* 1980; **32**:314–21.
24. Jeffreys AJ, Wilson V, Thein SL. Hypervariable 'minisatellite' regions in human DNA. *Nature* 1985; **314**:67–73.
25. Nakamura Y, Leppert M, O'Connell P et al. Variable number of tandem repeat (VNTR) markers for human gene mapping. *Science* 1987; **235**:1616–22.
26. Weber J, May PE. Abundant class of human DNA polymorphisms which can be typed using the polymerase chain reaction. *Am J Hum Genet* 1989; **44**:388–96.
27. Hoffman EP. The evolving genome project: current and future impact. *Am J Hum Genet* 1994; **54**:129–36.
28. Bently DR, Dunham I. Mapping human chromosomes. *Curr Opin Genet Dev* 1995; **5**:328–34.
29. Collins FS. Positional cloning moves from perditional to traditional. *Nature Genet* 1995; **9**:347–50.
30. Atkinson MA, Maclaren NK. Islet cell autoantigens in insulin-dependent diabetes. *J Clin Invest* 1993; **92**:1608–16.
31. Stern MP, Duggirala R, Mitchell BD et al. Evidence for linkage of regions on chromosomes 6 and 11 to plasma glucose concentrations in Mexican Americans. *Genome Res* 1996; **6**:724–34.
32. Hanis CL, Boerwinkle E, Chakraborty R et al. A genome-wide search for human non-insulin-dependent (type 2) diabetes genes reveals a major susceptibility locus on chromosome 2. *Nature Genet* 1996; **13**:161–6.
33. Hanson R. The Pima Diabetes Genes Group. Genomic scan for markers linked to type II diabetes in Pima Indians. *Diabetes* 1997; **46** (suppl. 1): 51A.
34. Haseman JK, Elston R. The investigation of linkage between a quantitative trait and a marker locus. *Behav Genet* 1972; **2**:3–9.
35. Aguilar-Bryan L, Bryan J. ATP-sensitive potassium channels, sulfonylurea receptors, and persistent hyperinsulinemic hypoglycemia of infancy. *Diabetes Rev* 1996; **4**:336–46.

4

Methods to Identify the Major Gene

M. McCARTHY

Reader in Molecular Genetics, Unit of Metabolic Medicine, Imperial College School of Medicine at St Mary's, Norfolk Place, London W2 1PG, UK

That current treatments for type 2 diabetes are unsatisfactory is clear to all those concerned – the physician, the scientist, the patient and the pharmaceutical industry. There is a need for novel preventive and therapeutic strategies that target the earliest stages in the development of type 2 diabetes, and for diagnostic tools to identify those individuals at the greatest risk of future diabetes. The main obstacle to both of these aims has been inadequate understanding of the basic pathophysiological processes. This has prevented a rigorous and logical approach to the identification of key molecules and critical metabolic processes suitable for manipulation. It is expected that current efforts to identify the major genes underlying the inherited susceptibility to type 2 diabetes will remedy this deficiency.

IS THERE A MAJOR GENE FOR TYPE 2 DIABETES?

The title of this chapter raises certain questions. What is meant by a 'major gene'? What is the evidence that major genes contribute to the development of type 2 diabetes? Are the methods that obtain in the identification of major genes qualitatively different to those employed in the detection of minor genetic effects?

It is tautology to define a major gene as 'a gene, variation in which accounts for a significant proportion of the variation in individual susceptibility to type 2 diabetes' but this represents the best description available. The concept is a relative one, because the proportion of the

Type 2 Diabetes: Prediction and Prevention. Edited by Graham A. Hitman

variance contributed by a given gene will depend on the extent of variation in other aetiological genes, as well as the variation in environmental susceptibility factors. Thus a gene may play a major role in one population, but not in another, and the importance of a gene may ebb and flow over the generations as environmental circumstances change. Records indicate scant evidence for diabetes among the Pima Indians of Arizona during the late nineteenth and early twentieth centuries, and consequently, no major genes for diabetes would have been detectable[1]. By the late twentieth century, the prevalence of diabetes has rocketed to 40% in this population and it is likely that a limited number of 'major' genes underlie the variation in glucose tolerance[2]. Variation within these major genes did not appear as if by magic over the course of a handful of generations. It seems reasonable to assume that relatively ancient polymorphisms in these aetiological genes have been maintained through selective advantage (perhaps through an enhanced ability to survive through periods of famine) and that their diabetogenic tendency has been unmasked by changes in lifestyle and diet[3,4].

Detecting major genetic effects is the province of segregation analysis, and several valiant attempts have been made to study segregation patterns in diabetic families to adduce evidence for their existence[2,5–7]. No consistent pattern has emerged. This may reflect the true state of affairs (i.e. major genes are seen in some populations but not others), but equally it may have resulted from the inherent methodological weaknesses of segregation analysis[8]. In practice, it is rarely possible to collect sufficient families to allow estimation of the multiple parameters required in any realistic model of the genetic architecture of type 2 diabetes and/or to test out feasible oligogenic alternatives to extreme single-gene and polygene models. Besides, accurate segregation analysis requires specification of the precise scheme under which the families were collected, to allow rigorous correction for that ascertainment scheme. For example, if families are ascertained only if they contain at least one diabetic subject, one needs to 'allow for' all those families with no diabetic subjects, if accurate estimates of gene frequencies and penetrances are to be obtained. It is difficult, if not impossible, to achieve this in most circumstances: one obvious source of bias is that motivational factors may lead to enhanced participation and, hence, over-representation, of families with strong family histories of diabetes.

Historically, distinction has been made between methods used to detect major genetic effects and those used to detect minor genetic effects. This distinction was always somewhat arbitrary and recent developments have blurred it further. Although this chapter principally charts the routes to the identification of major genes, many of the approaches described have broad application in the search for all types of type 2 diabetes loci.

WHAT ARE THE PROBLEMS WITH GENETIC DISSECTION?

To appreciate the decisions taken by researchers in their quest for the major susceptibility genes, it is vital to understand the obstacles that nature has placed in the way of this endeavour. Some of these are seen in other complex traits, whereas others are peculiar to, or particularly troublesome in, type 2 diabetes.

PROBLEMS WITH ANY COMPLEX TRAIT

As with any complex trait, the supposition is that susceptibility to type 2 diabetes results from the interaction of multiple genetic and environmental factors, some of which are 'major' and many 'minor' in both cases. Consequently, we expect the correlations between the clinical disease phenotype and genetic variation at any individual locus to be fairly weak, with obvious implications for the power of analyses that aim to detect individual genetic signals among (other) genetic and environmental noise.

Second, we have little idea about the characteristics of the loci that we are seeking. If the penetrances, dominance and allele frequencies at the most important susceptibility loci were known, we might wish to focus sample ascertainment among pedigrees that are presumed to be most informative for their detection[9]. If there were incontrovertible evidence for a single overweaning major gene for type 2 diabetes in a given population, our choice of methodology might change accordingly. If we knew which pathophysiological processes were critical for the maintenance of normal glucose tolerance, the choice of candidate genes might be more focused, and it might be clearer which intermediate trait parameters should be included in the phenotypic assessment of recruited families.

PROBLEMS SPECIFIC TO TYPE 2 DIABETES

Pathophysiology

It is disappointing to report that three decades of research into the physiological and metabolic basis of type 2 diabetes has seen only limited progress in the definition of the basic underlying defects[10,11]. In established type 2 diabetes, as well as in a variety of pre-diabetic subject groups, there are manifest abnormalities in both insulin action and insulin secretion, and there is evidence for an inherited basis for both, at least in Pima Indians[12,13]. However, disputes about the precise relationship between these two aspects of glucose metabolism have surfaced from time to time[10,11]. The inconsistency of physiological and metabolic studies in people with type 2 diabetes, as well as the diverse clinical features, suggest that the diagnostic umbrella of type 2 diabetes gathers together individuals who have arrived at a state of glucose intolerance through a variety of pathological mechanisms. This has obvious implications for genetic heterogeneity.

Diagnosis

The diagnosis of diabetes depends on threshold glucose levels that dichotomize a continuous distribution. These diagnostic thresholds were devised to reflect the risk of developing diabetic complications[14] and may not be relevant to genetic or environmental parameters that determine the development of hyperglycaemia; this may influence the entire range of glucose tolerance. The diagnostic procedure (the oral glucose tolerance test) is poorly reproducible and inaccurate[15]. Classification of the different subtypes of diabetes is largely empirical and currently under revision (see Table 1.1). Type 2 diabetes will remain essentially a diagnosis of exclusion, made after other, more readily identified causes of diabetes have been ruled out (e.g. type 1 diabetes; mitochondrial diabetes with deafness or MIDD). The boundaries between the types of diabetes are not precise: many subjects thought on clinical grounds to have type 2 diabetes show features more typical of slow-onset type 1[16].

Ethnic Variation

The 'thrifty genotype' hypothesis, in its broadest sense, suggests that diabetes-susceptibility alleles originally established themselves as variants to promote survival during times of nutrient scarcity[3,4]. It may well be that ethnic differences in prevalence and characteristics of type 2 diabetes result from the adoption of diverse mechanisms for metabolic efficiency during human history (in other words, convergent evolution). If so, it should be no surprise to find appreciable heterogeneity in the genetic basis of type 2 diabetes between ethnic groups.

Demographics

Type 2 diabetes usually arises late in life and is associated with premature mortality. This renders virtually impossible the collection of large multigenerational families segregating typical type 2 diabetes and even for sib-pair studies it makes it difficult to obtain parental DNA[17]. Furthermore, the information available from apparently unaffected relatives is compromised by the high rates of subclinical disease (such relatives may now be diabetic) and the age-related penetrance (they may become diabetic in the future).

Quantitative Traits

As the correlation between genotype and final disease phenotype (diabetes) is likely to be weak, it may be worthwhile to study intermediate traits (such as insulin secretion, insulin action and β-cell mass) which, it is presumed, lie proximal to the disease phenotype in the pathophysiological hierarchy[18]. Ideally, one would want to be able to measure such traits with high precision and low cost, and for them to provide useful information irrespective of the disease phenotype. Sadly, neither is true for type 2 diabetes. Notably, the intermediate trait information available from affected subjects (presumably, the very people most likely to be expressing susceptibility genes) is degraded by the effects of hyperglycaemia itself, and/or its treatment[19]. It may therefore be necessary to focus quantitative trait analyses among normoglycaemic individuals.

OVERVIEW OF APPROACHES EMPLOYED

Faced with this formidable array of obstacles and uncertainties, it is no surprise that different research groups have adopted different approaches to the identification of diabetes susceptibility genes; no single methodology can guarantee success. Ultimately, the success of each approach will depend on the extent to which the assumptions implicit in each strategy are a faithul reflection of the true state of affairs. For example, if it turns out that diabetes in rodents and that in humans have a completely different basis, then approaches that seek human genes through examination of regions syntenic to rodent susceptibility loci will not prove particularly rewarding. If there are no major genes for type 2 diabetes in a given population, a genome-wide scan for regions of excess allele sharing will have little power to pick out weak minor gene signals amidst the statistical noise. Perversely, these assumptions will only readily be tested when the genes have been found and the genetic architecture of the disease unravelled. This plurality of approaches enhances the chances that major genes will ultimately be found, whatever their nature or effects; however, the very diversity of datasets and methodologies may be a source of frustration and confusion when replication of positive findings is attempted.

The main steps to the identification of a major gene for type 2 diabetes in the late 1990s are summarized in Figure 4.1 and described in detail below.

SELECTING A SUITABLE CANDIDATE GENE

As Francis Collins has elegantly described[20,21], the simplistic distinction between 'forward' and 'reverse' genetics (the former proceeding from a

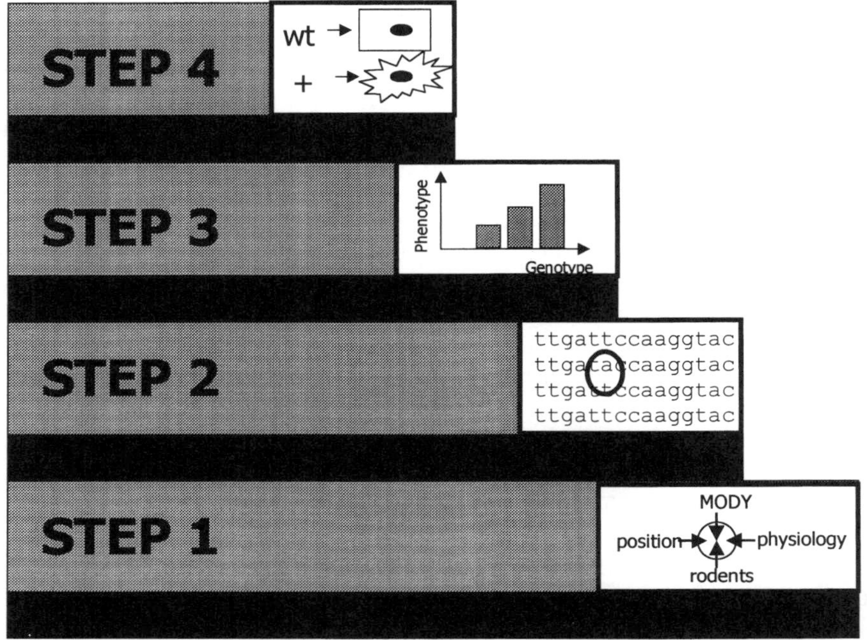

Figure 4.1. Steps on the way to identification of a type 2 diabetes susceptibility locus. For details, see the text.

knowledge of disease pathology to characterization of the genetic defect, the latter using identification of associated genetic defects as the basis for understanding disease pathophysiology) has probably outlived its usefulness. Increasingly, the clues that lead to identification of a complex trait susceptibility locus will come from a number of sources – positional information in humans, experiments in animal models of disease, and/or knowledge about the biology of the trait under examination

The term 'candidate gene' is here used in the widest sense – any gene that (on the basis of prior information) has a plausible claim to involvement in determining variation in the disease phenotype.

THE LIMITS OF CURRENT BIOLOGICAL KNOWLEDGE

The classic 'forward genetic' approach proceeds from an understanding of disease pathogenesis to characterization of the genetic defect. The limitations of this approach are obvious in type 2 diabetes. Although it is easy to identify a large number of processes that are evidently deranged in subjects with established diabetes, it is not clear which of these represent primary (potentially genetically determined) abnormalities and which are merely secondary. Loci influencing the inherited susceptibility to type 2 diabetes may therefore be operating in many diverse pathways and processes: β-cell glucose sensing, muscle insulin sensitivity, pancreatic development, incretin secretion, placental transport, to name but a few. Any gene implicated in the implementation or regulation of any of these processes could, if disrupted, contribute to the diabetic phenotype, and the list of potential candidates is consequently a long one. An increasing number of these biological candidates have been assessed for their role in type 2 diabetes, but this approach has produced only limited success thus far (see McCarthy and Hitman[22] for a review). Certainly, no major genes have been defined. This does not necessarily invalidate the purely biological approach (there is always the hope that the next gene chosen for study will hit the 'jackpot'), but it does increase the suspicion that many of the most important genes underlying type 2 diabetes susceptibility influence metabolic and developmental processes that are, as yet, poorly understood, and for which the major regulatory loci have not been identified.

USING POSITIONAL INFORMATION TO LOCATE SUSCEPTIBILITY GENES

A variety of strategies has developed over the past few years to tackle the problem of identifying susceptibility genes in the absence of prior biological candidates.

Strategy 1: Collect Small Multiplex Families and Search for Excess Allele Sharing

For both practical and theoretical reasons, the approach favoured by many groups has focused on the ascertainment of large numbers of small multiplex families, typically (though not exclusively) based around sibships with multiple diabetic siblings. Although such collections can be employed to test out candidate regions (for example, those arising out of linkage studies in rodent models of diabetes), the main value of these nuclear families lies in the implementation of genome-wide scans, i.e. unbiased global searches of the human genome. The rationale is simple. If one makes a collection of sibling pairs at random (i.e. the siblings are chosen without regard to their phenotype), we know, using simple rules of mendelian transmission, that the members of these pairs will, on average, share 50% of their genomes with each other. If, instead, the sib-pairs are selected so that they are correlated for some phenotype of interest (e.g. type 2 diabetes), and if we test them for a marker closely linked to a diabetes susceptibility locus, we expect to find them sharing somewhat more than 50% of their genomes. Put simply, sib-pairs displaying phenotypic correlations will show genotypic correlations around loci predisposing to that phenotype. Detection of such excess allele sharing is therefore the key to localization of the susceptibility genes.

In Figure 4.2 it is demonstrated that large numbers of families are required if one is to detect loci with the magnitude of effect expected in type 2 diabetes. The sibling relative risk (λ_S: the ratio obtained by dividing the prevalence of disease in the siblings of an affected individual with that in the population at large) for type 2 diabetes in European populations is around 3.5–4.0 (40% vs 10%)[23,24]. This figure gives some idea of the extent of familial aggregation of the trait, but, in the case of a complex trait such as type 2 diabetes, it incorporates the concerted action of several genes plus shared family environment. The component of this overall λ_s attributable to any individual locus will be considerably less (arbitrarily, we might expect a major gene for type 2 diabetes to have a locus-specific λ_s of 1.5–2.0). Figure 4.2 shows the power of sib-pair resources of differing sizes to detect linkage for trait loci with locus-specific sibling relative risks ranging from 1.1 (definitely a 'minor' gene) to 2.0 (undoubtedly a 'major' gene). It has been assumed that a genome-wide scan has been performed with sufficient microsatellites typed to extract 70% of the information content from the sib-pairs collected (this implies that a denser, more polymorphic map would be needed if the parents of the sib-pairs were not available)[25]. The threshold for detection of linkage is taken to be an MLS (maximised LOD score; a measure of the strength of the evidence for linkage) of 2.6 (this is the level associated with 'suggestive' evidence for genome-wide linkage advocated in recent guidelines)[26]. As expected, large genetic effects will be easier to detect

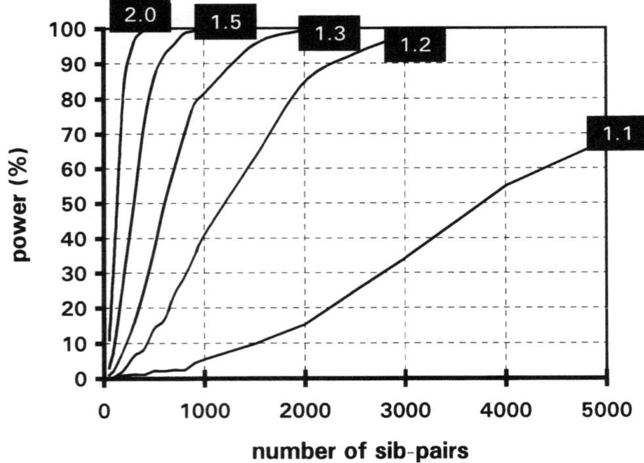

Figure 4.2. The power of affected sib-pairs to detect linkage to trait loci with sibling relative risks between 1.1 and 2.0. For a full description, see the text.

than small effects, but reliable detection of a major gene may require about 500 sib-pairs or more. Minor loci with a λ_s of less than 1.2 are not likely to be detected at all with this approach, whereas loci of modest effects (λ_s between 1.3 and 1.5) may escape detection unless extremely large clinical resources are deployed.

Uncertainties about the genetic architecture of type 2 diabetes mean that the researcher contemplating such a sib-pair study has to make several important decisions based on precious little information. The first concerns the population from which the families should be recruited. There are advantages in selecting sib-pairs from populations considered to be less ethnically heterogeneous – one may be dealing with a simpler genetic architecture in which certain loci are playing an inflated (and more easily detected) role in susceptibility to type 2 diabetes. Some of the earliest genome scans for type 2 diabetes have therefore been performed in Pima Indian and Finnish families[27,28]. Of course, the inevitable downside is that genes found in such 'atypical' populations may not be important determinants of diabetes in numerically more important populations. This need not concern us unduly, given our current state of ignorance; any locus contributing to susceptibility to type 2 diabetes is likely to provide profound biological insights irrespective of its numerical contribution worldwide.

The sib-pair collector also needs to consider which sib-pairs to ascertain. Not all sib-pairs will be equally informative for the detection of given locus, and it may be temping to pick out sib-pairs from families in which the apparent segregation pattern conforms to some idealized notion of trait locus segregation. For example, if a group were convinced that type 2 diabetes genes were dominantly transmitted in a given population, they might restrict ascertainment to sib-pairs from particular families (presumably, those with one parent affected and at least one unaffected sibling within the sib-ship) on the grounds that this will enhance power and reduce genotyping demands. It transpires that this is a risky procedure in the absence of precise information concerning the genetic architecture of the disease and the parameters of the loci to be detected. Families collected under such strict ascertainment schemes may indeed be more powerful if the segregation model has been accurately specified, but may prove woefully inadequate to the task of detecting loci with other characteristics. Strategies that are based around collecting all sib-pairs that meet diagnostic criteria for type 2 diabetes are, in contrast, robust under a wide range of genetic models[9,29].

With the advent of dense maps of well-characterized, highly polymorphic microsatellites[30], semi-automated high-throughput genotyping[31] and improved analytical techniques[32], implementation of a large genome scan has become a fairly routine, if expensive and time-consuming, procedure. Several genome scans for type 2 diabetes have reported their findings[27,33] and many more are under way[28,34,35].

The recent report of a possible diabetes susceptibility on chromosome 2q illustrates some of the problems with interpretation and replication that are arising as the results of these scans are published. Incidentally, these problems are by no means limited to the investigation of type 2 diabetes genetics[36–38]. In a collection of around 250 Mexican–American diabetic sibships, Hanis and colleagues[33] found suggestive evidence for linkage between type 2 diabetes and a region on chromosome 2q (the putative locus has been designated *NIDDM1*). Several other groups have subsequently examined this region in their respective datasets (including at least one other collection of Mexican–American families), but no replications have been forthcoming[33,35,39,40]. Reference to Figure 4.2 helps to explain why this might be. In the original positive study, the estimate of the locus-specific relative risk (λ_s) for *NIDDM1* was 1.37 with a wide confidence interval (1.13–1.74). Assume, for the moment, that this original study has indeed accurately pinpointed a susceptibility gene, but that the locus-specific relative risk of 1.37 somewhat overestimates the role played by *NIDDM1* outside Mexican–American populations. It is clear then from Figure 4.2 that these other replication studies (which have mostly employed in the region of 100–300 sib-pairs, and often used diagnostic criteria and ascertainment strategies different from those in the Hanis study) would have had relatively little power to detect *NIDDM1*. Replication of positive results obtained in one dataset is going to be difficult, not only because of implicit differences in the various clinical datasets available (with respect to ethnic group, diagnostic criteria and family structure), but also because most sib-pair resources (even those comprising a few hundred families) are relatively underpowered for the detection of loci of modest effect (λ_s between 1.3 and 1.5)[36,41].

If these underpowered replication studies represent 'false-negative' findings, there is perhaps even greater concern about the possibility of 'false positives', i.e. attribution of linkage where none exists. Some of the earliest efforts in tracking complex trait genes have ably demonstrated the confusion that can result[42,43] and Lander and Kruglyak[26] have more recently drawn attention to the implications for significance testing of the multiple analyses implicit in any genome-wide scan. In such an experiment, large numbers of markers are being typed (these represent semi-independent trials of linkage), and quite marked deviations in the direction of excess allele sharing are therefore to be expected on occasion, even in the absence of linkage. These 'spurious' peaks represent regions of excess allele sharing as a result of stochastic fluctuations in the allele-sharing statistic, and are indistinguishable from those 'real' peaks reflecting excess allele sharing caused by an underlying susceptibility gene. Of course, the larger the peak, the more probable that it is the result of true linkage, but, given the relative underpowering of most genome-wide scans, the likely outcome of many scans will be several peaks of modest significance (say, MLS scores of 1.5–3.0). This leaves the researcher with the unenviable task of prioritizing these for further analysis, in the knowledge that only a proportion of these peaks will ultimately yield susceptibility loci. It is at this point that the integration of information from other genome scans and/or other experimental paradigms will prove most useful. Any peak that coincides with positive findings from another genome scan and/or overlies a particularly promising biological candidate, becomes a priority for further examination.

A further limitation of these sib-pair scans is that they cannot be expected to provide precise mapping information; typically, the region within which the susceptibility locus is localized will span 10–20 cM ($1–2 \times 10^7$ basepairs). In simple Mendelian diseases, it is routine to examine further meioses in the expectation that additional recombination events will allow one to narrow the critical region containing the disease gene. However, in a complex trait such as type 2 diabetes, the uncertainties arising out of incomplete penetrance, genetic heterogeneity and the possibility of phenocopies mean that recombinants cannot be relied on to provide definitive localization, and the number of meioses needed to narrow the region appreciably is unrealistic[26]. In fact, getting from the large regions identified in genome scans to the smaller regions amenable to standard positional cloning techniques (say 1–2 cM) represents one of the major obstacles to progress in complex trait mapping (see below).

Strategy 2: Collect Larger Pedigrees and Use Traditional Positional Cloning Approaches

The standard paradigm for identifying the gene underlying a given Mendelian trait is well rehearsed[44,45]. A collection of mutigenerational families segregating the trait of interest is established and, in the absence of a good candidate gene, a genome-wise linkage scan is used to localize the underlying gene. Once an initial localization has been made, the critical region is narrowed through the mapping of additional recombinants while, in tandem, an inventory of the genes mapping to that region is made through cDNA selection and/or exon trapping. These genes are then prioritized for mutation detection to identify and characterize variants.

This approach has been successfully employed to identify the loci responsible in families that segregate maturity-onset diabetes of the young (MODY), an autosomal dominant form of early onset type 2 diabetes (see Chapter 6 for further details). Thus far, five MODY genes have been identified (hepatocyte nuclear factor-4α [*HNF-4α*], glucokinase, hepatocyte nuclear factors-1α and -1β [*HNF-1α*, HNF-1β], and insulin promoter factor-1), by a combination of traditional positional cloning and biological candidate approaches[45–49]. Similar strategies have been employed to locate the aetiological genes for several other inherited diseases that include type 2 diabetes within their phenotype (e.g. Friedreich's ataxia[50]).

Any gene found to have a role in such a condition becomes a strong candidate for involvement in more typical type 2 diabetes, and several groups have sought evidence of co-segregation between type 2 diabetes and MODY candidate regions. Mahtani et al.[27] presented evidence supporting a role for a gene in the *MODY3* region in defective insulin secretion in a collection of Botnian families from Finland. To date, no mutations in the *HNF-1α* gene have been reported in these families, and the significance of the original linkage findings has, to some extent, been revised downwards[51]. More intriguing are several reports of positive linkage in the region of the *MODY1* gene on chromosome 20q[52,53]. It remains to be seen if these are substantiated and, if so, whether the *HNF-4α* gene itself, or another gene in the vicinity, is implicated.

Some groups have set out to apply this 'traditional' approach directly to type 2 diabetes through ascertainment of large multigenerational pedigrees that appear to be segregating typical type 2 diabetes. Such families may, at first sight, appear rather attractive; individually they may be large enough to provide 'evidence' for or against linkage to a given locus, at least under a 'strict' single-gene parametric model (i.e. assuming high penetrance and a low phenocopy rate). However, if the family is truly segregating typical type 2 diabetes, intrafamilial heterogeneity is almost inevitable given the high population prevalence of this disease and the high frequency of diabetes-susceptibility genes; application of 'strict' parametric analysis models under such circumstances will generally be inaccurate. Selecting multigenerational families on the basis that the disease appears to be segregating as a dominant trait with high penetrance is no guarantee that the family is actually harbouring such a gene – polygenic inheritance (even random environment) will occasionally produce families with such appearances[54]. A further paradox is that, given the demographic constraints of typical type 2 diabetes, any family featuring multiple generations of living affected individuals, is, by that very fact, rather unusual. One possibility is that the family is segregating so many diabetes-susceptibility alleles that the power to detect linkage to any one of them will be commensurately poor[55,56] or that the family is segregating an atypical subtype of type 2 diabetes. Somewhat perversely, therefore, the 'large family approach' will probably be most useful when the latter is the case (an analogy would be with single-gene familial and polygenic forms of hypercholesterolaemia).

Whether or not the genes that underlie these 'atypical' forms of type 2 diabetes (such as MODY and other inherited syndromes) are important determinants of type 2 diabetes worldwide is not itself a major issue. These 'experiments of nature' enable us to characterize 'mission-critical' pathways, which, if disturbed, can set in motion the metabolic decompensation that leads to diabetes. Other genes in these pathways become prime candidates for a role in susceptibility to type 2 diabetes.

Strategy 3: Using Linkage Disequilibrium Methods to Map Disease Loci

The common basis of linkage disequilibrium methods is that they seek evidence for an association between the trait of interest and alleles at polymorphic sites[57]. Such genotype–phenotype associations can arise for a variety of reasons:

1. The allele concerned is a functional variant that directly influences disease susceptibility.
2. The allele does not directly influence disease susceptibility but is in linkage disequilibrium with a nearby variant that does. Linkage disequilibrium in the region of a disease-susceptibility locus is usually assumed to result from the fact that the aetiological mutation(s) originally entered the population on a limited number of ancestral chromosomes, for example, through a founder effect[58–60], or through a novel mutation that became widely established through selective advantage (as in the case of haemochromatosis).
3. The association between the allele and the disease does not reflect linkage between the two loci, but instead results from some artefact of population structure or history (e.g. population stratification).

On this basis, therefore, it is clear that, if we are able to demonstrate linkage disequilibrium between a particular allele (or haplotype) and a phenotype of interest, and provided that we can discount the possibility of population stratification and other causes of association that do not reflect linkage, this information should help in our efforts to localize and identify aetiological mutations. Furthermore, as linkage disequilibrium in many outbred populations is usually found to extend over quite short ranges (<1 cM), its detection implies quite precise localization of the actual susceptibility locus.

A number of different methodological approaches have been used for the detection of linkage disequilibrium. The simplest paradigm is the case–control study in which cohorts of cases (unrelated subjects with type 2 diabetes) and controls (usually, individuals with no personal or family history of diabetes) are compared for the frequency of some candidate polymorphism. The genetics literature for type 2 diabetes is replete with such studies, at least in part, because suitable clinical resources are relatively easy to ascertain[22]. However, the major disadvantage of this study design is the acute sensitivity to the effects of population stratification, which may manufacture 'false-negative' and 'false-positive' results ('false' in the sense that the association observed does not reflect linkage). In practice, there is no reliable way to ensure that cases and controls have been sampled from the same pool of chromosomes and as such, any differences observed in allele frequencies may reflect differences in ethnic background rather than in disease state. For example, Hager and colleagues[61] were first to report an association between type 2 diabetes and a Gly40Ser polymorphism in the glucagon receptor, seen in about 4% of diabetic subjects, but only 1% of 'ethnically matched' controls. Subsequent studies have replicated this finding that suggested that it was, in fact, an artefact of population stratification[62].

A second approach has been the 'cross-sectional' strategy exemplified by Pedersen and colleagues[63]. This group have obtained both DNA and detailed intermediate trait information from a large cohort of healthy young Danish subjects[63]. This allows the phenotypic correlates of genetic variation in candidate genes to be rapidly assessed, by analysing the intermediate trait measurements obtained from individuals according to genotype at any candidate polymorphism[64]. This has certainly proved an extremely useful strategy for screening polymorphisms before more detailed in vitro functional analysis; however, this strategy remains susceptible to the potentially disruptive effects of latent population structure.

In the past few years, it has become clear that family-based association methods hold one solution to the problems posed by latent population stratification[65–67]. By examining the transmission of variants from heterozygous parents to affected offspring, it is possible to derive measures of association that are positive only in the presence of linkage (i.e. positive under circumstances (1) and (2) above, but not under (3)). The basic substrate for such analyses are parent–offspring trios (families with one parent available can be used but are less powerful and certain 'safety warnings' operate)[68] and the most-frequently employed statistical test is the TDT (transmission/disequilibrium test)[65]. In the absence of segregation distortion, one expects a parent heterozygous for a given variant to have an equal chance of passing on either allele to any offspring; if we find transmission in excess of expectation to offspring with a particular phenotype, this must reflect the fact that the variant and the disease are (1) linked and (2) in linkage disequilibrium[66]. Although extensively deployed in the study of type 1 diabetes[69], the TDT has been little used in type 2 diabetes to date, for the simple reason that the substrate configuration (both parents of an affected offspring) is difficult to collect in a late-onset disease such as type 2 diabetes. One way round this is to identify individuals with a high future risk of type 2 diabetes, at an age when both parents are likely to be alive – for example, ascertaining through women with gestational diabetes or polycystic ovarian disease[70–72].

With such clinical resources, linkage disequilibrium mapping is proving an increasingly useful tool in a variety of scenarios relevant to the mapping of complex trait loci.

Evaluation of Promising Polymorphisms Uncovered in Candidate Genes

Once a candidate locus has been defined and an inventory of variants within the gene compiled, these variants need to be tested for possible involvement in determining disease susceptibility. Note, however, that a positive result for any single variant (even with a robust method like TDT) will not determine whether that variant plays a directly functional role, or is merely a marker in linkage disequilibrium. 'Cross-match' haplotype analysis, transracial mapping and in vitro and in vivo functional studies will be needed to distinguish between these two options (see below).

Demonstrating Evidence for Linkage Disequilibrium Within a Region of Excess Allele-sharing Previously Identified in a Sib-pair Dataset

Such a finding provides an independent confirmation of the initial linkage result and may be particularly important when the original linkage finding was not conclusive[73].

Fine-mapping of Susceptibility Loci

Genome-wide scans in sib-pairs provide only approximate localization of the underlying susceptibility locus. Typically, these regions will be of the order of 10–20 cM and, on average, can be expected to encompass 20 000 000 base-pairs and over 500 genes. Regions of this size are not amenable to standard positional cloning strategies and, in the absence of some red-hot biological candidate known to map to the vicinity, the task of finding the single causative mutation among the 20 000 polymorphisms within such a region represents a forbidding challenge. However, finding evidence for LD within the region not only supports the original linkage result, but also narrows the region within which the gene lies. In effect, rather than relying on recombinations within families to narrow the critical region[74], one is exploiting the power obtained from the many recombination events that have befallen the ancestral chromosome(s) during the population's history. The extent of linkage disequilibrium in any given situation depends on a large number of factors, most of which will be unknowable in advance, such as the proportion of diseased individuals who carry descendent copies of any particular ancestral chromosome and the number of generations since the introduction of the founder mutation. There are several examples of the use of linkage disequilibrium mapping to localize Mendelian disease genes in isolated founder populations[59,75]; what has surprised (and delighted) many researchers is evidence that linkage disequilibrium can be detected under less auspicious circumstances (to detect complex trait loci in outbred populations)[73,76].

Genome-wide Scans for Linkage Disequilibrium

It has been appreciated for some time that tests of linkage disequilibrium are often more powerful than tests of linkage[77]. The main impediment to exploiting this approach for genome-wide analyses at present appears to be technical rather than theoretical. As linkage disequilibrium effects occur over short ranges (<1 cM) in most populations, the density of markers required for such a scan is considerably greater than that currently available (particularly as it may be preferable to employ biallelic markers that are more stable, but less informative, than microsatellites). In many outbred populations, one may need to test up to 10^6 markers in order to cover the genome (compared with 400 or so in a sib-pair linkage study). This leads to an appreciable multiple-testing problem, and it has been suggested that genome-wide significance would require a point-wise threshold for linkage of around 5×10^{-8} [77]. Consequently, large samples would be required in order to reach this target. The overall number of genotypes required to complete such a linkage disequilibrium scan in an outbred population is therefore likely to be three to four orders of magnitude greater than that for the equivalent linkage scan, and it is likely to be a few years until this becomes achievable.

Strategy 4: Using Quantitative Trait Information to Map Diabetes Genes

Current knowledge allows us to identify certain intermediate traits likely to be of relevance to the development of type 2 diabetes, such as insulin secretion and insulin action. As described above, researchers hoping to use such intermediate trait information in the search for type 2 diabetes genes face particular difficulties, which have impeded efforts to use such data[78]. However, recent improvements in the tools for the genetic analysis of quantitative traits in human pedigrees have reactivated interest in this approach[39,79].

Several approaches to the anlysis of quantitative traits related to type 2 diabetes have been employed to date. The Phoenix group has been able to use extensive longitudinal data in their Pima Indian population to analyse quantitative trait data from individuals before the development of diabetes thereby circumventing the degradation of intermediate trait information once hyperglycaemia occurs[28]. In contrast, the approach taken by the San Antonio group has been to ascertain and intensively phenotype a collection of large Mexican–American families, most of which were not selected for any particular phenotype. As the background prevalence of type 2 diabetes in this population is high, but the pedigrees have not been ascertained for a high density of type 2 diabetes, these families seem to provide an ideal substrate in which to examine the segregation of quantitative trait loci (QTLs) underlying a variety of traits related to diabetes and cardiovascular disease[39,79]. The cross-sectional approach employed by the Steno group has been discussed earlier.

It may be that concerns about the value of intermediate trait data from subjects with established diabetes are overstated. In 1996, Mahtani and colleages[27] reported their findings from a genome-wide scan for type 2 diabetes loci conducted on 30 moderately sized Finnish families. When the genome-wide genotypes were analysed taking type 2 diabetes as the phenotype, no regions of significant excess allele sharing were seen. However, when families were stratified according to measurements of insulin secretion among the diabetic individuals, evidence for linkage to the region of the *MODY3* gene on chromosome 12 emerged among the families with the lowest insulin secretion. Given that the key physiological characteristic of *MODY3* is defective insulin secretion, this may indicate that a proportion of these Finnish families have a mutation either in the *MODY3* (*HNF-1*α) gene[45] itself or in some other gene in the neighbourhood.

A number of other strategies for QTL analyses in diabetes may be envisaged, including: (1) focusing on sib-pairs chosen to be discordant for intermediate traits of interest[80]; (2) use of twin data (one potential advantage here is that comparisons between monozygotic and dizygotic twins might identify the most strongly inherited intermediate traits); and (3) in low-prevalence populations, such as Europeans, the examination of unaffected relatives from families enriched for susceptibility genes (e.g. the offspring of conjugal diabetic parents, or the siblings of an affected sib-pair).

Collecting extensive and accurate QTL information in type 2 diabetes is costly and demanding for the participating families. As such, there is an inherent conflict between the desire for 'breadth' (large numbers of families with only minimal intermediate trait information) and 'depth' (fewer but more intensively phenotyped families). As we have repeatedly seen, it is not possible to determine which of these two extreme strategies is the more likely to succeed. We simply do not know which intermediate traits (of the many known to be associated with type 2 diabetes) will display the strongest genotype–phenotype correlations (in other words, which are the most strongly inherited and which have the simplest genetic architecture).

Strategy 5: Use Rodent Models of Diabetes to Pull out Human Genes

As discussed in Chapter 5, it is likely that animal models will increasingly play a role in defining human type 2 diabetes genes. Provided that suitable animal models exist, mapping susceptibility loci is generally a much more feasible activity in rodents than in humans, and tools such as congenic strains and transgenic technology facilitate the tasks of fine-mapping, gene identification and genotype–phenotype correlation. Given the extensive syntenic relationships between rodents and humans, it is usually a trivial exercise to define the human region likely to contain the homologue of any rodent susceptibility locus, and to submit that human region to direct analysis (for example, in affected sib-pairs). This approach has already proved useful in studies of human obesity[81–83].

Integrating Information From Different Sources

We can expect the methods described above, over the next few years, to deliver the chromosomal locations of most, if not all, of the major genes for type 2 diabetes. In some cases, linkage disequilibrium mapping will have provided close localization of the underlying susceptibility gene, allowing the implementation of standard positional cloning methods and/or extensive direct sequencing; in others, strong biological candidates will be known to map to the regions implicated, allowing direct examination. In many circumstances, however, neither will be true, and other strategies will be required if the most promising loci from the region of interest are to be identified.

Of course, within the next decade, the full genome sequence will be available and, with it, the sequence and location of all genes in any given region. In the meantime, hopes are pinned on the rapid development of the human transcript map[84,85]. Currently, something like 40% of all human transcripts have been localized, and this proportion is expected to increase sharply over the next 2–3 years. Many of these transcripts are not particularly well characterized at present, consisting of little more than a partial sequence and a record of the tissue from which the cDNA was extracted. For these databases to be useful to prioritize regional transcripts for further examination, the amount of biological information attached to each needs to undergo similar expansion.

FINDING THE FUNCTIONAL MUTATION

Once a candidate has been identified, an inventory of genetic variation in that gene and its regulatory elements must be compiled[86]. In most cases, this search will focus on coding regions of the gene and immediate regulatory regions, but there is the possibility that significant variation may occur in more remote *cis*-regulatory regions, in the 3′ untranslated region (perhaps influencing message stability) or buried within introns (cryptic splice acceptor and donor sites producing abnormal message). Finding a polymorphism in a gene of interest proves little – the human genome is rife with polymorphisms, and few of these are likely to have functional significance. To demonstrate that a variant plays a functional role, one needs (1) to show some correlation between the genotype and the phenotype and (2) to show that the variant itself is responsible, rather than simply being in linkage disequilibrium with a nearby mutation.

Most of the methods appropriate for the former task have already been discussed (see Strategy 3) and here we need consider only some of the ways in which the functional mutation can be identified. This may not be a trivial exercise; the very linkage disequilibrium that may have acted as a beacon to the location of the susceptibility locus may obscure the identity of the main aetiological mutation. This point is well illustrated by the difficulties encountered in locating the specific type 1 diabetes susceptibility locus within the HLA region, a chromosomal segment displaying extremely strong linkage disequilibrium[87].

Some of the ways in which this obstacle can be overcome are illustrated by studies on another type 1 diabetes susceptibility locus, *IDDM2* (see the literature[88] for a detailed account). Broadly speaking, the strategy includes:

1. Completion of an inventory of all variants mapping to the region of linkage disequilibrium.
2. Construction of a linkage disequilibrium map across the region to pinpoint the most-strongly associated polymorphism.
3. Determining haplotypes across the region of interest, and characterizing them in terms of susceptibility profile (protective, neutral or disease associated).
4. Excluding those polymorphisms that were represented on both protective and susceptibility haplotypes, on the basis that these cannot be conferring disease risk.
5. Using data from several different ethnic groups (transracial mapping) in order to dissect those linkage disequilibrium relationships that are too tight to separate within a single population.

By these (and other means) the aetiological polymorphism at the *IDDM2* locus was narrowed down to the VNTR (variable number tandem repeat) polymorphism which lies just 5′ to the insulin gene[89].

In part, these indirect methods were only required in the case of *IDDM2* because of the nature of the VNTR (the repetitive sequence proved difficult for use of the polymerase chain reaction, making genetic manipulation of the functional element problematic). Increasingly, under similar circumstances, and given a polymorphism with strong credentials for a functional role (for example, one that results in a non-conservative residue change at a critical point in a key regulatory protein), more direct functional assessments of the variant would be appropriate (for example, transfection and binding studies in the case of a receptor; reporter gene constructs in the case of a promoter mutation; transgenic manipulation in rodents).

STRUCTURE AND FUNCTION

Gene-hunting is only a means to an end. Having found a susceptibility locus, the scene is set for the intensive exploration of the biological consequences of the disease mutation. We need to understand what effect the variant has on gene transcription and translation, on the structure of the protein encoded and on the expression patterns of the product, and the downstream consequences for the cell, relevant organs, and the organism as a whole. We may find that these sequelae are not constant over time, or between individuals, and may therefore need to embark on searches for other genes with which our susceptibility locus interacts, or for environmental factors that influence the phenotypic expression of the variant.

By these means, we would hope to understand how it is that type 2 diabetes comes about, and to use that knowledge to achieve the goal of improved prevention and treatment.

REFERENCES

1. Knowler WC, Pettitt DJ, Saad MF, Bennett PH. Diabetes mellitus in the Pima Indians: incidence, risk factors and pathogenesis. *Diabetes/Metab. Rev* 1990; **6**:1–27.
2. Hanson RL, Elston RC, Pettitt DJ, Bennett PH, Knowler WC. Segregation analysis of non-insulin-dependent diabetes melitus in Pima Indians: evidence for a major-gene effect. *Am J. Hum Genet* 1995; **57**:160–70.
3. Neel JV. The thrifty genotype revisited. In Köbberling J, Tattersall R eds. *The Genetics of Diabetes Mellitus*, London: Academic Press, 1982; 283–93.
4. Robinson S, Johnston DG. Advantage of diabetes? *Nature* 1995; **375**:640.
5. Elston RC, Namboodiri KK, Nino HV, Pollitzer WS. Studies on blood and urine glucose in Seminole Indians: indications for segregation of a major gene. *Am J Hum Gen* 1974; **26**:13–34.
6. McCarthy MI, Hitman GA, Shields DC et al. Family studies of non-insulin-dependent diabetes mellitus in South Indians. *Diabetologia* 1994; **37**:1221–30.
7. Cook JTE, Shields DC, Page RCL et al. Segregation analysis of type 2 diabetes in Caucasian families. *Diabetologia* 1994; **37**:1231–40.
8. Ott J. Invited editorial: cutting a Gordian knot in the linkage analysis of complex human traits *Am J Human Genet* 1990; **4**:219–21.
9. McCarthy MI, Kruglyak L, Lander ES. Sibpair collection strategies for complex diseases. *Genet Epidemiol* 1998; **15**:317–40.
10. Turner R, O'Rahilly S, Levy J, Rudenski A, Clark A. Does type II diabetes arise from a major gene defect producing insulin resistance or β-cell dysfunction? In: Nerup J, Mandrup-Poulsen T, Hökfelt B eds. Amsterdam: Elsevier, *Genes and Gene products in the Development of Diabetes Mellitus* 1989; 171–183.
11. Taylor SI, Accili D, Imai Y. Insulin resistance or insulin deficiency? Which is the primary cause of NIDDM? *Diabetes* 1994; **43**:735–40.
12. Janssen RC, Bogardus C, Takeda J, Knowler WC, Thompson DB. Linkage analysis of acute insulin secretion with GLUT2 and glucokinase in Pima Indians and the identification of a missense mutation in GLUT2. *Diabetes* 1994; **43**:558–63.
13. Bogardus C, Lillioja S, Nyomba BL et al. Distribution of in vivo insulin action in Pima Indians as mixture of three normal distributions. *Diabetes* 1989; **38**:1423–32.
14. World Health Organisation Study Group. *Diabetes Mellitus. WHO Technical Report Service*, no. 727. Geneva: WHO, 1985.
15. Swai ABM, McLarty DG, Kitange HM et al. Study in Tanzania of impaired glucose tolerance. Methodological Myth? *Diabetes* 1991; **40**:516–20.
16. Tuomi T, Groop LC, Zimmet PZ, Rowley MJ, Knowles W, Mackay IR. Antibodies to glutamic acid decarboxylase reveal latent autoimmune diabetes

mellitus in adults with a non-insulin-dependent onset of disease *Diabetes* 1993; **42**:359–62.
17. Cook JTE, Hattersley AT, Levy JC et al. Distribution of type II diabetes in nuclear families *Diabetes* 1993; **42**:106–13.
18. Sing CF, Haviland MB, Templeton AR, Zerba KE, Reilly SL. Biological complexity and strategies for finding DNA variations responsible for inter-individual variation in risk of a common chronic disease, coronary artery disease. *Ann Med* 1992; **24**:539–48.
19. Rossetti L, Giaccori A, De Fronzo RA. Glucose toxicity. *Diabetes Care* 1990; **13**:610–30.
20. Collins, FS. Positional cloning: let's not call it reverse anymore. *Nature Genet* 1992; **1**:3–6.
21. Collins FS. Positional cloning moves from the perditional to traditional. *Nature Genet* 1995; **9**:347–50.
22. McCarthy M, Hitman GA. The genetic aspects of non-insulin dependent diabetes mellitus. In: Leslie RDG, ed. *Causes of Diabetes: Genetics and Environmental Factors*. London: John Wiley 1993: 157–183.
23. Rich SS. Mapping genes in diabetes: genetic epidemiological perspective. *Diabetes* 1990; **39**:1315–19.
24. Risch N. Linkage strategies for genetically complex traits. I. Multilocus models. *Am J Hum Genet* 1990; **46**:222–8.
25. Bishop DT, Williamson JA. The power of identity-by-state methods for linkage analysis. *Am J Hum Genet* 1990; **46**:254–65.
26. Lander E, Kruglyak L. Genetic dissection of complex traits: guidelines for interpreting and reporting linkage results. *Nature Genet* 1995; **11**:241–7.
27. Mahtani MM, Widén E, Lehto M et al. Mapping of a gene for NIDDM associated with an insulin secretion defect by a genome scan in Finnish families. *Nature Genet* 1996; **14**:90–5.
28. Pratley RE, Thompson DB, Prochazka M et al. Genome scan for linkage to prediabetic traits in Pima Indians. *Diabetologia* 1997; **40 (suppl1)**: A158 (abstract).
29. McCarthy MI, Kruglyak L, Lander ES. Sibpair collection strategies in complex trait analysis. *American Journal of Human Genet* 1996; **59 (Suppl)**: A227 (abstract).
30. Dib C, Fauré S, Fizames C et al. A comprehensive genetic map of the human genome based on 5,264 microsatellites. *Nature* 1996; **380**:152–4.
31. Reed PW, Davies JL, Copeman JB et al. Chromosome-specific microsatellite sets for fluorescence-based, semi-automated genome mapping. *Nature Genet* 1994; **7**:390–5.
32. Kruglyak L, Daly MJ, Reeve-Daly MP, Lander ES. Parametric and non-parametric linkage analysis: a unified multipoint approach. *Am J Hum Genet* 1996; **58**:1347–63.
33. Hanis CL, Boerwinkle E, Chakraborty R et al. A genome-wide search for human non-insulin-dependent (type 2) diabetes genes reveals a major susceptibility locus on chromosome 2. *Nature Genet* 1996; **13**:161–71.
34. Ghosh S, Hauser ER, Magnuson VL et al. for the Finland–United States Investigation of NIDDM (FUSION) Study. Multipoint linkage analysis of NIDDM in 534 Finnish families in the Fusion Study. *Diabetologia* 1997; **40 (suppl)**, A158 (abstract).
35. Cassell P, Saker PJ, Armstrong M et al. No evidence for excess allele-sharing on chromosome 2q (region of NIDDM1) in a large sibship collection. *Diabetologia* 1997; **40 (suppl 1)**:A157 (abstract).
36. Bell JL, Lathrop GM. Multiple loci for multiple sclerosis. *Nature Genet* 1996; **13**:377–8.

37. Moldin SO. The maddening hunt for madness genes. *Nature Genet* 1997; **17**: 127–9.
38. Risch N, Botstein D. A manic depressive history. *Nature Genet* 1996; **12**:351–353.
39. Stern M, Duggirala R, Mitchell B et al. Evidence for linkage of regions on chromosomes 6 and 11 to plasma glucose concentrations in Mexican Americans. *Genome Res* 1996; **6**:724–34.
40. Hani E, Hager J, Philippi A, Demenais F, Froguel P, Vionnet N. Mapping NIDDM susceptibility loci in French families. Studies with markers in the region of NIDDM1 on chromosome 2q. *Diabetes* 1997; **46**:1225–6.
41. Suarez BK, Hampe CL, van Eerdewegh P. In: Gershon ES, Cloninger CR, eds. *Genetic Approaches to Mental Disorders*. Washington DC: American Psychiatric Press, 1994: 23–46.
42. Egeland JA, Gerhard DS, Pauls DL et al. Bipolar affective disorders linked to DNA markers on chromosome 11. *Nature* 1987; **325**:783–7.
43. Kelsoe JR, Ginns EI, Egeland JA et al. Re-evaluation of the linkage relationship between chromosome 11p loci and the gene for bipolar affective disorder in the Old Order Amish. *Nature*:1989; **342**:238–43.
44. Menzel S, Yamagata K, Trabb JB et al. Localization of MODY3 to a 5-cM region of human chromosome 12. *Diabetes* 1995; **44**:1408–13.
45. Yamagata K, Oda N, Kaisaki PJ et al. Mutations in the hepatocyte nuclear factor-1α gene in maturity-onset diabetes of the young (MODY3). *Nature* 1996; **384**:455–8.
46. Froguel Ph, Vaxillaire M, Sun F et al. Close linkage of glucokinase locus on chromosome 7p to early-onset non-insulin-dependent diabetes mellitus. *Nature* 1992; **356**:162–5.
47. Hattersley AT, Turner RC, Permutt MA et al. Linkage of type 2 diabetes to the glucokinase gene. *Lancet* 1992; **339**:1307–10.
48. Yamagata K, Furuta H, Oda N et al. Mutations in the hepatocyte nuclear factor-4α gene in maturity-onset diabetes of the young (MODY1). *Nature* 1996; **384**: 458–60.
49. Stoffers DA, Ferrer J, Clarke WL, Habener JF. Early-onset type-II diabetes mellitus (MODY4) linked to IPF1. *Nature Genet* 1997; **17**:138–9.
50. Carvajal JJ, Pook MA, dos Santos M et al. The Friedreich's ataxia gene encodes a novel phosphatidylinositol-4-phosphate 5-kinase. *Nature Genet* 1996; **14**:157–62.
51. Kong A, Frigge M, Bell GI, Lander ES, Daly MJ, Cox NJ. Diabetes, dependence, asymptotics, selection and significance. *Nature Genet* 1997; **17**:148.
52. Bowden D, Howard T, Sale M et al. Linkage of genetic markers in the MODY1 region of chromosome 20 to NIDDM in families enriched for nephropathy. *Diabetes* 1996; **45** (suppl 2): 79A (abstract).
53. Ji L, Yang Y, Rich SS, Warram JH, Krolewski AS. Linkage of NIDDM to the MODY 1 gene region on chromosome 20. *Diabetes* 1996; **45 (suppl 2)**: 77A (abstract).
54. McGuffin P, Huckle P. Simulation of Mendelism revisited: the recessive gene for attending medical school. *American J Hum Genet* 1990; **46**:994–9.
55. O'Rahilly S, Turner R. Early onset type 2 diabetes vs. maturity onset diabetes of youth: evidence for the existence of two distinct diabetic syndromes. *Diabetic Med* 1988; **5**:224–9.
56. O'Rahilly S, Spivey RS, Holman RR, Nugent Z, Clark A, Turner RC. Type II diabetes of early onset: a distinct clinical and genetic syndrome? *BMJ* 1987; **294**:923–8.
57. Lander ES, Schork NJ. Genetic dissection of complex traits. *Science* 1994; **265**:2037–48.

58. Norio R, Nevanlinna HR, Perheentupa J. Hereditary diseases in Finland. *Ann Clin Res* 1973; **5**:109–41.
59. Hästbacka J, de la Chapelle A, Kaitila I, Sistonen P, Weaver A, Lander E. Linkage disequilibrium mapping in isolated founder populations: diastrophic dysplasia in Finland. *Nature Genet* 1993; **2**:204–11.
60. Stephens JC, Briscoe D, O'Brien SJ. Mapping by admixture linkage disequilibrium in human populations: limits and guidelines. *Am J Hum Genet* **55**:809–24.
61. Hager J, Hansen L, Vaisse C et al. A missense mutation in the glucagon receptor gene is associated with non-insulin-dependent diabetes mellitus. *Nature Genet* 1995; **9**:299–304.
62. Gough SCL, Saker PJ, Pritchard LE et al. Mutation of the glucagon receptor gene and diabetes mellitus in the UK: association or founder effect? *Hum Mol Genet* 1995; **4**:1609–12
63. Clausen J, Borch-Johansen K, Ibsen H et al. Insulin sensitivity index, acute insulin response, and glucose effectiveness in a population-based sample of 380 young healthy caucasians. *J Clin Invest* 1996; **98**:1195–209.
64. Urhammer SA, Clausen JO, Hansen T, Pedersen O. Insulin sensitivity and body weight changes in young white carriers of the codon 64 amino acid polymorphism of the β_3-adrenergic receptor gene. *Diabetes* 1996; **45**:1115–20.
65. Spielman RS, McGinnis RE, Ewens WJ. Transmission test for linkage disequilibrium: the insulin gene region and insulin-dependent diabetes mellitus (IDDM). *Am J Hum Genet* 1993; **52**:506–16.
66. Spielman RS, Ewens WJ. The TDT and other family-based tests for linkage disequilibrium and associaton. *Am J Hum Genet* 1996; **59**:983–9.
67. Schaid DJ, Sommer SS. Comparison of statistics of candidate-gene association studies using cases and parents. *Am J Hum Genet* 1994; **55**:402–9.
68. Curtis D, Sham PC. A note on the application of the transmission disequilibrium test when a parent is missing. *Am J Hum Genet* 1995; **56**:811–12.
69. Todd JA. Genetic analysis of type 1 diabetes using whole genome approaches. *Proc Nat Acad Sci USA* 1995; **92**:8560–65.
70. Ali Z, Alexis SD. Occurrence of diabetes mellitus after gestational diabetes mellitus in Trinidad. *Diabetes Care* 1990; **13**:527–9.
71. Franks S. Polycystic ovary syndrome. *N Eng J Med* 1995; **333**:853–61.
72. Waterworth DM, Bennett ST, Gharani N et al. Association of class III alleles at the insulin gene VNTR with polycystic ovary syndrome (PCOS). *Lancet* 1997; **349**: 986–990.
73. Merriman T, Twells R, Merriman M et al. Evidence by allelic association-dependent methods for a type 1 diabetes polygene (IDDM6) on chromosome 18q21. *Hum Mol Genet* 1997; **6**:1003–10.
74. Kruglyak L, Lander ES. Complete multipoint sib-pair analysis of qualitative and quantitative traits. *Am J Hum Genet* 1995; **57**:439–54.
75. Sulisalo T, Klockers J, Mäkitie O et al. High-resolution linkage-disequilibrium mapping of the cartilage-hair hypoplasia gene. *Am J Hum Genet* 1994; **55**:937–45.
76. Lucassen AM, Julier C, Beressi JP et al. Susceptibility to insulin dependent diabetes mellitus maps to a 4.1 kb segment of DNA spanning the insulin gene and associated VNTR. *Nature Genet* 1993; **4**:305–10.
77. Risch N, Merikangas K. The future of genetic studies of complex human diseases. *Science* 1996; **273**:1516–17.
78. Ghosh S, Schork NJ. Genetic analysis of NIDDM. The study of quantitative traits. *Diabetes* 1996; **45**:1–14.

79. Commuzzie AG, Hixson JE, Almasy L et al. A major quantitative trait locus determining serum leptin levels and fat mass is located on human chromosome 2. *Nature Genet* 1997; **15**:273–76.
80. Risch N, Zhang H. Extreme discordant sib pairs for mapping quantitative trait loci in humans. *Science* 1995; **268**:1584–9.
81. Zhang Y, Proenca R, Maffel M, Barone M, Leopold L, Friedman JM. Positional cloning of the mouse *obese* gene and its human homologue. *Nature* 1994; **372**:425–32.
82. Clément K, Garner C, Hager J et al. Indication for linkage of the human OB gene region with extreme obesity. *Diabetes* 1996; **45**:687–90.
83. Montague CT, Farooqi IS, Whitehead JP. Congenital leptin deficiency is associated with severe early-onset obesity in humans. *Nature* 1997; **387**:903–8.
84. Boguski MS, Schuler GD. Establishing a human transcript map. *Nature Genet* 1995; **10**:369–71.
85. Schuler GD, Boguski MS, Stewart EA et al. A gene map of the human genome. *Science* 1996; **274**:540–546.
86. Grompe M. The rapid detection of unknown mutations in nucleic acids. *Nature Genet* 1993; **5**:111–17.
87. Todd JA. The emperor's new genes: 1993 RD Lawrence Lecture. *Diabetic Med* 1994; **11**:6–16.
88. Bennett ST, Todd JA. Human Type 1 diabetes and the insulin gene: principles of mapping polygenes. *Ann Rev Genet* 1996; **30**:343–70.
89. Bennett ST, Lucassen AM, Gough SCL et al. Susceptibility to human type 1 diabetes at IDDM2 is determined by tandem repeat variation at the insulin gene minisatellite locus. *Nature Genet* 1995; **9**:284–92.

5

Insulin Resistance: The Evidence for a Genetic Component

O. PEDERSEN

Steno Diabetes Center, Niels Steensens Vej 2, DK 2820 Gentofte, Denmark

Over the past 10–15 years there has been a great deal of interest in insulin resistance as a potential risk factor in the pathogenesis of several widespread disorders, including type 2 diabetes mellitus[1–7]. Do we really know, however, what we are referring to when we use the term insulin resistance?

In the literature, insulin resistance is often defined qualitatively as an abnormally high concentration of circulating insulin needed to ensure metabolic homeostasis. However, despite the fact that several methods for measuring whole body insulin sensitivity of glucose metabolism, including the euglycaemic, hyperinsulinaemic clamp[8] and the intravenous glucose tolerance test with mathematical modelling[9], have been validated, there is no accepted consensus for a definition of insulin resistance on a quantitative basis. Therefore, if insulin resistance is to be more than a mere taxonomic convention, prospective studies are needed to define the possible prognostic significance of impaired insulin sensitivity in the risk profile of common diseases.

As a starting point, it may be relevant to use a statistical definition of insulin resistance in cross-sectional studies. By applying the lowest sex-specific fifth of the insulin sensitivity index, measured by the intravenous glucose tolerance test in a population sample of 380 young healthy Caucasians, as an arbitrary cut-off value, we recently showed that subjects within this fifth were characterized by being significantly more obese and less glucose tolerant, with elevated fasting serum levels of lipids and a dysfunction of the fibrinolytic system, and with higher blood pressure, compared with the other subjects in the population sample[10].

Type 2 Diabetes: Prediction and Prevention. Edited by Graham A. Hitman

At present there are no results from longitudinal studies that answer the question of whether insulin resistance in the young general population predicts increased risk of developing android obesity, type 2 diabetes, essential hypertension, dyslipidemia or premature atherosclerosis later in life; numerous cross-sectional studies do, however, point to subgroups of these common disorders being associated with a relative decrease in whole-body insulin sensitivity of glucose metabolism (for review, see the literature[1–7]). Several of the phenotypes tend to cluster, e.g. about 80% of Causcasian type 2 diabetic patients are obese, 40% have essential hypertension and an equal number may have dyslipidemia. The observational studies have raised the fundamental question of whether insulin resistance, including both acquired and genetic components is a common underlying factor in the pathogenesis subsets of these diseases.

The present chapter focuses primarily on current evidence for genetic determinants in the multifactorial basis of insulin resistance, with a special reference to the pathogenesis of type 2 diabetes.

DETERMINANTS OF INSULIN SENSITIVITY IN A YOUNG NORMAL POPULATION

Lifestyle factors such as lack of physical activity[11], cigarette smoking[12] and diet (both excessive intake of food and especially a diet with a high content of saturated fatty acids)[13] have in some studies been reported to cause impairments of insulin sensitivity and they may obviously alter the degree and timing of expression of associated insulin-resistant disorders. Moreover, each disorder in the cluster of prevalent insulin-resistant states increases in prevalence as the population ages. In patients with morbid obesity, type 2 diabetes, hypertension or premature ischaemic cardiovascular disorders, the level of insulin resistance risk factors, e.g. decreased maximal aerobic capacity ($\dot{V}O_{2\,max}$) is also influenced by the disease state. Therefore, studies examining the impact of various factors that modulate insulin sensitivity might ideally be undertaken in young healthy subjects.

We examined the distribution of the insulin sensitivity index, as estimated by the intravenous glucose tolerance test in combination with injection of tolbutamide in a population sample of 380 healthy subjects aged 18–32 years[10]. The distribution of the insulin sensitivity index was skewed to the right for both sexes but the insulin sensitivity did not differ between men and women. This finding may be the result of women, compared to men, having less abdominal fat but also less muscle mass. In both sexes there was a huge variation (about tenfold) in the insulin sensitivity index. In univariate analysis, significantly negative associations with measures of body fat mass, body mass index (BMI), body fat percentage and waist circumference were found in both men and women. Of the variation in the insulin sensitivity index 29% and 12% could be explained by BMI in men and women, respectively.

The variation in the insulin sensitivity index (defined as the coefficient of variation) was, however, highest among the leanest subjects, suggesting the existence of other strong regulators of whole-body sensitivity to insulin operating under normal conditions[10]. In the obese subjects, the variation in insulin sensitivity index was low partly as a result of the absolute value of the insulin sensitivity index being lowest in this group and partly because of a lower coefficient of variation.

Further analysis of this population sample demonstrated that $\dot{V}O_{2\,max}$ was the other major modulator of the insulin sensitivity index[10]. Thus, a graded positive association response was found between $\dot{V}O_{2\,max}$ and the insulin sensitivity in both sexes. In univariate analysis, 19% and 10% of the variation in the insulin sensitivity index could be explained by $\dot{V}O_{2\,max}$ in men and women, respectively. In contrast, consumption of alcohol or smoking was not associated with any significant difference in the insulin sensitivity index in men or women[10]. Intake of saturated fat was negatively correlated to the insulin sensitivity in men but not in women. In women, use of oral contraceptives was associated with a considerable lowering of the insulin sensitivity index (decreased by 27%)[10].

Multiple regression analysis including age, sex, $\dot{V}O_{2\,max}$, BMI, waist circumference, intake of alcohol, intake of saturated fat, smoking and use of oral contraceptives, confirmed that variables measuring obesity and body fat distribution, $\dot{V}O_{2\,max}$ and use of oral contraceptives were the most important determinants of the insulin sensitivity index[10]. Obviously, both measures of obesity and $\dot{V}O_{2\,max}$ as determinants of insulin sensitivity, have genetic and lifestyle components. However, only 37% of the total variation in the insulin sensitivity index could be explained by the measured variables[10]. This leaves open a large component for unmeasured variables, including genetic effects on the overall variance in the insulin sensitivity index in the young, healthy population.

FEATURES OF INSULIN RESISTANCE IN OVERT TYPE 2 DIABETES

In poorly controlled type 2 diabetes characterized by a relative or absolute insulin deficiency, severe hyperglycaemia and elevated circulating concentrations of free fatty acids, impaired insulin sensitivity of all target tissues for insulin action is a universal finding[7].

Of course, modulators of insulin sensitivity known from studies of the normal population, such as amount and composition of food, level of physical activity and smoking, are also operating in diabetes; in decompensated cases of type 2 diabetes, however, the major factors causing insulin resistance appear to be glucose and free fatty acids (FFAs). Normalization or near normalization of the circulating levels of glucose and FFAs are irrespective of the type of therapeutic intervention associated with a considerable improvement in whole-body insulin senstivity[7].

Accordingly, recent reviews[14–16] underline that a number of studies in humans and rodents have demonstrated that chronic hyperglycaemia can lead to the development of what is called metabolic or secondary insulin resistance, which results from downregulation of the insulin-regulated glucose transport system, as well as from post-glucose transport steps. Diabetic patients have increased tissue glucose uptake in the basal state compared with control subjects, and normal glucose uptake in the postprandial state as a result of the mass action effect of glucose[17]. Increased activity of the hexosamine pathway in muscle tissue appears to be a crucial factor for the toxic effects of glucose on insulin action[18]. When glucose flux is artificially elevated, insulin-stimulated glucose disposal is impaired and associated with increases in flux through the glucosamine pathway[17]. The impairment in insulin-regulated glucose uptake can be reproduced by giving glucosamine to non-diabetic rats[19]. Also, when the rate-limiting enzyme for hexosamine production (glucosamine fructose aminotransferase or GFAT) is overexpressed in transgenic mice, this produces insulin resistance[20]. In humans, GFAT activity in skeletal muscle from type 2 diabetic patients is increased and correlates closely with the impairment of whole-body insulin sensitivity[21].

Another key feature of decompensated type 2 diabetes is an increased lipolysis resulting in 'toxic' effects of FFAs on insulin-stimulated glucose uptake in skeletal muscles[22]. As discussed in this recent review the elevated plasma levels of FFAs enhance its uptake in muscle cells by mass action and stimulate lipid oxidation. In muscle, the accelerated rate of lipid oxidation impairs insulin-mediated glucose transport/phosphorylation, resulting in an insulin resistance to both glucose oxidation and glycogen synthesis.

From a quantitative standpoint, impaired glycogen synthesis in skeletal muscle represents the major pathway responsible for the insulin resistance in type 2 diabetes[7]. However, although the in vivo studies are suggestive of a major role for the elevated levels of FFAs and glucose in mediating the insulin resistance of type 2 diabetes, in vitro studies point to possible intrinsic abnormalities in the insulin-regulated glycogen synthesis pathway. Thus, cultured fibroblasts[23] or muscle cells[24] isolated from patients with insulin-resistant type 2 diabetes exhibit a poor glycogen synthesis rate in response to insulin, when compared with findings obtained in cultured cells from normal control subjects.

Evidence is also emerging that, in obese patients with type 2 diabetes, autocrine and/or paracrine effects of the cytokine, tumour necrosis factor-α (TNF-α), secreted from adipose cells may be involved in the pathogenesis of insulin resistance. Studies in animals suggest that TNFα inhibits insulin-stimulated glucose uptake in adipose and muscle tissue by inhibiting the activity of several proximal key proteins in the cellular insulin-signalling cascade[25].

It is beyond the scope of this chapter to discuss the numerous studies of biochemical abnormalities of cellular insulin action and glucose metabolism in patients with type 2 diabetes (for a review, see De Fronzo[7]). It appears that multiple dysfunctions in insulin signalling to glucose transport, glucose phosphorylation and glycogen synthesis are responsible for cellular insulin resistance in frank type 2 diabetes. These abnormalities include decreased expression and/or activity of the insulin receptor tyrosine kinase, insulin receptor substrate-1, phosphatidylinositol-3-kinase and glycogen synthase, as well as increased activity and/or expression of proteins with inhibitory impact on insulin signalling, such as the insulin receptor serine/threonine receptor kinase and phosphotyrosine phosphatases, Rad and PC-1. Some of these abnormalities are most probably acquired, although studies in glucose-tolerant first-degree relatives of patients with type 2 diabetes indicate that impaired insulin activation of muscle glycogen synthase may represent an inherited defect[26,27].

INSULIN RESISTANCE IN GLUCOSE-TOLERANT SUBJECTS AT HIGH RISK OF DEVELOPING TYPE 2 DIABETES

As a result of the detrimental effects of high plasma levels of glucose and FFAs on both insulin action and insulin secretion by the time type 2 diabetes is fully established, several groups of investigators have performed measurements of whole-body insulin sensitivity in glucose-tolerant, non-obese, first-degree relatives of type 2 diabetic parents. These studies show that, under the given experimental conditions, the insulin sensitivity of the non-oxidative glucose metabolism in the peripheral tissue of the offspring is characteristically decreased by about 30% when compared with the findings in carefully matched control subjects[26,27]. Insulin-stimulated glucose oxidation is also impaired, but this is a minor part of total glucose disposal. Therefore, quantitatively, the major abnormality appears to be accounted for by decreased insulin-stimulated glycogen synthesis in skeletal muscle.

In studies combining nuclear magnetic resonance (NMR) spectroscopy and the hyperinsulinaemic clamp technique, it was furthermore demonstrated that the increases in muscle glucose 6-phosphate levels in both people with type 2 diabetes[28] and their glucose-tolerant relatives[29] were significantly below those of normal insulin-sensitive control subjects, indicating that glucose transport and/or phosphorylation is impaired in glucose-tolerant, but insulin-resistant, offspring of type 2 diabetic parents. In contrast, studies of the inhibitory effects of insulin on the hepatic glucose production appears to be normal in these subjects. Also studies of monozygotic twins discordant for type 2 diabetes have shown that both the non-diabetic and the diabetic twin have impaired insulin-stimulated, non-oxidative glucose metabolism of their peripheral tissues[30], again suggesting that insulin resistance of glucose metabolism of skeletal muscle may represent an early and probably inherited abnormality in the pathogenesis of many cases of type 2 diabetes.

Of crucial interest are the reports on prospective studies of first-degree relatives of type 2 diabetic patients. Thus, longitudinal studies of the offspring of two Caucasian parents with type 2 diabetes demonstrate that insulin resistance is an important predictor for later development of type 2 diabetes[31]. Likewise, prospective studies in Pima Indians and Mexican–Americans have shown that the first step in the pathogenesis of type 2 diabetes is likely to be resistance to insulin-stimulated glucose uptake in skeletal muscle[32,33]. Insulin resistance can initially be overcome by elevated plasma insulin concentrations, but after a period of time this mechanism is no longer able to compensate sufficiently and hyperglycaemia occurs.

Our knowledge of the molecular mechanisms that trigger the early insulin resistance of glucose-tolerant subjects is sparse. One possibility that is to be discussed in more detail in this chapter, is inherited defects in genes that control critical proteins in either the insulin-signalling network or energy metabolism. However, hypothetically, causes of inherited insulin resistance are innumerable, e.g. genetic abnormalities causing decreased synethsis or control of proteins involved in the secretion or action of insulin, counter-regulatory hormone systems, or overexpression of other proteins with negative regulatory impact on insulin action might well be candidates for a primary insulin resistance.

The insulin resistance of type 2 diabetic offspring might also reflect other underlying dysfunctions known to be associated with reduced insulin sensitivity. For instance, it has been shown that subjects at risk of developing type 2 diabetes have decreased $\dot{V}O_{2\,max}$[34], increased number of type IIb fibres in skeletal muscle[35], an increased number of muscle capillaries[36] and increased waist : hip ratio without a significant increase in total body fat[30]. The last finding suggests that type 2 diabetes inheritance may favour triglyceride accumulation in the abdominal viscera[37]. An increase in intra-abdominal fat would result in an increased availability of FFAs for oxidation in skeletal muscle because the intra-abdominal fat deposit is very sensitive to the lipolytic effects of catecholamines, but relatively resistant to the antilipolytic effects of insulin[37]. In this scenario of events, the impaired insulin action on muscle glycogen synthesis in the pre-diabetic state would be secondary to an increased activity in the triglyceride-storing system of intra-abdominally localized adipose cells.

LESSONS FROM ANIMAL MODELS OF GENETICALLY ENGINEERED INSULIN RESISTANCE

Over the last few years, several groups of investigators have attempted to create models of type 2 diabetes by eliminating expression of one or two proteins known to play a major role in glucose homeostasis; until now, more than 30 reports of genetic manipulation of insulin action and glucose metabolism have been published (for a review, see Patti and Kahm[38]). Within the remit of this chapter the biological consequences of the knock-out of three proteins – the major insulin-sensitive glucose transporter (GLUT4), the insulin receptor (IR) and the insulin receptor substrate-1 (IRS-1) – are of particular interest. Experimentally these studies were designed as either one-hit homozygous, one-hit heterozygous or two-hit (compound) heterozygous knockout models. Each of the experiments tested the hypothesis that has been generated from the longitudinal studies of first-degree relatives of type 2 diabetic patients; impaired insulin action on glucose uptake is the earliest and primary event, which is accompanied by an adaptive hypersecretion of insulin. However, according to this hypothesis, the secondary hyperinsulinaemia cannot be sustained indefinitely and, as the capacity for insulin secretion declines, overt diabetes eventually develops. In fact heterozygous knockout of either GLUT4 or IR, and compound heterozygous knockout of IR and IRS-1, in mice can initiate a series of metabolic dysfunctions that lead to insulin resistance and, in some animals, to frank diabetes.

ONE-HIT HOMOZYGOUS OR HETEROZYGOUS KNOCKOUTS

Mice homozygous for the targeted disruption of the *IR* gene are severely insulin resistant and die from diabetic ketoacidosis within 3–7 days of birth[39,40], whereas mice lacking IRS-1 are severely growth retarded as well as insulin resistant[41,42]. Mice that are heterozygous for the *IR* gene knockout are moderately insulin resistant and hyperinsulinaemic, and about 10% of the animals develop overt diabetes at the age of 4–6 months. By contrast, mice that are heterozygous for the IRS-1 knockout do not exhibit any obvious clinical phenotype.

Homogyzous disruption of the GLUT4 gene[43] results in mice that are growth retarded with hypertrophic hearts and shortened lifespan. These animals are not diabetic and it has been shown that GLUT4 null mice develop various mechanisms to compensate for the lack of GLUT4, including an increase in postprandial insulin levels which stimulates glucose uptake in skeletal muscles. However, interestingly, a recent paper showed that male mice that are heterozygous for the GLUT4 knockout and are phenotypically normal at birth develop progressive hyperinsulineamia[44]. At the age of 2–4 months, 14% of male mice are hyperglycaemic and, during the next 4–5 months, most become diabetic. The phenotype of these diabetic mice is also characterized by hypertension and cardiac hypertrophy – findings that are often seen in human type 2 diabetes.

Thus, deletion of one allele of IR or GLUT4 provides proof of concept for the hypothesis that subclinical alteration in the expression of a key molecule in insulin signalling or glucose uptake can trigger a series of events that result in insulin resistance, hyperinsulinaemia and diabetes in later life (monogenic models of insulin resistance and diabetes).

TWO-HIT HETEROZYGOUS (COMPOUND) KNOCKOUTS

Based on the idea that the genetics of insulin resistance or type 2 diabetes in humans are not caused in most cases by one major defect in a single gene, other researchers recently created an oligogenic mice model of insulin resistance and diabetes. Mice were made doubly heterozygous for null allelles in the *IR* and the $IRS-1$ genes[45]. Shortly after birth and at the age of 2 months, these animals were phenotypically normal, but with time they developed progressive hyperinsulinaemia and, by 4–6 months, 40% of the mice were diabetic. Similar to the findings in the heterozygous GLUT4 knockout mice, sexual dimorphism was present with a preponderance of males progressing to frank diabetes. Thus, this animal model clearly shows that two relatively mild genetic defects within the same signalling pathway can interact to provoke insulin resistance, marked hyperinsulinaemia and eventually diabetes, in the absence of pancreatic β-cell failure and of an environmental pressure from, for example, lack of exercise or hyperalimentation. A comparable proof of concept for an oligogenic model of type 2 diabetes has been given by Terauchi et al.[46], who produced mice that were doubly heterozygous for null alleles of the insulin receptor and glucokinase genes.

The complexity of the human gene pool and the possibility that, even within relatively homogeneous populations, different genes may interact in the pathogenesis of various forms of insulin resistance and type 2 diabetes make the relevance of the specific mouse models questionable for the human genetic studies. However, the beauty and strength of the findings in the mouse models are the clear message that relatively subtle changes in the expression of one or two molecules with critical impact on insulin action or glucose metabolism, if present from birth, may start a process that leads to metabolic disorders, insulin resistance and diabetes in adult life. This paradigm is helpful in the ongoing elucidation of the puzzle behind the presumed non-Mendelian inheritance of most cases of insulin resistance or type 2 diabetes in humans.

LESSONS FROM A CANDIDATE GENE APPROACH

In parallel with the advances in the understanding of the cellular insulin-signalling network[4,47] and the pathophysiological and potentially pathogenic characteristics of insulin action in glucose-tolerant offspring of type 2 diabetic parents, a series of mutational analyses have been conducted in genes that are involved in the insulin transduction pathway in skeletal muscle from the insulin receptor to glycogen synthase. The working hypothesis for these studies has been that it is likely that the genetic component of insulin resistance is the result of a polygenic interaction involving the simultaneous inheritance of several widespread mutations (polymorphisms); each of these has subtle or minor effects on the development of insulin resistance. The sum of effects of these genetic variants will be the basis on which environmental risk factors act[48].

THE INSULIN RECEPTOR GENE

Mutational analyses of the insulin receptor gene have revealed more than 50 different mutations in the coding part of the gene[49]. Most of this genetic variability has been found in patients with extreme insulin resistance, many of whom have a type 2 diabetes-like disorder[50]. The variety of clinical syndromes caused by mutations in the insulin receptor includes:

1. Leprechaunism characterized by intrauterine and postnatal growth retardation, acanthosis nigricans, aged facies appearance and early death.
2. Type A insulin resistance with hyperandrogenism, acanthosis nigricans and, in some cases, lipoatrophy.
3. Rabson–Mendenhall syndrome with hyperplasia of the pineal gland, features of type A insulin resistance, dental dysplasia and dysmorphic features.
4. Congenital muscle fibre dysproportion myopathy and severe insulin resistance.

Transfection studies have shown that the identified mutations in the insulin receptor gene can cause insulin resistance by interfering with all known steps in the biosynthesis and function of the protein[49]. Most patients suffering from the mentioned severe insulin resistance syndromes have either compound heterozygous or homozygous mutations. Heterozygous gene variants in the tyrosine kinase domain of the β subunit of the receptor often result in a pronounced insulin resistance compatible with a dominant negative effect.

A Val985Met variant was first reported in sporadic form in cohorts of type 2 diabetic patients and later in control subjects[51]. When studied in type 2 diabetic pedigrees this Val985Met insulin receptor variant did not segregate with type 2 diabetes, although carriers of the polymorphism tended to have higher levels of oral post-glucose load values of plasma glucose[52]. Transfection studies failed to demonstrate any negative impact of this variant on insulin signalling[53]. A recent study in a Dutch population sample[54] has, however, shown an association between the codon 985 polymorphism and type 2 diabetes (carrier frequency of 5.6% vs 1.3%). This finding could not be replicated in an association study of 254 Danish Caucasian type 2 diabetic patients and 243 matched control subjects where the genotype frequency in both groups averaged 2%[55]. Nor did we find any relationship between the codon 985 variant and the insulin sensitivity index in a population sample of 380 young healthy Caucasians. Taken together, mutations in the *IR* gene cause several phenotypes of extreme insulin resistance, whereas at present there is no convincing evidence that variability in the structural part of the *IR* gene is involved in the pathogenesis of insulin resistance in the general population or in the more common forms of idiopathic type 2 diabetes.

INSULIN RECEPTOR SUBSTRATE-1

As *IR* mutations are unlikely to add to the genetic predisposition of the widespread forms of insulin resistance, *IRS-1* was considered to be a logical candidate gene[56]. Several amino acid substitutions in *IRS-1* have been discovered and transfection studies have demonstrated that all the tested *IRS-1* variants cause impaired insulin signalling when expressed in 32 D cells, ranging from a 25% to a 50% decrease in cellular insulin action[62,63]. The most common polymorphism, Gly972Arg, has a carrier prevalence of about 9% in the young healthy Caucasian population, and genotype–phenotype interaction studies in a random sample of 380 young healthy subjects show that this gene variant, in its heterozygous form, has no testable impact on whole-body insulin sensitivity in lean subjects, whereas it was shown to potentiate obesity-linked insulin resistance[48]. Multivariate analysis substantiated that the combination of obesity and the codon 972 variant was associated with a 50% reduction in the insulin sensitivity index. The same obese subjects were characterized by a clustering of metabolic cardiovascular risk factors with a relative rise in fasting levels of plasma glucose, serum triglyceride, plasma tPA (tissue plasminogen activator) and plasma PAI-1 (plasminogen-activator inhibitor-1) activity[48]. The molecular mechanisms behind this interaction between the *IRS-1* gene variant and obesity are unknown, but might involve an increased sensitivity of the mutated IRS-1 protein to obesity-associated factors that are known to be toxic to the insulin transduction pathway such as TNFα. If the results of the genotype–phenotype studies in obese individuals can be replicated, they may suggest that the codon 972 variant is involved in the pathogenesis of insulin resistance in the general population.

Small association studies performed in various ethnic groups clearly demonstrate that the prevalence of the codon 972 variant of *IRS-1* is not increased in random type 2 diabetic patients when compared with control subjects[57–61,64–66]. A recent British study[67] showed, however, that the prevalence of the codon 972 polymorphism is doubled in a subset of patients with insulin-resistant type 2 diabetes. This finding may point to the possibility that the Gly972Arg polymorphism of *IRS-1* interacts with other insulin-resistance genes to increase the risk of developing an insulin-resistant form of type 2 diabetes.

STUDIES OF OTHER GENES IN THE INSULIN-REGULATED GLYCOGEN SYNTHESIS PATHWAY

Phosphatidylinositol-3-kinase (PI3-K) is a proximal component of the insulin signalling pathway of several growth factor and polypeptide hormone receptors, including the insulin receptor[68–71]. This signalling protein is a heterodimer consisting of a regulatory subunit (various isoforms with molecular weights of 45–85 kDa) and a catalytic subunit with a molecular weight of 110 kDa. Phosphatidylinositol-3-kinase appears to regulate the basal plasma membrane glucose transporter recycling and the organization of the transporter intracellular pool, in addition to being an insulin signal for translocation of glucose transporters to the plasma membrane[72,73]. Variations in the genes encoding PI3-K might therefore be involved not only in the pathogenesis of insulin resistance, but also in the pathogenesis of the impaired insulin-independent glucose turnover?

In this context, it is interesting that longitudinal studies of the offspring of two parents with type 2 diabetes show that both a low insulin sensitivity and a reduced glucose effectiveness[31] predict an increased risk of type 2 diabetes. Glucose effectiveness, as defined from a minimal model analysis of data obtained from an intravenous glucose tolerance test, is the relative effect of glucose, at basal insulin, in increasing net glucose disappearance (i.e. enhancing glucose utilization and suppressing glucose output)[9,74].

Mutational analysis of the gene encoding the p85α regulatory subunit of PI3-K revealed a prevalent (31% of the general Caucasian population) Met326Ile polymorphism[75]. The same variant is predicted to be present in the smaller regulatory subunits of PI3-K. The codon 326 variant was not, in its heterozygous form, associated with any measurable phenotype. However, homozygous carriers of this polymorphism (about 2% of the Caucasian population) are characterized by significant reductions in whole body glucose effectiveness and in the intravenous glucose disappearance constant. Moreover, a non-significant ($p = 0.08$) reduction was observed in whole-body insulin sensitivity. Therefore, if the in vivo findings can be replicated and substantiated by in vitro structure–function analysis, they may suggest that homozygosity for the codon 326 polymorphism of the regulatory subunits of PI3-K is a subtle risk factor for impairments of insulin- and non-insulin-regulated glucose metabolism. In combination with other genetic or environmental risk factors, the PI3-K variant might confer an increased susceptibility to glucose intolerance.

Variability has also been reported in the gene encoding the glycogen-associated form of protein phosphatase-1 (PP1), derived from skeletal muscle. This enzyme complex is also a heterodimer composed of a 124-kDa regulatory subunit (PP1G) and various isoforms of 37-kDa catalytic subunits[76–80]. Insulin stimulates glycogen synthesis through activation of PP1G and inhibition of glycogen synthase kinase-3 (GSK-3)[81–83]. So far, no functional variants have been identified in three catalytic (α, β, γ) subunits of glycogen-associated PP1[84,85] or in the two isoforms (α, β) of GSK-3[86]. However an Asp905Tyr polymorphism has been detected in the regulatory subunit of PP1 which has a carrier prevalence of 18% among Caucasians[87,88]. This variant, which in itself is not associated with an increased prevalence of type 2 diabetes, occurs in healthy control subjects, together with a normal insulin-stimulated glucose disposal rate, but with an impaired insulin-stimulated, non-oxidative, glucose metabolism. Replication studies and transfection experiments are now needed to evaluate the potential impact of this PP1G variant on the pathogenesis of insulin resistance in the general population.

More genes coding for proteins in the insulin-stimulated glycogen synthesis, including GLUT4[89–92], hexokinase II[93–98], insulin-stimulated protein kinase-1[84] and glycogen synthase[92,99], have been examined for variability. These studies have failed to reveal any common polymorphisms that could be associated with insulin resistance, impaired glucose tolerance of type 2 diabetes. Yet, recently a Met416Val polymorphism in the glycogen synthase gene was found with an allele frequency of 9.7% in the general Japanese population[100]. This genetic variant was not associated with diabetes, but heterozygous carriers of the polymorphism were characterized by a 40% reduction in whole-body insulin sensitivity. This finding was recently challenged by a Finnish study showing no impact of the met416Val variant on whole-body insulin sensitivity[101]. Previous marker studies have indicated an association between type 2 diabetes and the glycogen synthase locus in Finnish people and Pima Indians[102,103], but it remains to be shown whether this coupling is the result of alterations in the glycogen synthase gene or a gene in its vicinity.

CANDIDATE GENES IN ENERGY METABOLISM

As many obese subjects appear to be insulin resistant, genetically determined obesity might be an obvious cause of insulin resistance. Also the successful studies of naturally occurring monogenic animal models, such as the ob/ob and db/db mouse[104,105], in which obesity accompanied by secondary insulin resistance and diabetes result from mutations of the gene for leptin and its receptor, have stimulated studies of the corresponding human genes. Genetic dissection of the human leptin and leptin receptor molecules have, however, failed to show any variation that is linked to an increased prevalence of common forms of human obesity[106–112].

A recent report on one homozygous carrier of a nonsense mutation in the leptin gene has, however, provided proof of the concept that severe congenital abnormalities in leptin – even though extremely rare – are able to cause childhood-onset obesity in humans[113].

Uncoupling proteins (UCPs) are important regulators of thermogenes is and genetic abnormalities might easily be envisioned to contribute to an increased fat storage. Mutational examination of the coding regions of the genes for human UCP1–2 has, however, excluded these candidates as common causes of human obesity[114,115].

The β_3-adrenergic receptor is a candidate protein that holds an important role in the control of the lipolysis of visceral fat. A Trp64Arg polymorphism has been reported with a carrier prevalence of about 20%[115–117]. In some, but not all, examined populations, this variant – especially in its homozygous form – may be asosciated with an increased amount of abdominal fat tissue, hyperinsulinaemia and insulin resistance[116–124].

RANDOM GENOME MAPPING APPROACH AND INSULIN RESISTANCE

The random genome search has so far been used only to a very limited extent as a complementary approach in the hunt for genetic risk factors that predispose to insulin resistance. One example is shown in studies in Pima Indians who, as a group, are morbid obese and insulin resistant and with about a 40% prevalence of type 2 diabetes in adulthood. Random genome mapping in this ethnic group demonstrated a genetic linkage of the quantitative trait, insulin resistance and a locus on chromosome 4q[125]. Subsequent mutational analyses of candidate genes within the identified locus showed an amino acid substitution in an intestinal fatty acid-binding protein, FABP2[126]. In in vitro studies, the mutated protein has an increased affinity for long-chain fatty acids, and physiological studies showed that Pima Indians who carried the polymorphism were more insulin resistant and had a higher rate of lipid oxidation when compared with non-carriers. Based on these findings, it has been suggested that the mutated FABP2 protein causes an increase in the intestinal absorption and processing of the dietary long-chain fatty acids, which cause a secondary enhanced lipid oxidation and insulin resistance.

GENETIC COMPONENTS OF INSULIN RESISTANCE: CHALLENGES FOR TOMORROW

To address the question of whether there is any evidence for genetic components in the multifactorial basis of insulin resistance, the short answer is yes; there is evidence from family studies that a relative resistance to insulin is an inherited trait which in some subjects may predispose for type 2 diabetes. Similar longitudinal studies in families at high risk of developing other insulin-resistant phenotypes are lacking. By contrast, when looking at the present knowledge about the precise genetic defects behind the inherited components of insulin resistance, the results are sparse and rather meager. However, based on the experiences gained up to now from studies in both humans and mouse models, it may be hypothesized that the aetiological platform of insulin resistance in a given ethnic group is made up of multiple subtle genetic variants; these interact with each other, as well as with lifestyle factors, in a variety of combinations to cause insulin-resistant phenotypes with a much lesser degree of clinical heterogeneity.

In other words, it is likely that the discussion of the molecular genetic defects involved in insulin resistance will be a tremendous task that calls on the combined efforts of collaborating international research consortia. To increase the chance for making substantial progress, several issues might be considered:

1. Prospective studies of large samples of the general population of specified ethnicity with careful phenotype characterizations are needed for a quantitative definition of insulin resistance based on its impact as a pathogenic factor.
2. The pathophysiology-driven candidate gene approach should to a large extent be complemented by a positional candidate gene search. The quantitative trait loci for insulin resistance might be derived from comprehensive family studies with extensive characterization of the insulin sensitivity at the whole-body level.
3. For performing gene-to-gene and gene-to-environment interaction studies, large and carefully characterized human cohorts (encompassing many thousands of individuals) are necessary.
4. To evaluate the whole-body level impact of single or combined genetic defects that are associated with insulin resistance in humans, transgenics and knock-in expression studies in animal models will be instrumental. The more homogeneous gene pool of an animal model will hopefully

make it possible to eliminate the 'noise' from the extremely heterogeneous genetic background of humans.

REFERENCES

1. Reaven GM. Pathophysiology of insulin resistance in human disease. *Physiol. Rev* 1996; **75**:473–86.
2. Olefsky JM. Insulin resistance in non-insulin dependent diabetes mellitus. *Curr Opin Endocrinol Diabetes* 1995; **2**:290–9.
3. Moller DE, Flier JS. Insulin resistance – mechanisms, syndromes, and implications. *Engl J. Med* 1991; **325**:938–48.
4. Kahn CR. Insulin action, diabetogenes, and the cause of type II diabetes. *Diabetes* 1994; **43**:1066–84.
5. Yki-Järvinen H. Role of insulin resistance in the pathogenesis of NIDDM. *Diabetologia* 1995; **38**:1378–88.
6. Beck-Nielsen H, Groop LC. Metabolic and genetic characterization of prediabetic states. Sequence of events leading to non-insulin-dependent diabetes mellitus. *J Clin Invest* 1994; **94**:1714–21.
7. DeFronzo RA. Pathogenesis of type 2 diabetes: metabolic and molecular implications for identifying diabetes genes. *Diabetes Rev* 1997 **3**:177–269.
8. DeFronzo RA, Tobin JD, Andres R. Glucose clamp technique: a method for quantifying insulin secretion and resistance. *Am J Physiol* 1979; **6**:E214–33.
9. Bergman RN. Towards physiological understanding of glucose tolerance: minimal–model approach. *Diabetes* 1989; **38**:1512–27.
10. Clausen JO, Borch-Johnsen K, Ibsen H et al. Insulin sensitivity index, acute insulin response, and glucose effectiveness in a population-based sample of 380 young healthy Caucasians. *J Clin Invest* 1996; **98**:1195–209.
11. Erikson J, Taimela S, Koivisto VA. Exercise and the metabolic syndrome. *Diabetologia* 1997; **40**:125–35.
12. Attvall S, Fowelin J, Lager I, Von Schenck H, Smith U. Smoking induces insulin resistance – a potential link with the insulin resistance syndrome. *J Intern Med* 1993; **233**:327–32.
13. Storlien LH, Bauer LA, Kriketos AD et al. Dietary fats and insulin action. *Diabetologia* 1996; **39**:621–631.
14. Rossetti L. Glucose toxicity: the implications of hyperglycaemia in the pathophysiology of diabetes mellitus. *Clin Invest Med* 1995; **18**:255–60.
15. Yki-Järvinien H. Glucose toxicity. *Endocr Rev* 1992; **13**:415–31.
16. McClain DA, Crook ED. Hexosamines and insulin resistance. *Diabetes* 1996; **45**:1003–9.
17. Vaag A, Damsbo P, Hother-Nielsen O, Beck-Nielsen H. Hyperglycemia compensates for the defect in insulin-mediated glucose metabolism and in the activation of glycogen synthase in the skeletal muscle of patients with type 2 (non-insulin-dependent) diabetes mellitus. *Diabetologia* 1992; **35**:80–8.
18. Marshall S, Bacote V, Traxinger RR. Discovery of a metabolic pathway mediating glucose-induced desensitization of the glucose transport system. *J Biol Chem* 1991; **266**:4706–12.
19. Baron AD, Zhu J, Zhu J, Weldon H, Maianu L, Garvey WT. Glucosamine induces insulin resistance in vivo by affecting GLUT4 translocation in skeletal muscle. *J Clin Invest* 1995; **96**:2792–801.

20. Hebert LF Jr, Daniels MC, Zhou J et al. Overexpression of glutamine: fructose-6-phosphate amidotransferase in transgenic mice leads to insulin resistance. *J Clin Invest* 1996; **98**:930–6.
21. Yki-Järvinen H, Daniel MC, Virkamaki A, Makimatila S, DeFronzo RA, McClain D. Increased glutamine:fructokinase-6-phosphate aminotransferase activity in skeletal muscle of patients with NIDDM. *Diabetes 1996;* **45**:302–7.
22. Boden G. Role of fatty acids in the pathogenesis of insulin resistance and NIDDM. *Diabete* 1997; **46**:3–10.
23. Wells AM, Sutcliffe IC, Johnson AB, Taylor R. Abnormal activation of glycogen synthesis in fibroblasts from NIDDM subjects: evidence for an abnormality specific to glucose metabolism. *Diabetes* 1993; **42**:583–9.
24. Henry RR, Ciaraldi TP, Abrams-Carter L, Mudaliar S, Park KS, Nikoulina SE. Glycogen synthase activity is reduced in cultured skeletal muscle cells of non-insulin-dependent diabetes mellitus subjects. *J Clin Invest* 1996; **98**:1231–6.
25. Saghizadeh M, Ong JM, Garvey WT, Henry RR, Kern PA. The expression of TNFα by human muscle. Relationship to insulin resistance. *J Clin Invest* 1995; **97**:1111–16.
26. Schalin-Jantti C, Harkonen M, Groop LC. Impaired activation of glycogen synthase in people at increased risk for developing NIDDM. *Diabetes* 1992; **41**:598–604.
27. Vaag A, Henriksen JE, Beck-Nielsen H. Decreased insulin activation of glycogen synthase in skeletal muscles in young non-obese Caucasian first-degree relatives of patients with non-insulin-dependent diabetes mellitus. *J. Clin Invest* 1992; **89**:782–88.
28. Rothman DL, Shulman RG, Shulman GI. 31P nuclear magnetic resonance measurements of muscle glucose-6-phosphate: evidence for reduced insulin-dependent muscle glucose transport or phosphorylation activity in non-insulin-dependent diabetes mellitus. *J Clin Invest* 1992; **89**:1069–75.
29. Rothman DL, Magnusson I, Cline G et al. Decreased muscle glucose transport/phosphorylation is an early defect in the pathogenesis of non-insulin-dependent diabetes mellitus. *Proc Natl Acad Sci USA* 1995; **92**:983–7.
30. Vaag A, Henriksen JE, Madsbad S, Holm N, Beck-Nielsen H. Insulin secretion, insulin action, and hepatic glucose production in identical twins discordant for non-insulin-dependent diabetes mellitus. *J Clin Invest* 1995; **95**:690–8.
31. Martin BC, Warran JH, Krolewski AS, Bergman RN, Soeldner JS, Kahn CR. Role of glucose and insulin resistance in development of type II diabetes mellitus: results of a 25-year follow-up study. *Lancet* 1992; **340**:925–9.
32. Lillioja S, Mott DM, Spraul M et al. Insulin resistance and insulin secretory dysfunction as precursors of non-insulin-dependent diabetes mellitus: prospective studies of Pima Indians. *N Engl J Med* 1993; **329**:1988–92.
33. Haffner SM, Miettinen H, Gaskill SP, Stern MP. Decreased insulin secretion and increased insulin resistance are independently related to the 7-year risk of NIDDM in Mexican-Americans. *Diabetes* 1995; **44**:1386–91.
34. Nyholm B, Mengel A, Nielsen S et al. Insulin resistance in relatives of patients with non-insulin dependent diabetes mellitus: the role of physical fitness and muscle metabolism. *Diabetologia* 1996; **39**:813–22.
35. Nyholm B, Qu Z, Kaal A et al. Evidence of an increased number of Type 2 b muscle fibres in insulin resistant first degree relatives of patients with NIDDM. *Diabetes* 1997; **47**:1822–8.
36. Erikson KF, Saltin B, Lindegärde F. Increased skeletal muscle capillary density precedes diabetes development in men with impaired glucose tolerance: a 15-year follow-up. *Diabetes* 1994; **43**:805–8.

37. Roden M, Price TB, Perseghin G et al. Mechanism of free fatty acid-induced insulin resistance in humans. *J Clin Invest* 1996; **97**:2859–65.
38. Patti ME, Kahm CR. Lessons from transgenic and knockout animals about non-insulin-dependent diabetes mellitus. *Trends Endocrinol Metab* 1996; **7**:311–19.
39. Accili D, Drago J, Lee EJ et al. Early neonatal death in mice homozygous for a null allele of the insulin receptor gene. *Nature Genet* 1996; **12**:106–9.
40. Joshi RL, Lamothe B, Cordonnier N et al. Targeted disruption of the insulin receptor gene in the mouse results in neonatal lethality. *EMBO J* 1996; **15**: 1542–7.
41. Araki E, Lipes MA, Patti ME et al. Alternative pathway of insulin signalling in mice with targeted disruption of the IRS-1 gene. *Nature* 1994; **372**:186–90.
42. Tamemoto H, Kadowaki T, Tobe K et al. Insulin resistance and growth retardation in mice lacking insulin receptor substrate-1. *Nature* 1994; **372**:812–16.
43. Katz EB, Stenbit AE, Hatton K, DePinho R, Charron MJ. Cardiac and adipose tissue abnormalities but not diabetes in mice deficient in GLUT4. *Nature* 1995; **377**:151–5.
44. Stenbit AE, Tsao T-S, Li J et al. GLUT 4 heterzygous knockout mice develop muscle insulin resistance and diabetes. *Nature Med* 1997; **3**:1096–101.
45. Brünning JC, Winnay J, Bonner-Weier S, Taylor SI, Accili D, Kahn CR. Development of a novel polygenic model of NIDDM in mice heterozygous for IR and IRS-1 null alleles. *Cell* 1997; **88**:561–72.
46. Terauchi Y et al. Development of non-insulin-dependent diabetes mellitus in double knockout mice with disruption of insulin receptor substrate-1 and beta cell glucokinase genes: genetic reconstitution of diabetes as a polygenic disease. *J Clin Invest* 1997; **99**:861–6.
47. Cheatham B, Kahn CR. Insulin action and the insulin signalling network. *Endoc Rev* 1995; **16**:117–142.
48. Clausen JO, Hansen T, Bjørbæk C et al. Insulin restistance: interactions between obesity and a common variant of insulin receptor substrate-1. *Lancet* 1995; **346**:397–402.
49. Taylor SI. Molecular mechanisms of insulin resistance: lessons from patients with mutations in the insulin receptor gene (Lilly Lecture). *Diabetes* 1992; **41**:1473–90.
50. Moller DE, O'Rahilly S. Syndromes of severe insulin resistance: clinical and pathophysiological features. In: Moller DE, eds. *Insulin Resistance*. Chichester: John Wiley & Sons, 1993: 49–81.
51. O'Rahilly S, Choi WH, Patel P, Turner RC, Flier JS, Moller DE. Detection of mutations in the insulin receptor gene in non-insulin dependent diabetic patients by analysis of single-stranded conformation polymorphism. *Diabetes* 1991; **40**:777–82.
52. Elbein SC, Sørensen LK, Schumacher MC. Methionine for valine substitution in exon 17 of the insulin receptor gene in a pedigree with familial NIDDM. *Diabetes* 1993; **42**:429–34.
53. Flier JS, Moller DE, Moses AC et al. Insulin-mediated pseudoacromegaly: clinical acid biochemical characterization of a syndrome of selective insulin resistance. *J Clin Endocrinol Metab* 1993; **76**:1533–41.
54. Van't Hart LM, Stolk RP, Heinse RJ, Grobber DE, van der Does FEE, Maassen JA. Association of the insulin receptor variant Met-985 with hyperglycemia and non-insulin-dependent diabetes mellitus in the Netherlands: a population-based study. *Am J Human Genet* 1996; **59**:1119–25.
55. Hansen L, Hansen T, Clausen JO et al. The Val 985 Met insulin receptor variant in the Danish Caucasian population: lack of associations with non-insulin

dependent diabetes mellitus or insulin resistance. *Am J Hum Genet* 1997; **60**:1532–35.

56. Sun XJ, Rothenberg PL, Kahn CR et al. The structure of the insulin receptor substrate IRS-1 defines a unique signal transduction protein. *Nature* 1991; **352**:73–77.
57. Almind K, Bjøorbæk C, Vestergaard H, Hansen T, Echwald S, Pedersen O. Amino acid polymorphisms of insulin receptor substrate-1 in non-insulin dependent diabetes mellitus. *Lancet* 1993; **342**:828–32.
58. Hitman GA, Hawrami K, McCarthy MI et al. Insulin receptor substrate-1 gene mutations in NIDDM: implications for the study of polygenic disease. *Diabetologia* 1995; **38**:481–6.
59. Laakso M, Malkki M, Kekalainen P, Kuusisto J, Deeb SS. Insulin receptor substrate-1 variants in non-insulin-dependent diabetes. *J Clin Invest* 1994; **94**: 1141–6.
60. Ura S, Araki E, Kishikawa H et al. Molecular scanning of the IRS-1 gene in Japanese patients with non-insulin-dependent diabetes mellitus: identification of five novel mutations in IRS-1 gene. *Diabetologia* 1996; **39**:600–8.
61. Imai Y, Fusco A, Suzuki Y et al. Variant sequences of insulin receptor substrate 1 in patients with non-insulin-dependent diabetes mellitus. *J Clin Endocrinol Metab* 1994; **79**:1655–8.
62. Almind K, Inous G, Pedersen O, Kahn CR. A common amino acid polymorphism in insulin receptor substrate-1 causes impaired insulin signalling. Evidence from transfection studies. *J Clin Invest* 1996; **97**:2569–75.
63. Yoshimura R, Araki E, Ura S et al. Impact of natural IRS-1 mutations on insulin signals. Mutations of IRS-1 in the PTB domain and near SH2 protein binding sites result in impaired function at different steps of IRS-1 signaling. *Diabetes* 1997; **46**:929–36.
64. Shimokawa K, Kadowaki H, Sakura H et al. Molecular scanning of the glycogen synthase and insulin receptor substrate 1 genes in Japanese subjects with non-insulin-independent diabetes mellitus. *Biochem Biophys Res Commun* 1994; **202**:463–9.
65. Hager J, Zouli H, Velho G, Froguel P. Insulin receptor substrate 1 (IRS-1) gene polymorphisms in French NIDDM families. *Lancet* 1993; **342**:1430.
66. Sigal RJ, Doria A, Warran JH, Krolewski AS. Codon 972 polymorphism in the insulin receptor substrate-1 gene, obesity and risk of non-insulin-dependent diabetes mellitus. *J Clin Endocrinol Metab* 1996; **81**:1657–9.
67. Zhang Y, Wat N, Stratton IM et al. UKPDS19: Heterogeneity in NIDDM. Separate contributions of IRS-1 and β_3-adrenergic-receptor mutations to insulin resistance and obesity respectively with no evidence for glycogen synthase gene mutations 1996; **39**:1505–11.
68. Skolnik EY, Margolis B, Mohammadi et al. Cloning of PI-3 kinase-associated p85 utilizing a novel method for expression/cloning of target protein for receptor tyrosine kinases. *Cell* 1991; **65**:83–90.
69. Cantley LC, Auger KR, Carpenter C et al. Oncogenes and signal transduction. *Cell* 1991; **64**:281–302.
70. Shepherd PR, Reaves BJ, Davidson HW. Phosphoinositide 3-kinase and membrane traffic. *Cell Biol* 1996; **6**:92–7.
71. Cheatham B, Vlahos CJ, Cheatham L, Wang L, Blenis J, Kahn CR. Phosphatidylinositol 3-kinase activation is required for insulin stimulation of pp70 S6-kinase. DNA synthesis, and glucose transporter translocation. *Mol Cell Biol* 1994; **14**:4902–11.

72. Tsakiridis T, McDowell HE, Walker T et al. Multiple roles of phosphatidylinositol 3-kinase in regulation of glucose transport, amino acid transport, and glucose transport in L6 skeletal muscle cells. *Endocrinology* 1995; **136**:4315–322.
73. Young AT, Dahl J, Hausdorff SF, Bauer PH, Birnbaum MJ, Benjamin TL. Phosphatidylinositol 3-kinase binding to polyoma virus middle tumor antigen mediates elevation of glucose transport by increasing translocation of the Glut 1 transporter. *Proc Natl Acad Sci USA* 1995; **92**:11613–17.
74. Kahn SE, Prigeon RL, McCulloch DK et al. The contribution of insulin-dependent and insulin-independent glucose uptake to intravenous glucose tolerance in healthy human subjects. *Diabetes* 1994; **43**:587–92.
75. Hansen T, Andersen CB, Echwald SM et al. Identification of a common amino acid polymorphism in the p85α regulatory subunit of phosphatidylinositol 3-kinase. *Diabetes* 1997; **46**:494–501.
76. Tang PM, Bondor JA, Swidereck KM, De Paolli-Roach AA. Molecular cloning and expression of the regulatory $R_{G1)}$ subunit of the glycogen associated protein phosphatase. *J Biol Chem* 1991; **266**:15782–9.
77. Barker HM, Jones TA, da Cruz e Silva EF, Spurr NK, Sheer D, Cohen PTW. Localization of the gene encoding a type 1 protein phosphatase catalytic subunit to human chromosome band 11q13. *Genomics* 1990: **7**:159–66.
78. Barker HM, Brewis ND, Street AJ, Spurr NK, Cohen PTW. Three genes for protein phosphatase 1 map to different human chromosomes: Sequence, expression and gene localization of protein serine/threonine phosphatase 1 beta (PP1CB). *Biochim Biophys Acta* 1994; **1220**:212–8.
79. Barker HM, Graig SP, Spurr NK, Cohen PTW. Sequence of protein serine/threonine phosphatase 1 gamma and localization of the gene (PP1CC) encoding it to chromosome bands 12q24.1-q24.2. *Biochim Biophys Acta* 1993; **1178**:228–33.
80. Alessi DR, Street AJ, Cohen PTW. Inhibitor-2 functions like a chaperone to fold three expressed isoforms of mammalian protein phosphatase-1 into a conformation with the specificity and regulatory properties of the native enzyme. *Eur J Biochem* 1993; **213**:1055–66.
81. Lawrence JC Jr, Roach PJ. New insights into the role and mechanism of glycogen synthase activation by insulin. *Diabetes* 1997; **46**:541–7.
82. Sutherland C, Leighton IA, Cohen P. Inactivation of glycogen synthase kinase 3β by phosphorylation: New kinase connection in insulin and growth factor signalling. *Biochem J* 1993; **296**:15–19.
83. Cross DAE, Alessi DR, Vandenheede JR, McDowell HE, Hundal HS, Cohen P. The inhibition of glycogen synthase kinase-3 by insulin or insulin-like growth factor 1 and the rat skeletal muscle cell line L6 is blocked by worthmannin, but not by rapamycin: evidence that worthmannin blocks activation of the mitogen-activated protein kinase pathway in L6 cells between Ras and Raf. *Biochem J* 1994; **303**:21–36.
84. Bjørbæk C, Vik TA, Echwald SM et al. Cloning of a human insulin-stimulated protein kinase (ISPK-1) gene and analysis of coding regions and mRNA levels of the ISPK-1 and the protein phosphatase-1 genes in muscle from NIDDM patients. *Diabetes* 1995; **44**:90–7.
85. Prochazka M, Mochizuki H, Baier LJ, Cohen PTW, Bogardus C. Molecular and linkage analysis of type-1 protein phosphatase catalytic beta-subunit gene: lack of evidence for its major role in insulin resistance in Pima Indians. *Diabetologia* 1995; **38**:461–6.
86. Hansen L, Arden KC, Rasmussen SB et al. Chromosomal mapping and mutational analysis of the coding region of the glycogen synthase kinase 3α and β isoforms in patients with NIDDM. *Diabetologia* 1997; **40**:940–6.

87. Chen YH, Hansen L, Chen MX et al. Sequence of the human glycogen associated regulatory subunit of type I protein phosphatase and analysis of its coding region and mRNA level in muscle from patients with NIDDM. *Diabetes* 1994; **43**:1234–41.
88. Hansen L, Hansen T, Vestergaard H. A widespread amino acid polymorphism at codon 905 of the glycogen-associated regulatory subunit of protein phosphatase-1 is associated with insulin resistance and hypersecretion of insulin. *Hum Mol Genet* 1995; **4**:1313–20.
89. Kusari J, Verma US, Buse JB, Henry RR, Olefski JM. Analysis of the gene sequences of the insulin receptor and the insulin-sensitive glucose transporter (Glut-4) in patients with common type non-insulin dependent diabetes mellitus. *J Clin Invest* 1991; **88**:1323–30.
90. Choi W-H, O'Rahilly S, Buse JB et al. Molecular scanning of insulin-responsive glucose transporter (Glut4) gene in NIDDM subjects. *Diabetes* 1991; **40**:1712–18.
91. O'Rahilly S, Krook A, Morgan R, Rees A, Flier JS, Moller DE. Insulin receptor and insulin-responsive glucose transporter (GLUT4) mutations and polymorphisms in a Welsh type 2 (non-insulin-dependent) diabetic population. *Diabetologia* 1992; **35**:486–9.
92. Bjørbæk C, Echwald S, Hubricht P et al. Genetic variants in promoters and coding regions of the muscle glycogen synthase and the insulin-responsive GLUT4 genes in NIDDM. *Diabetes* 1994; **43**:976–83.
93. Laakso M, Malkki M, Deeb SS. Amino acid substitutions in hexokinase II among patients with NIDDM. *Diabetes* 1995; **44**:330–4.
94. Vidal-Puig A, Printz RL, Stratton IM, Granner DK, Moller DE. Analysis of the hexokinase II gene in subjects with insulin resistance and NIDDM and detection of a Gln^{142} →His substitution. *Diabetes* 1995; **44**:340–6.
95. Echwald SM, Bjørbæk C, Hansen T et al. Identification of four amino acid substitutions in hexokinase II and studies of relationship to NIDDM, glucose effectiveness and insulin sensitivity. *Diabetes* 1995; **44**:347–53.
96. Lehto M, Huang X, Le Bean MM et al. Human hexokinase II gene: exon–intron organization, mutation screening in NIDDM, and its relationship to muscle hexokinase activity. *Diabetologia* 1995; **38**:1466–74.
97. Laakso M, Malkiki M, Kekälainen P, Kuusisto J, Deeb SS. Polymorphisms of the human hexokinase II gene: lack of association with NIDDM and insulin resistance. *Diabetologia* 1995; **38**:617–22.
98. Malkki M, Laakso M, Deeb SS. The human hexokinase II gene promoter: functional characterization and detection of variants among patients with NIDDM. *Diabetologia* 1997; **40**:1461–9.
99. Orho M, Nikula-Tjas P, Schalin-Jantti C, Permutt A, Groop LC. Isolation and characterization of the human muscle glycogen synthase gene. *Diabetes* 1995; **44**:1099–105.
100. Shimomura H, Sanke T, Weda K, Hanabusa T, Sakagashira S, Nanjo K. A missense mutation of the muscle glycogen synthase gene (M416V) is associated with insulin resistance in the Japanese population. *Diabetologia* 1997; **40**:947–52.
101. Rissanen J, Pihlajamäki J, Heikkinen S et al. New variants in the glycogen synthase gene (Gln71His, Met416Val) in patients with NIDDM from eastern Finland. *Diabetologia* 1997; **40**:1313–19.
102. Groop LC., Kankuri M, Schalin-Hantti C et al. Association between polymorphism of the glycogen synthase gene and non insulin dependent diabetes mellitus. *N Engl J Med* 1993; **328**:10–14.
103. Majer M, Mott DM, Mochizuki H et al. Association of the glycogen synthase locus on 19q13 and NIDDM in Pima Indians. *Diabetologia* 1996; **39**:314–21.

104. Chen H, Charlat O, Tartaglia LA et al. Evidence that the db/db gene encodes the leptin receptor: identification of a mutation in the leptin receptor gene in db/db mice. *Cell* 1996; **84**:491–5.
105. Chua SC, Jr, Chung WK, Wu-Peng XS et al. Phenotypes of mouse diabetes and rat fatty due to mutations in the OB (Leptin) receptor. *Science* 1996; **271**:994–6.
106. Considine RV, Considine EL, Williams CJ et al. Evidence against either a premature stop codon or the absence of obese gene mRNA in human obesity. *J Clin Invest* 1995; **95**:2986–8.
107. Echwald SM, Rasmussen SB, Sørensen TIA et al. Identification of two novel missense mutations in the human OB gene. *Int J Obesity* 1997; **21**:321–6.
108. Considine RV, Considine EL, Williams CJ, Hyde TM, Caro JF. The hypothalamic leptin receptor in humans: identification of incidental sequence polymorphisms and absence of the db/db mouse and fa/fa rat mutations. *Diabetes* 1996; **45**:992–4.
109. Echwald SM, Sørensen TD, Sørensen TIA et al. Amino-acid variants in the human leptin receptor: lack of association to juvenile-onset obesity. *Biochem Biophys Res Commun* 1997; **233**:248–52.
110. Chung WK, Power-Kehoe L, Chua M et al. Exonic and intronic sequence variation in the human leptin receptor gene (LE PR). *Diabetes* 1997; **46**:1509–11.
111. Gotoda T, Manning BS, Goldstone AP et al. Leptin receptor gene variation and obesity: lack of association in a white British male population. *Hum Mol Gen* 1997; **6**:869–6.
112. Matsuoka N, Ogawa Y, Hosoda K et al. Human leptin receptor gene in obese Japanese subjects: evidence against either obesity causing mutations or association of sequence variants with obesity. *Diabetologia* 1997; **40**:1204–10.
113. Montague CT, Faroogi IS, Whitehead JP et al. Congenital leptin deficiency is associated with severe early-onset obesity in humans. *Nature* 1997; **387**:903–8.
114. Urhammer SA, Friedberg M, Sørensen TIA et al. Studies of genetic variability of the uncoupling protein 1 gene in Caucasian subjects with juvenile onset obesity. *J Clin Endocrinol Metab* 1997; **82**:4069–74.
115. Urhamemr SA, Dalgaard LT, Sørensen TIA et al. Mutational analysis of the coding region of the uncoupling protein 2 gene in obese NIDDM patients: impact of a common amino acid polymorphism on juvenile and maturity onset forms of obesity and insulin resistance. *Diabetologia* 1997; **40**:1227–30.
116. Waiston J, Silver K, Bogardus C et al. Time of onset of non-insulin-dependent diabetes mellitus and genetic variation in the $\beta 3$-adrenergic-receptor gene. *N Engl J Med* 1995; **333**:343–7.
117. Widen E, Letho M, Kanninen T, Waston J, Shuldiner AR, Groop LC. Association of a polymorphism in the $\beta 3$-adrenergic receptor gene with features of the insulin resistance syndrome in Finns. *N Engl J Med* 1995; **333**:348–51.
118. Clement K, Vaisse C, Manning BSJ et al. Genetic variation in the $\beta 3$-adrenergic receptor and an increased capacity to gain weight in patients with morbid obesity. *N Engl J Med* 1995; **333**:352–4.
119. Kadowaki H, Yasuda K, Iwamoto K et al. A mutation in the $\beta 3$-adrenergic receptor gene is associated with obesity and hyperinsulinemia in Japanese subjects. Biochem Biophys Res Commun 1995; **215** 555–60.
120. Arner P. Phenotype characterization of the Trp 64 Arg polymorphism in the beta3-adrenergic receptor gene in normal weight and obese subjects. *Diabetologia* 1996; **39**:857–60.
121. Urhammer SA, Clausen JO, Hansen T, Pedersen O. Insulin sensitivity and body weight changes in young white carriers of the codon 64 amino acid polymorphism of the $\beta 3$-adrenergic receptor gene. *Diabetes* 1996; **45**:1115–20.

122. Sakane N, Yoshida T, Umekawa T, Kondo M, Sakai Y, Takahashi T. β3-adrenergic receptor polymorphism: a genetic marker for visceral obesity and the insulin resistance syndrome. *Diabetologia* 1997; **40**:200–4.
123. Fujisawa T, Ikegami H, Yamato E et al. Association of Trp 64 Arg mutation of the β3-adrenergic receptor with NIDDM and body weight gain. *Diabetologia* 1996; **39**:349–52.
124. Sipiläinen R, Uusitupa M, Heikkinen S, Rissannen A, Laakso M. Polymorphism of the β3-adrenergic receptor gene affects basal metabolic rate in obese Finns. *Diabetes* 1997; **46**:77–80.
125. Prochazka M, Lillioja S, Tait J et al. Linkage of chromosomal markers at 4q with a putative gene determining maximal insulin action in Pima Indians. *Diabetes* 1993; **42**:514–19.
126. Baier LJ, Sacchettini JC, Knowler WC et al. An amino acid substitution in the human intestinal fatty acid binding protein is associated with increased fatty acid binding, increased fat oxidation and insulin resistance. *J Clin Invest* 1995; **95**:1281–7.

6

Maturity-onset Diabetes of the Young: A Monogenic Model of Diabetes

T. FRAYLING, F. BEARDS AND A.T. HATTERSLEY

Division of Molecular Genetics, Department of Clinical Science, Postgraduate School of Medicine and Health Sciences, University of Exeter, Barrack Road, Exeter EX2 5AX, UK

Prediction and prevention of diabetes are always much easier when the cause of diabetes is known. The cause of diabetes is now known in most patients with maturity-onset diabetes of the young (MODY), a genetic subgroup of type 2 diabetes. There are many important lessons to be learned from MODY that are relevant to the more common types of type 2 diabetes. The results of the genetic analysis of MODY have emphasized that, even when a tightly defined phenotype is used, there is considerable genetic heterogeneity and the genes involved may not be obvious candidates. Predictions of the likely clinical course in patients with MODY is now possible after genetic analysis and this has a clear use. Prediction in unaffected family members is now possible, in some types of MODY, but the precise role for this in a clinical setting is uncertain in the absence of a successful preventive strategy. Prevention of MODY by correction of a genetic defect is still a long way off, although early results suggest that alteration of the diet may delay the onset of diabetes. MODY offers an important model for understanding the possibilities of prediction and prevention in type 2 diabetes.

DEFINITION

Maturity-onset diabetes of the young is a subtype of type 2 diabetes characterized by an early onset, usually under 25 years; autosomal dominant

---

Type 2 Diabetes: Prediction and Prevention. Edited by Graham A. Hitman

inheritance and β-cell dysfunction[1,2] (Figure 6.1 gives an example). If defined by strict criteria it is a monogenic condition, i.e. the inheritance of a mutation in a single gene will cause type 2 diabetes. Hence the identification of that mutation allows a definitive diagnosis of the cause of the diabetes to be made. Environmental factors play a small role in determining whether a subject will develop diabetes.

Maturity-onset diabetes of the young is genetically heterogeneous because it can result from mutations in five genes: the pancreatic 'glucose-sensing' enzyme glucokinase (*MODY2*)[3,4], and the transcription factors hepatic nuclear factor 4α (HNF-4α) (*MODY1*)[5], HNF-1α (*MODY3*)[6], insulin promoter factor-1 (IPF1) (*MODY4*)[7] and HNF1-β (*MODY5*)[8]. There are other MODY families in which none of the known genes plays a role, so there must be at least one other gene[9]. This chapter concentrates on the lesson learned from the study of the three most common genetic subtypes: glucokinase, HNF-1α and HNF-4α. The methodology leading to the discovery of these genes and their discrete phenotype has important lessons for type 2 diabetes, and is summarized in Figure 6.2.

MODY: THE START OF THE GENETIC ANALYSIS OF TYPE 2 DIABETES

WHY STUDY MODY?

Maturity-onset diabetes of the young was the ideal place to begin the study of the genetics of type 2 diabetes. The characteristics of MODY made the collection of large, multi-generational families and the subsequent search for genes relatively easy. In contrast, the study of late-onset type 2 diabetes has been described as a 'geneticist's nightmare'[10]. The late age of onset and the association with increased mortality have made the collection of large families very difficult; parents of affected individuals are not usually alive and offspring are usually too young to develop the condition. In addition, evidence suggests that, in most individuals, type 2 diabetes results from the combined effect of variants in many genes (polygeneity) and that it is not a single disease, but rather a collection of diseases with different genetics (heterogeneity)[11]. These factors greatly increase the difficulty in identifying the genes involved in late-onset type 2 diabetes. The study of MODY has therefore enabled the identification of at least some genes that cause type 2 diabetes. This has provided clues about the types of genes, and hence the pathophysiological pathways that could be involved in non-MODY type 2 diabetes.

Finally, the importance of studying MODY as a disease in its own right should not be underestimated. MODY affects about one in 3000 individuals in the UK[12] and hence is one of the most common monogenic disorders in

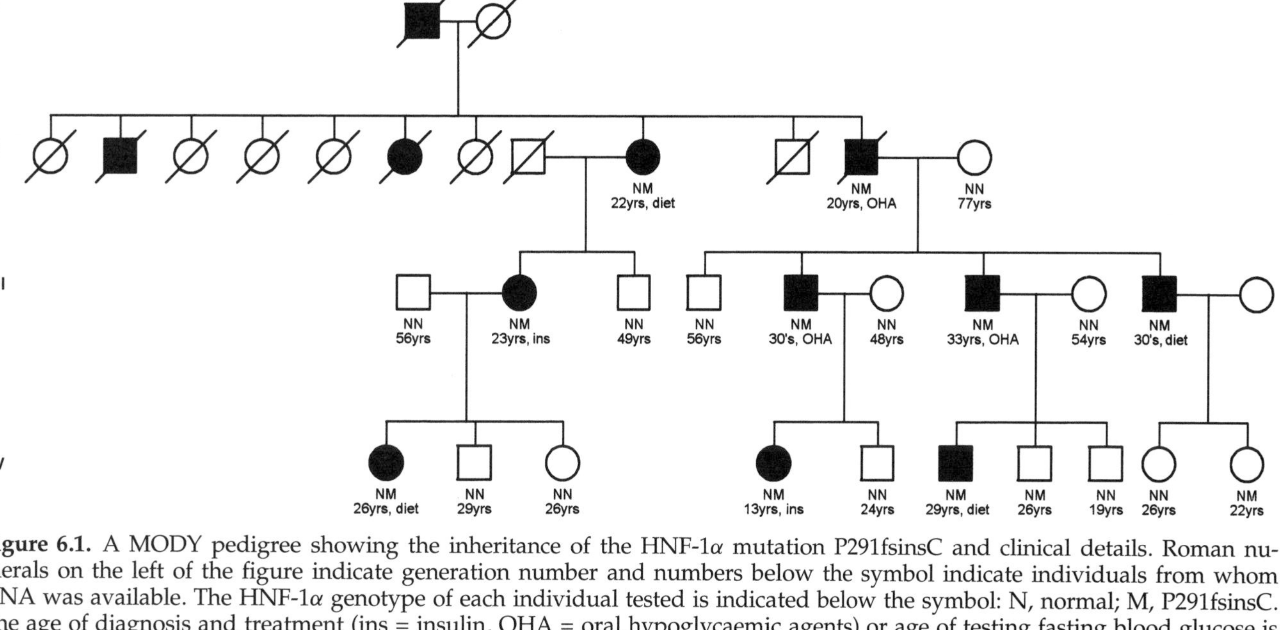

Figure 6.1. A MODY pedigree showing the inheritance of the HNF-1α mutation P291fsinsC and clinical details. Roman numerals on the left of the figure indicate generation number and numbers below the symbol indicate individuals from whom DNA was available. The HNF-1α genotype of each individual tested is indicated below the symbol: N, normal; M, P291fsinsC. The age of diagnosis and treatment (ins = insulin, OHA = oral hypoglycaemic agents) or age of testing fasting blood glucose is shown below the genotype information. Reproduced, with the permission of the American Diabetes Association, from Frayling et al.[48].

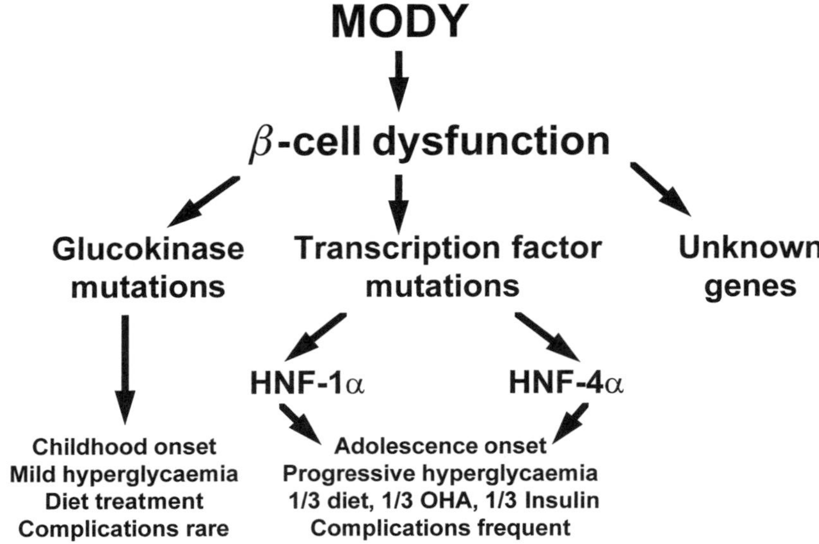

Figure 6.2. Summary of the genetic heterogeneity in MODY and the associated clinical features.

which the gene is known. If a preventive strategy can be developed, this would be important for a considerable number of people.

THE SEARCH FOR GENES CAUSING MODY

The search for MODY genes has been successful as a result of a combination of approaches. The analysis of genes with an obvious role in β-cell function (candidate genes) resulted in the identification of glucokinase mutations[3,4]. Positional cloning or 'reverse genetics', which aims to locate a gene whose protein product is unknown, resulted in the identification of HNF-1α as a MODY gene[6]. This approach relies on the identification of genetic markers that segregate, i.e. are linked, with the condition within a family. Once the locality of the gene within the human genome has been established and a physical map developed, then genes within this region can be systematically analysed.

Genes predisposing to type 2 diabetes are likely to be identified using a similar combination of approaches. However, the discovery that two transcription factors thought to be primarily expressed in the liver can cause type 2 diabetes suggests that many of the genes involved in late-onset type 2 diabetes will not be obvious candidates for study.

GLUCOKINASE MUTATIONS

GLUCOKINASE AS A CANDIDATE GENE FOR MODY

The role of glucokinase in insulin secretion makes it an ideal candidate gene for MODY. Glucokinase is one of four hexokinase enzymes that catalyse the first step in the metabolism of glucose: the phosphorylation of glucose to glucose-6-phosphate. It is principally expressed in pancreatic β cells and in hepatocytes. In β cells this step is closely linked with the initiation of insulin secretion[13,14]. Unlike the other hexokinases, glucokinase has a low affinity for glucose (Michaelis constant or K_m of 5 mmol/1 plasma glucose concentration) and is not inhibited by its product. These features allow β cells and hepatocytes to change glucose phosphorylation rates at physiological glucose concentrations (4–15 mmol/l). Glucokinase has consequently been termed the 'glucose sensor'.

LINKAGE STUDIES

Linkage studies provide a simple method of determining whether candidate genes are likely to be involved in a disorder. If DNA markers close to a candidate gene segregate with diabetes within families, such a gene merits further investigation, i.e. it should be screened directly for mutations. Using markers close to the glucokinase gene on chromosome 7, two group demonstrated linkage to MODY in 1992[3,4].

MUTATION STUDIES

The demonstration of linkage between MODY and the glucokinase gene was quickly followed by the characterization of the human gene and the detection of mutations[15–18]. The first mutation was reported in 1992[15] and over 40 mutations of the glucokinase gene have now been described in many populations, although the vast majority have been found in France[15–17,19–25]. All these mutations were associated with hyperglycaemia. Interestingly, one recently reported mutation is associated not with hyperglycaemia, but with the opposite phenotype, hyperinsulinaemia[26]. This is caused by the mutation resulting in an activation of the enzyme, which then results in overproduction of insulin in response to glucose.

Reported glucokinase mutation frequencies are very variable. In France, the prevalence of glucokinase mutations was estimated at 56%[22] but in the British MODY pedigrees it is only 12.5%[4,27,28] and, in Japanese early-onset type 2 diabetes, less than 1%[29]. These differences are likely to be the result of racial genetic differences and the different approaches to selecting families used in different studies. British and Japanese patients were recruited from clinic appointments, presumably once they showed symptoms of diabetes. In contrast, French patients responded to nationwide publicity for a study, which then involved the screening of asymptomatic children[30]. The French collection would therefore have included a larger proportion of pedigrees that contained younger patients with no symptoms. Glucokinase mutations are associated with this mild phenotype and so the French study would have been more likely to find mutations of this gene. Screening studies have shown that glucokinase mutations have been detected in 0.5–2% of patients with type 2 diabetes[17,31] and 1–5% of those with gestational diabetes[20,31,32].

PHENOTYPE

Different mutations of the glucokinase gene result in a remarkably similar phenotype[33,34]. Patients with glucokinase mutations have mild (6–9 mmol/l) fasting hyperglycaemia from early childhood and probably from birth[22]. There is a small increment during an oral glucose tolerance test[35]; only 46% of a large French series had diabetes according to WHO criteria[22]. In keeping with the mild hyperglycaemia found in these patients, diabetic complications, particularly microvascular ones, are rare and treatment with diet is usually adequate[22,25,36]. One exception is during pregnancy when most patients need, or are given, insulin to obtain strict glycaemic control[36].

β-Cell dysfunction has been seen in glucokinase-deficient subjects through the use of a wide variety of methods of physiological testing[4,36–38]. This β-cell defect is an abnormality of glucose sensing as was elegantly demonstrated by Byrne et al.[38] who measured insulin secretion during a slow stepped glucose infusion. In glucokinase-deficient subjects, the maximum rate of change of insulin secretion was at a glucose value of 7 mmol/l, rather than the 5.5 mmol/l seen in controls. This is consistent with the idea of a resetting of the pancreatic glucose sensor as a result of glucokinase mutations. The increase in the plasma glucose threshold for insulin secretion by the β-cell results in mild hyperglycaemia throughout life. A slight deterioration of β-cell function is seen with age, but the rate of decline is similar to that for people who are not diabetic[36].

Insulin resistance is not an important feature of glucokinase mutations. In a large family, insulin resistance was similar in glucokinase-deficient subjects and controls[36], although a larger series from France did show a slight increase in insulin resistance, particularly in those with WHO criteria for type 2 diabetes[39]. Standard tests of insulin resistance do not sensitively detect a reduction in glucose uptake by the liver. Using nuclear magnetic resonance and labelled glucose isotopes, Velho et al. demonstrated a significant reduction in hepatic glycogen synthesis in glucokinase-deficient patients[40]. This result supports the idea that hepatic glucose uptake is reduced, but it is uncertain what contribution this makes to the hyperglycaemia seen in patients with glucokinase mutations.

MUTATIONS OF THE GLUCOKINASE GENE AS A CAUSE OF DIABETES

Mutations are distributed throughout the glucokinase gene, although there is apparent clustering around exon 7. This pointed to an obvious mechanism by which the enzyme's function is disrupted. The protein consists of two domains – large and small – separated by a deep cleft, at the bottom of which is the glucose-binding site[41]. Exon 7 encodes this active site, with the surrounding exons encoding those regions of the protein that form the cleft. Mutations in this region would be expected to inhibit the normal interaction of glucokinase with glucose and to reduce enzyme activity.

The expression of mutant forms of glucokinase in *Escherichia coli* confirmed that enzyme activity was significantly reduced in the mutants found in association with hyperglycaemia[41]. These findings were consistent with the hypothesis that glucokinase mutations lead to hyperglycaemia by a gene-dosage mechanism. This infers that the reduced quantity of normal enzyme as such causes β-cell dysfunction, rather than the mutant protein itself exerting any pathogenic effect.

Nonsense, frameshift and splice mutations result in incomplete protein synthesis. Missense mutations may result in hyperglycaemia by many methods. These were classified by Velho et al.[25]:

1. Mutations altering conserved active site residues in the active site cleft separating the two domains, as well as in surface loops leading into the cleft; this results in a large reduction in enzyme activity and has a severe effect on catalytic activity.
2. Mutations located far from the active site, in a region predicted to undergo a substrate-induced conformational change and resulting in distortion of the active site cleft, produce less reduction in enzyme activity.
3. Mutations of surface residues that eliminate conserved interactions with residues, and may reduce the structural stability or affect the conformational change seen on glucose binding, only slightly reduce enzyme activity and are unlikely to affect catalysis.

HNF-1α MUTATIONS

HNF-1α: A CANDIDATE GENE FOR MODY?

Unlike glucokinase, the transcription factor HNF-1α was not an obvious candidate gene for MODY. As a DNA-binding protein regulating gene with expressed in many tissues[42–44], it is not obviously linked to a pancreatic β-cell defect. Mutations of HNF-1α were therefore found to cause MODY by a far less direct route of investigation than that used to identify glucokinase as a MODY gene.

POSITIONAL CLONING

A search of the entire human genome, in those MODY families that are not linked to glucokinase of the *MODY1* region on chromosome 20, identified in six of the twelve families a 10-cM locus on the long arm of chromosome 12[45]. This region was termed *MODY3*. Further genetic and physical mapping information[46] was used to narrow this region down and start a systematic search of all the genes within it that are expressed in the pancreas. A C-insertion mutation in exon 4 of HNF-1α, in a Scottish MODY family, indicated that this gene was the cause of MODY3. Characterization of further mutations, all segregating with diabetes in six other families, confirmed HNF-1α as a MODY gene[6].

HNF-1α MUTATIONS: A COMMON CAUSE OF MODY

HNF-1α mutations are likely to be the most common cause of MODY, at least in Caucasians. Over 50 HNF-1α mutations have already been described in many populations, giving support to this as the most common cause of MODY[6,47–51]. Screening of MODY families in the UK has shown that 60–70% of them have an HNF-1α mutation[48]. In a French series, HNF-1α mutations are estimated to account for 25–50% of MODY families[52]. As with glucokinase, the difference between the UK and the French estimates of mutation frequency may be attributable to ascertainment bias during recruitment of families.

MUTATION HOTSPOTS

Although mutations occur throughout the HNF-1α gene, two regions are common sites for mutation: 20 families have been described with mutations at amino acid position 291 in exon 4[6,47,48,50] (T Frayling, M Bulman, S Ellard, AT Hattersley unpublished observations), whereas six families have a mutation at amino acid position 379 in exon 6[6,48,49,51,52]. Studies have shown that families with the same mutation are not related by a distant ancestor and so these regions are prone to recurring mutations[47,48,50]. Both of these mutation 'hotspots' occur within stretches of repetitive DNA. Such sequences are thought to be more unstable during DNA replication and hence have an increased likelihood of mutating. The occurrence of these repetitive tracts of DNA in the HNF-1α gene may therefore, partially account for the high frequency of HNF-1α mutations in MODY. Screening for these mutations in MODY probands in the UK suggests that those at position 291 occur in 12% of those with MODY, whereas those at position 379 occur in 2%[53]. These relative frequencies might have been expected given that the repetitive DNA sequence around residue 291 is longer than that around residue 379 (eight or nine cytosines compared with five cytosines) and therefore, presumably, more unstable and more prone to mutation.

PHENOTYPE

There are striking differences between the phenotype of patients with HNF-1α and that of those with glucokinase mutations. Patients with HNF-1α mutations are normoglycaemic initially and usually develop diabetes in adolescence or early adulthood. Their presentation is usually symptomatic with osmotic symptoms in more than 50% of patients[54] at a mean age of diagnosis of 22 years[48]. Mutations are highly penetrant, with only 7% of individuals with mutations over the age of 25 years not being diabetic[48]. Patients have a progressive deterioration in β-cell function, resulting in increased hyperglycaemia and/or increased treatment requirements with age. In a large UK series, 25% were treated by diet, 44% with tablets and 31% with insulin[48]. Patients with a long duration of diabetes frequently suffer from complications, particularly retinopathy and nephropathy[55], so it is as important to aim for as tight a glycaemic control as there is in other types of diabetes.

The predominant pathophysiology is β-cell dysfunction although, unlike glucokinase, this is not a failure of glucose sensing. In contrast to most type 2 diabetes, insulin resistance is not a feature of diabetes in these patients. Non-diabetic subjects with HNF-1α mutations show normal insulin responses at normal blood glucose concentrations but, once levels exceed 8 mmol/l, a reduced insulin secretion response (ISR) is seen[56]. β-cell function progressively deteriorates with age and patients become increasingly hyperglycaemic. This contrasts with subjects with glucokinase mutations who always have a fasting plasma glucose above normal but with a β-cell dysfunction that is relatively stable throughout life.

HNF-4α MUTATIONS

As with HNF-1α, the functionally related transcription factor HNF-4α was not an obvious candidate gene for MODY. HNF-4α is present in a 13-cM region on chromosome 20q, which had been identified as a MODY gene locus (*MODY1*) by linkage analysis in one large North American MODY pedigree[57]. No other MODY families were linked to this region, however, making further localization of the gene difficult and a systematic search of all the genes within it impractical.

Once HNF-1α had been identified as a MODY gene, HNF-4α became an obvious candidate for investigation. Sequence analysis of the HNF-4α gene in members of the linked North American family revealed a mutations, Q268X, that results in a truncated HNF-4α protein. This mutation was found to co-segregate with type 2 diabetes confirming it as the gene for MODY1[5].

HNF-4α MUTATIONS: A RARE CAUSE OF MODY

Mutations of HNF-4α are likely to be a rare cause of MODY. So far seven mutations in eight families have been described in a range of populations[5,58,59].

PHENOTYPE

Subjects with HNF-4α mutations show a very similar phenotype to those with HNF-1α mutations. This may be a reflection of the similar functions and expression patterns of the two proteins. Indeed mutations in HNF-4α may produce diabetes by reducing the activity of HNF-1α. The only difference is seen in the response to low-dose glucose infusion in pre-diabetic subjects. Asymptomatic subjects with an HNF-4α mutation show a loss of the priming effect of glucose on the insulin secretion rate[60], whereas those with an HNF-1α mutation maintain this response until the onset of overt diabetes[56]. This is based on data from just one HNF-4α family, however, and remains to be confirmed in other families.

MUTATIONS IN TRANSCRIPTION FACTOR GENES: A CAUSE OF TYPE 2 DIABETES

Unlike glucokinase mutations, there is no obvious role for HNF-1α and HNF-4α defects in β-cell dysfunction. Both regulate the expression of many genes in the liver, kidney and pancreas[42,44,61], including some of the genes involved in glucose metabolism, such as PEPCK (phosphoenolpyruvate carboxykinase) and pyruvate kinase[62–64]. Both HNF-1α and HNF-4α are also involved in the regulation of gene expression during development[65]. HNF-4α is expressed at earlier stages of development and, interestingly, it is involved in the regulation of HNF-1α[65]. HNF-4α mutations may therefore be pathogenic as a result of their altered effect on HNF-1α regulation.

The functions of HNF-1α and HNF-4α are clearly complex and numerous, and much study is likely to be required before the exact pathophysiological pathways linking mutations to β-cell dysfunction are identified. The first step is to determine how mutations affect the structure and function of the proteins that they encode. Both proteins have several functional domains common to most transcription factors:

1. The dimerization domain allows two of the proteins to bind to each other. HNF-1α proteins, for example, will bind to other HNF-1α proteins, as well as to the related HNF-1β proteins[43].
2. The DNA-binding domain: as a dimer, the protein complex can bind to DNA-regulatory sequences, the 'promoter' sequences close to the 5′ end of genes, via DNA-binding domains.
3. The transactivation domain: the gene regulation process involves the interaction of additional transcription factors and cofactors with HNF-1α and HNF-4α through this domain[66,67].

In addition, HNF-4α encodes a ligand-binding domain that facilitates the binding of a steroid hormone[68], an additional interaction necessary before the HNF-4α protein complex can bind to DNA and affect gene regulation (this hormone is currently unknown, and hence HNF-4α is known as an 'orphan receptor').

Missense mutations have been described that would alter all of the functional regions of HNF-1α and most of the functional regions of HNF-4α. This indicates that defects in all parts of the resulting proteins can cause β-cell dysfunction.

A number of proposals have been put forward about how altered HNF-1α and HNF-4α proteins function. Mutant proteins may cause a dominant negative effect, in which the dimerization of mutant and normal proteins results in an additional, pathogenic effect to the normal function of protein dimers formed from two normal proteins. Mouse models lacking one copy of HNF-1α support this hypothesis; these mice have half the quantity of normal HNF-1α protein but no mutant protein, yet they are phenotypically normal. However, studies looking at the function of disrupted HNF-1α proteins suggest that different mutations may alter the protein's function in different ways. Some mutations appear to have a dominant negative effect whereas others result in a gene-dosage effect, in which the reduced quantity of normal HNF-1α protein itself causes β-cell dysfunction (Vaxillaire, Froguel communication at Genetics of Diabetes conference, Ystad, 1997).

Studies looking at the effects of the HNF-4α mutation Q268X have shown that at least this mutation does not have a dominant negative effect, because the truncated protein loses all its binding activity. An artificial mutation, resulting in a shortened protein of 360 amino acids, does, however, exert a dominant negative effect[69]. This suggests that, as for HNF-1α mutations, different HNF-4α mutations have different effects on the protein.

Another important issue is how mutated HNF-1α and HNF-4α proteins affect the genes that they regulate. Expression of the HNF-4α mutation Q268X in cultured cell lines results in the downregulation of many genes, including L-type pyruvate kinase and the glucose transport gene *GLUT2* (but not *GLUT1* and *GLUT3*). HNF-1α is also downregulated, but this effect is relatively small[70]. The interaction between HNF-1α and HNF-4α may yet prove important, however, because a mutation in the HNF-4α-binding site of the HNF-1α promoter region has been found in one MODY family[71].

As more MODY families are identified, the number of HNF-1α and HNF-4α mutations characterized will increase. Further studies examining the effects of these, together with mutations already published, should then provide additional insight into the mechanisms involved in β-cell dysfunction in MODY.

OTHER GENES IN MODY

MODY4 AND MODY5

A heterozygous mutation in the insulin promoter factor-1 (IPF1 gene) was shown to cause early onset type 2 diabetes in one Caucasian family in the USA. In the same family, a homozygous mutation resulted in pancreatic agenesis. Mutations in *IPF1* are not common causes of MODY[9], although we have found functionally significant mutations in subjects with early onset type 2 diabetes who do not conform with strict MODY criteria (S Ellard, T Frayling, M Bulman, AT Hattersley, unpublished observations). As there is no published physiological or clinical details and only one published family, it is hard to discuss genotype–phenotype relationships in *MODY4*.

HNF-1β was always likely to be an excellent candidate gene because it forms a functional dimer with HNF-1α. At present information about only one Japanese family that has a mutation in this gene has been published[8]. One fascinating feature was that, in addition to relatively severe type 2 diabetes requiring insulin, there was also severe renal impairment. In two European families with HNF-1β mutations, there was also severe renal impairment (T Linden, GI Bell 1998, unpublished data; AT Hattersley, S Ellard, T Frayling, M Bulman unpublished data). It seems possible that, although this is a rare cause,[9] there may be a discrete phenotype that will represent a new clinical syndrome.

FUTURE GENES CAUSING MODY

As some families that fit the diagnostic criteria for MODY are not linked to any of the five known MODY genes, at least one further gene remains to be found[9]. Genome-wide searches and positional cloning are likely to be the methods used to identify this gene(s) and rapid advances in technology should make this a short-term project. As with the search for late-onset type 2 diabetes genes, however, the candidate gene approach should not be forgotten. This involvement of two transcription factors in the pathogenesis of type 2 diabetes has now resulted in a long list of genes that could be studied. These will include other genes in the HNF-1α and HNF-4α

regulatory pathway[6] and genes involved in the regulation of pancreas development.

CLINICAL APPLICATIONS OF GENETIC INFORMATION IN DIABETES

The identification of a MODY gene mutation in a diabetic patient allows an accurate prediction of the course of that diabetes, in both the patient and other affected relatives who have the same mutation (Figure 6.3). In addition, there is an opportunity for early prediction and possibly for prevention of diabetes in non-diabetic family members at risk of inheriting the mutation. The identification of late-onset type 2 diabetes genes will benefit patients and their clinicians in a similar way, although prediction of the course of a patient's diabetes will not be as definite as a result of the multifactorial nature of the condition. It is interesting that, in MODY, the low effect of environmental influences makes accurate prediction possible, although it makes prevention by manipulation of the environment difficult. In contrast, in type 2 diabetes, environmental factors play a key role in determining who is diabetic, making prediction more difficult but prevention easier (Figure 6.4).

Glucokinase mutations result in relatively mild diabetes. The identification of a mutation in a diabetic patient therefore provides a good prognosis. The elimination of the other MODY genes and type 1 diabetes as potential diagnoses represents one of the few cases in which the discovery of a genetic defect is good news for the patient. Genetic counselling, together with molecular genetic testing for at-risk subjects who are asymptomatic, has little role

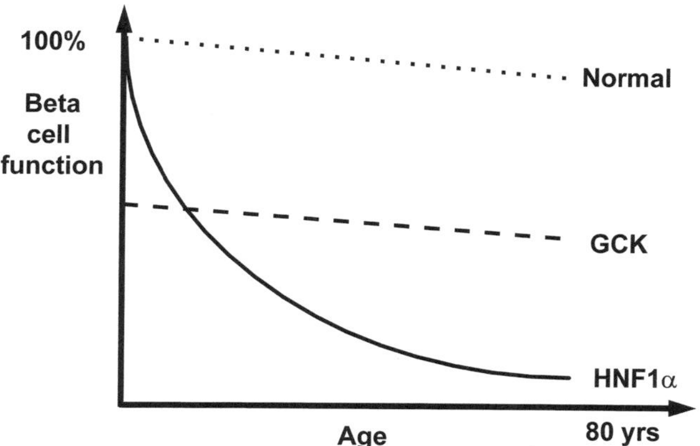

Figure 6.3. Diagrammatic representation of the variation in β-cell function with age in normal subjects and MODY patients with glucokinase and HNF-1α mutations.

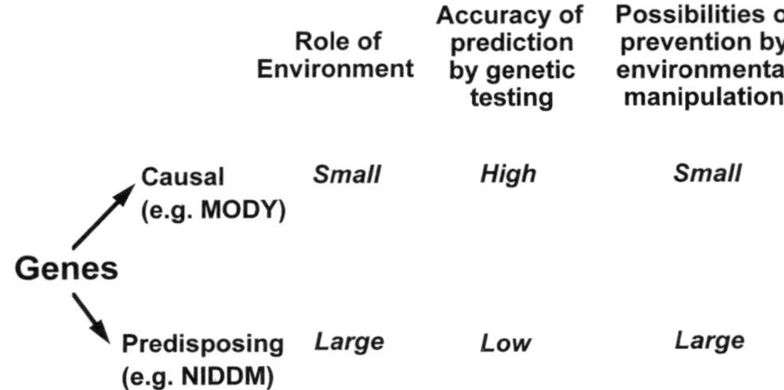

Figure 6.4 Summary of how prediction using genetic studies and prevention by environmental manipulation alters in conditions with causal (e.g. MODY) and predisposing genes (e.g. type 2 diabetes).

in families in which diabetes results from a glucokinase mutation. All that is needed is a fasting blood glucose to see whether a family member is affected.

In most cases, HNF-1α and HNF-4α mutations cause MODY before the age of 25. It is therefore often misdiagnosed as type 1 diabetes, and hence inappropriate treatment and advice may be given to the patient. Although diabetes is often severe, insulin therapy may not be required for many years after diagnosis. This knowledge may reassure patients and encourage them to maintain good glycaemic control, to delay the need for insulin treatment. The identification of an HNF-1α or HNF-4α mutation will, however, prepare patients and their clinicians for progressive β-cell dysfunction with age and the resulting increased treatment requirements.

PREVENTION IN MODY: THE FUTURE

ENVIRONMENTAL MANIPULATION

The mutations in HNF-1α and HNF-4α are highly penetrant, with over 95% of subjects aged over 25 developing overt diabetes. Despite this, the feasibility of preventing the onset of diabetes in at-risk individuals should be thoroughly investigated. Preliminary evidence suggests that asymptomatic subjects with HNF-1α mutations have a lower body mass index (BMI) than those with diabetes (Table 6.1) (AT Hattersley, unpublished data). This suggests that staying slim could delay the onset of MODY. If further studies confirm these findings, at-risk individuals can be offered genetic counselling and a mutation test. Such counselling could become an ethically contentious issue, however, especially if it remains unclear whether helping patients to modify their lifestyles prevents the onset of diabetes. In the absence of an effective treatment, some authorities suggest that subjects under the age of

Table 6.1. Characteristics of subjects who have inherited HNF-1α mutations

	Normoglycaemic subjects[a] with HNF-1α mutations ($n = 10$)	Diabetic subjects with HNF-1α mutations ($n = 84$)	Significance
Fasting plasma glucose	5.1 ± 0.62	9.2 ± 3.9	$p < 0.01$
HbA_{1c}	4.0 ± 0.5	6.7 ± 0.65	$p < 0.0001$
Age	26 ± 13	45 ± 20	$p < 0.02$
BMI	21.6 ± 3.8	24.4 ± 3.9	$p < 0.05$
Percentage on diet/OHA insulin	–	24/46/30	
Age at diagnosis (years)	–	23 ± 12	

[a]Fasting plasma glucose <6 mmol/l.
HbA_{1c}, glycated haemoglobin.
OHA, oral hypoglycaemic agent.

16 should not be tested for genetic defects, yet in MODY diabetes has often occurred by this age.

GENE THERAPY

The identification of genes that if mutated, cause type 2 diabetes will lead to a greater understanding of the biological processes involved in this complex disorder. This will, in turn, result in improved drug therapies because the definitive causes of the disease can be targeted. With MODY, a further possibility exists: gene therapy, in which the defective genes themselves are modified or replaced in an attempt to prevent or treat the disease.

There are several possible approaches to gene therapy. One is to introduce normal genes into cells where the loss of function of a gene has caused disease. This is termed 'gene augmentation therapy'. Such an approach may be applicable to the treatment or prevention of diabetes caused by glucokinase mutations, where only half the normal level of glucokinase enzyme is available for pancreatic and hepatic 'glucose-sensing'. The addition of normal glucokinase genes to the β cell and liver may increase these levels towards normal and so correct the defect.

If a mutated gene causes disease by altering the function of the protein, targeted inhibition of the expression of that gene is likely to be the best approach. In dominant conditions, this may require allele-specific inhibition, in which expression of the mutated copy of the gene is inhibited but not that of the normal copy. This approach may be required to provide gene therapy for HNF-1α and HNF-4α mutations if they cause disease through a dominant negative effect. For these genes, however, the possibility that mutations cause MODY through abnormal β-cell development complicates the potential for gene therapy. Targeted intervention is likely to be required well before birth, possibly at a very early stage of embryogenesis.

Gene therapy, even at the fetal level, will become a realistic option for the treatment of many single-gene disorders, but the timescale of this is uncertain. For some conditions, including MODY, this prospect is still an extremely distant one. The first diseases in which this type of treatment has been used have been life-threatening recessive diseases where the affected tissue is easily accessed, e.g. immunodeficiency resulting from adenosine deaminase (ADA) deficiency. MODY is a non-life-threatening, dominant disorder affecting the inaccessible pancreas, so the need for tight regulation of insulin secretion will be a low priority and technically very difficult.

CONCLUSION

Maturity-onset diabetes of the young, as a monogenic subtype of type 2 diabetes has been ideal for genetic analysis. This analysis has found five casual genes: the pancreatic 'glucose-sensing' enzyme glucokinase (*MODY2*), and the transcription factors HNF-4α (*MODY1*), HNF-1α (*MODY3*), *IPF1* (*MODY4*) and HNF-1β (*MODY5*). Identifying the cause of diabetes in most MODY families makes prediction of the future clinical course possible in both diabetic and non-diabetic family members. Prevention of diabetes is not possible at present, although even in this genetic subtype maintaining a low BMI may significantly delay the onset of diabetes.

ACKNOWLEDGEMENTS

The work reported in this review was supported by the Northcott Trust, British Diabetic Association, the Medical Research Council, DIRECT, The Royal Devon and Exeter NHS Trust, Applied Biosystems and Exeter University.

REFERENCES

1. Tattersall RB, Fajans SS. A difference between the inheritance of classical juvenile-onset and maturity-onset type diabetes of young people. *Diabetes* 1975; 24:44–53.
2. Hattersley AT. Maturity-onset diabetes of the young. *Ballière's Clinical Paediatrics* 1996; **4**:663–80.
3. Froguel P, Vaxillaire M, Sun F et al. Close linkage of glucokinase locus on chromosome 7p to early-onset non-insulin-dependent diabetes mellitus. *Nature* 1992; **356**(6365):162–4.
4. Hattersley AT, Turner RC, Permutt MA et al. Linkage of type 2 diabetes to the glucokinase gene. *Lancet* 1992: **339**(8805):1307–10.

5. Yamagata K, Furuta H, Oda N et al. Mutations in the hepatocyte nuclear factor 4 alpha gene in maturity-onset diabetes of the young (MODY1). *Nature* 1996; **384**:458–60.
6. Yamagata K, Oda N, Kaisaki PJ et al. Mutations in the hepatic nuclear factor 1 alpha gene in maturity-onset diabetes of the young (MODY3). *Nature* 1996; **384**:455–8.
7. Stoffers DA, Ferrer J, Clarke WL, Habener JF. Early-onset type-II diabetes mellitus (MODY4) linked to IPF1. *Nature Genet* 1997; **17**:138–9.
8. Horikawa Y, Iwasaki N, Hara M et al. Mutation in hepatocyte nuclear factor-1b gene (TCF2) associated with MODY. *Nature Genet* 1997; **17**:384–5.
9. Beards F, Frayling T, Bulman M et al. Mutations in hepatocyte nuclear factor 1beta are not a common cause of maturity-onset diabetes of the young in the UK. *Diabetes* 1998: **47**:1152–4.
10. O'Rahilly S, Wainscoat JS, Turner RC. Type 2 (non-insulin-dependent) diabetes. New genetics for old nightmares. *Diabetologia* 1988; **31**:407–14.
11. McCarthy MI, Froguel P, Hitman GA. The genetics of non-insulin-dependent diabetes mellitus: tools and aims. [Review]. *Diabetologia* 1994; **37**:959–68.
12. Appleton M, Hattersley AT. Maturity onset diabetes of the young: a missed diagnosis. *Diabetic Med* 1996; suppl. 2: Ap3.
13. Meglasson MD, Matschinsky FM. Pancreatic islet glucose metabolism and regulation of insulin secretion. *Diabetes/Metab Rev* 1986; **2**:163–214.
14. Matschinsky FM. Glucokinase as glucose sensor and metabolic signal generator in pancreatic β-cell and hepatocytes. *Diabetes* 1990: **30**:647–752.
15. Vionnet N, Stoffel M, Takeda J et al. Nonsense mutation in the glucokinase gene causes early-onset non-insulin-dependent diabetes mellitus. *Nature* 1992; **356**(6371):721–2.
16. Stoffel M, Froguel P, Takeda J et al. Human glucokinase gene: isolation, characterization, and identification of two missense mutations linked to early-onset non-insulin-dependent. *Proc Nat Acad Sc USA* 1992; **89**:7698–702.
17. Stoffel M, Patel P, Lo YM et al. Missense glucokinase mutation in maturity-onset diabetes of the young and mutation screening in late-onset diabetes. *Nature Gene* 1992; **2**:153–6.
18. Tanizawa Y, Matsutani A, Chiu KC, Permutt MA. Human glucokinase gene: isolation, structural characterization, and identification of a microsatellite repeat polymorphism. *Mol Endocrinol* 1992; **6**:1070–81.
19. Sun F, Knebelmann B. Pueyo ME et al. Deletion of the donor splice site of intron 4 in the glucokinase gene causes maturity-onset diabetes of the young. *J Clin Investi* 1993; **92**:1174–80.
20. Stoffel M, Bell K, Blackburn C et al. Identification of glucokinase mutations in subjects with gestational diabetes mellitus. *Diabetes* 1993; **42**:937–40.
21. Shimada F, Makino H, Hashimoto N et al. Type 2 (non-insulin-dependent) diabetes mellitus associated with a mutation of the glucokinase gene in a Japanese family. *Diabetologia* 1993; **36**:433–7.
22. Froguel P, Zouali H, Vionnet N et al. Familial hyperglycemia due to mutations in glucokinase. Definition of a subtype of diabetes mellitus. *N Engl J Med* 1993; **328**:697–702.
23. Hager J, Blanche H, Sun F et al. Six mutations in the glucokinase gene identified in MODY by using a nonradioactive sensitive screening technique. *Diabetes* 1994; **43**:730–3.
24. Eto K, Sakura H, Shimokawa K et al. Sequence variations of the glucokinase gene in Japanese subjects with NIDDM. *Diabetes* 1993; **42**:1133–7.

25. Velho G, Blanche H, Vaxillaire M et al. Identification of 14 new glucokinase mutations and description of the clinical profile of 42 MODY-2 families. Diabetologia 1997; **40**:217–24.
26. Glaser B, Kesavan P, Heyman M et al. Familial hyperinsulinism caused by an activating glucokinase mutation. *N Engl J Med* 1998; **338**:226–30.
27. Dow E, Gelding SV, Skinner E et al. Genetic analysis of glucokinase and the chromosome 20 diabetes susceptibility locus in families with type 2 diabetes. *Diabetes Med* 1994; 11:856–61.
28. Zhang Y, Warren-Perry MG, Saker PJ et al. Candidate genes study in pedigrees with Maturity-onset diabetes of the young not linked with glucokinase. *Diabetologia* 1995; **38**:1055–60.
29. Katagiri H, Asano T, Ishihara H et al. Nonsense mutation of glucokinase gene in late-onset non-insluin-dependent diabetes mellitus. *Lancet* 1992; **340**(8831): 1316–17.
30. Frougel P, Velho G, Cohen D, Passa P. Strategies for the collection of sibling-pair data for genetic studies in type 2 (non-insulin-dependent) diabetes mellitus [letter]. *Diabetologia* 1991; **34**:685.
31. Zouali H, Vaxillaire M, Lesage S et al. Linkage analysis and molecular scanning of glucokinase gene in NIDDM families. *Diabetes* 1993; **42**:1238–45.
32. Saker PJ, Hattersley AT, Barrow et al. High prevalence of a missense mutation of the glucokinase gene in gestational diabetic patients due to a founder-effect in a local population. *Diabetologia* 1996; **39**:1325–8.
33. Hattersley AT, Turner RC. Mutations of the glucokinase gene and type 2 diabetes [Review]. *Q J Med* 1993; **86**:227–32.
34. Hattersley AT. Glucokinase mutations and Type 2 diabetes. In: Lightman S, ed. *Horizons in Medicine*, vol. 7. Bristol: Blackwell Science, 1996; 440–9.
35. O'Rahilly S, Hattersley A, Vaag A, Gray H. Insulin resistance as the major cause of impaired glucose tolerance: a self-fulfilling prophesy? *Lancet* 1994; **344**(8922): 585–9.
36. Page RC, Hattersley AT, Levy JC et al. Clinical characteristics of subjects with a missense mutation in glucokinase. *Diabetic Med* 1995: **12**:209–17.
37. Velho G, Froguel P. Clement K et al. Primary pancreatic beta-cell secretory defect caused by mutations in glucokinase gene in kindreds of maturity onset diabetes of the young. *Lancet* 1992; **340**(8817): 444–8.
38. Byrne MM, Sturis J, Clement K et al. Insulin secretory abnormalities in subjects with hyperglycemia due to glucokinase mutations. *J Clin Invest* 1994; **93**: 1120–30.
39. Clement K, Pueyo ME, Vaxillaire M et al. Assessment of insulin sensitivity in glucokinase-deficient subjects. *Diabetologia* 1996; **39**:82–90.
40. Velho G, Hwang J-H, Petersen K et al. Altered hepatic glycogen synthesis in glucokinase deficient subjects [abstract]. *Diabetologia* 1994; **37**:A131.
41. Gidh-Jain M, Takeda J, Xu LZ et al. Glucokinase mutations associated with non-insulin-dependent (type 2) diabetes mellitus have decreased enzymatic activity: implications for structure/function relationships. *Proc Nat Acad Sci USA* 1993; **90**:1932–6.
42. Frain M, Swart G, Monaci P et al. The liver-specific transcription factor LF-B1 contains a highly diverged homeobox DNA binding domain. *Cell* 1989; **59**: 145–57.
43. Mendel DB, Hansen LP, Graves MK, Conley PB, Crabtree GR. HNF-1α and HNF-1β (vHNF-1) share dimerisation and homeo domains, but not activation domains, and form heterodimers in vitro. *Genes Dev* 1991; **5**:1042–56.

44. Miquerol L, Lopez S, Cartier N, Tulliez M, Raymondjean M, Kahn A. Expression of the L-type pyruvate kinase gene and the hepatocyte nuclear factor 4 transcription factor in exocrine and endocrine pancreas. *J Biol Chem* 1994; **269**: 8944–51.
45. Vaxillaire M, Boccio V, Philippi A et al. A gene for maturity onset diabetes of the young (MODY) maps to chromosome 12q. *Nature Gene* 1995; **9**:418–23.
46. Menzel S, Yamagata K, Trabb J et al. Localization of MODY3 to a 5-cM region of human chromosome 12. *Diabetes* 1995; **44**:1408–13.
47. Kaisaki PJ, Menzel S, Lindner T et al. Mutations in the Hepatocyte Nuclear Factor 1α Gene in MODY and Early-onset NIDDM: Evidence for a Mutational Hotspot in Exon 4. *Diabetes* 1997: **45**:528–35.
48. Frayling T, Bulman MP, Ellard S et al. Mutations in the Hepatocyte Nuclear Factor 1 Alpha gene are a common cause of maturity-onset diabetes of the young in the United Kingdom. *Diabetes* 1997; **46**:720–5.
49. Hansen T, Eiberg H, Rouard M et al. Novel MODY3 Mutations in the Hepatic Nuclear Factor-1α Gene. *Diabetes* 1997; **46**:726–30.
50. Glucksmann MA, Lehto M, Tayber O et al. Novel mutations and a mutational hotspot in the MODY3 gene. *Diabetes* 1997; **46**:1081–6.
51. Iwasaki N, Oda N, Ogata M et al. Mutations in the Hepatocyte Nuclear Factor-1α/MODY3 gene in Japanese subjects with early- and late-onset NIDDM. *Diabetes* 1997; **46**:1504–8.
52. Vaxillaire M, Rouard M, Yamagata K et al. Identification of nine novel mutations in the hepatocyte nuclear factor 1 alpha gene associated with maturity onset diabetes of the young (MODY3). *Hum Mol Gene* 1997; **6**:583–6.
53. Frayling TM, Bulman MP, Appleton M, Bain SC, Hattersley AT, Ellard S. A rapid screening method for hepatocyte nuclear factor 1 alpha; prevalence in Maturity-onset Diabetes of the Young and late-onset non-insulin dependent diabetes. *Hum Genet* 1997; **101**:351–4.
54. Appleton M, Ellard S, Bulman M, Frayling T, Page R, Hattersley AT. Clinical characteristics of the HNF1α (MODY3) and glucokinase mutations. *Diabetologia* 1997; **40**:A161.
55. Velho G, Vaxillaire M. Boccio V. Charpentier G, Froguel P. Diabetes complications in NIDDM kindreds linked to the MODY3 locus on chromosome 12q. *Diabetes Care* 1996; **19**:915–19.
56. Byrne MM, Sturis J, Menzel S et al. Altered insulin secretory responses to glucose in diabetic and nondiabetic subjects with mutations in the diabetes susceptibility gene MODY3 on Chromosome 12. *Diabetes* 1996; **45**:1503–10.
57. Bell GI, Xiang KS, Newman MV et al. Gene for non-insulin-dependent diabetes mellitus (maturity-onset diabetes of the young subtype) is linked to DNA polymorphism on human chromosome 20q. *Proc Nat Acad Sci USA* 1991; **88**:1484–8.
58. Bulman M, Dronsfield MJ, Frayling T et al. A missense mutation in the hepatocyte nuclear factor 4 alpha gene in a UK pedigree with maturity-onset diabetes of the young. *Diabetologia* 1997; **40**:859–63.
59. Moller AM, Urhammer SA, Dalgaard LT et al. Studies of the genetic variability of the coding region of the hepatocyte nuclear factor-4α in Caucasians with maturity onset NIDDM. *Diabetologia* 1997; **40**:980–3.
60. Byrne MM, Sturis J, Fajans SS et al. Altered insulin secretory responses to glucose in subjects with a mutation in the MODY1 gene on chromosome 20. *Diabetes* 1995; **44**:699–704.
61. Pontoglio M, Barra J, Hadchouel M et al. Hepatocyte nuclear factor 1 inactivation results in hepatic dysfunction, phenylketonuria, and renal fanconi syndrome. *Cell* 1996; **84**:575–85.

62. Vaulont SaK A. Transcriptional control of metabolic regulation genes by carbohydrates. *FASEB J* 1994; **8**:28–35.
63. Diaz-Guerra M-JM, Bergot M-O, Martinze A, Cuif M-H, Kahn A, Raymondjean M. Functional characterization of the L-type pyruvate kinase gene glucose response complex. *Mol Cell Biol* 1993; **13**:7725–33.
64. Bergot M-O, Diaz-Guerra M-JM, Puzenat N, Raymondjean M, Kahn A. Cis-regulation of the L-type pyruvate kinase gene promoter by glucose, insulin and cyclic AMP. *Nucleic Acids Res* 1992; **20**:1871–8.
65. Kuo CJ, Conley PB, Chen L, Sladek FM, Darnell Jr JE, Crabtree GR. A transcriptional hierarchy involved in mammalian cell-type specification. *Nature* 1992; **355**:457–61.
66. Bach I, Pontoglio M, Yaniv M. Structure of the gene encoding hepatocyte nuclear factor 1 (HNF1). *Nucleic Acids Res* 1992; **20**:4199–204.
67. Hadzopoulou-Cladaras M, Kistanova E, Evagelopoulou C, Zeng S, Cladaras C. Ladias JAA. Functional domains of the nuclear receptor hepatocyte nuclear factor 4. *J Biol Chem* 1997; **272**:539–50.
68. Sladek FM, Zhong W, Lai E, Darnell Jr JE. Liver-enriched transcription factor HNF-4 is a novel member of the steroid hormone receptor superfamily. *Genes Dev* 1990; **4**:2353–65.
69. Stoffel M, Vaisse C, Kim J, Dundan SA. Molecular characterisation of the HNF-4α Q268X (MODY1) Mutation. *Diabetes* 1997; **6**(suppl 1): 51A.
70. Stoffel M, Duncan SA. Identification of target genes of Hepatocyte Nuclear Factor 4 (HNF-4α). *Diabetes* 1997; **46**(suppl 1): 51A.
71. Gragnoli C, Lindner T, Marozzi G, Andreani D. Disruption of the HNF-4α promoter in an Italian family with MODY. *Diabetologia* 1997; **40**(suppl 1): A7.

7

Relevance of Animal Models to Humans

P. HAVEL[1], N. SCHONFELD-WARDEN[2] AND C.H. WARDEN[2]

[1]Department of Nutrition; [2]Department of Pediatrics, University of California at Davis, Davis, CA 95616, USA

The number of animal models of type 2 diabetes increases every year, with each model having unique advantages and disadvantages. There are scores of models, as well as many different classes of models: genetic, non-genetic, viral, knockout, and transgenic. Many excellent reviews provide details on the specific comparisons of individual animal models with human type 2 diabetes[1]. Novel models are introduced and regularly discussed at Lessons for Animal Diabetes Workshops[2]. However, to date, no animal model completely mimics human type 2 diabetes. In this chapter, we discuss: (1) the advantages and disadvantages of a few different animal models, as well as recent contributions to the understanding of type 2 diabetes; (2) several recent developments in model development of type 2 diabetes and older models in which recent findings have imparted renewed interest; and (3) the future prospects for exploring the basis of human type 2 diabetes using animal model systems.

In any disease, there are several genes, gene modifiers, and other biochemical factors that influence disease phenotypes. The differences in phenotypes between same-species individuals with the same disease can be large. The complexity of phenotype and genotype relationships is even greater in complex diseases, because more genes, biochemical, and physiologic factors are involved.

Species, strain, and ethnicity further complicate studies in complex diseases. Thus, correlated traits in each model are so strongly influenced by the background and modifier genes that it may be impossible to draw conclusions about cause-and-effect relationships. This may also help explain why

Type 2 Diabetes: Prediction and Prevention. Edited by Graham A. Hitman

there are so many different models, as each appears to provide some novel information.

ADVANTAGES AND LIMITATIONS OF ANIMAL MODELS

Animal models provide many advantages for gene discovery, especially for complex traits, such as type 2 diabetes. We discuss advantages and disadvantages in the following animal models: rodents, nonhuman primates, and the nematode, *Caenorhabditis elegans*[3]. Rodents have been the most studied animal models of type 2 diabetes because there are an extensive number of specific models that exhibit a type 2 diabetes phenotype: fasting hyperglycemia and insulin resistance. Nonhuman primates provide models that may be especially relevant because of the similarities of the progressive nature of type 2 diabetes in humans and nonhuman primates. *C. elegans* will be the first animal to have its genome completely sequenced[4]. Therefore, this animal might provide tools for rapid discovery of genes in pathways for complex traits, such as type 2 diabetes, provided that *C. elegans* exhibits phenotypes that are characteristic. Animal model studies require that the model exhibit phenotypes that are similar to the human disease, even though advances in DNA-sequencing and analysis software make discovery of homologous genes routine. Besides the characteristics of some animal models, we also address some recent contributions to the understanding of type 2 diabetes.

Advantages common to all animal models, along with those present in some models, but not in others, are summarized in Table 7.1. Control of environmental and breeding, tissue collection, and hypothesis testing are common advantages of all models, but diet, mutants, and genome sequencing are advantages specific to only some models.

RODENTS

ADVANTAGES

Rodent colonies are relatively inexpensive to maintain. More importantly, however, rodents have short generation times that are crucial for conducting genetic studies. A high degree of control over experimental variables is another major advantage of rodent studies: control of heterogeneity, breeding, physiologic studies, nutritional studies, and control of germline transmission for hypothesis testing (Table 7.1). These advantages allow several approaches to identifying genes that cause diabetes, including the use of

Table 7.1. Advantages of animal models

Advantages common to all animal models	
Environmental control	Temperature and population density can be varied as required
Breeding control	Animals can be mated as needed
Tissue collection	Surgery and sacrifices can be used for hypothesis testing and biochemical studies in mice and primates
	Whole *C. elegans* can be sacrificed as needed
Hypothesis testing	Transgenic and knockout animals can be made for mice and *C. elegans*
	Gene and drug therapy can be used to test hypotheses in primates
The following advantages apply to some but not all models	
Diet control	Primates and rodents can be fed diets similar to human diets
	One can control the amount and content of the diet and observe the effects on disease phenotypes
	In contrast, *C. elegans* eats bacteria, so its diet is difficult to relate to human nutrition
Mutants	Mice and *C. elegans* colonies have many spontaneous mutants with a wide variety of phenotypes
	This advantage does not apply to primates because they are outbred, like humans, and thus exhibit fewer spontaneous mutants
Genome sequencing	*C. elegans* sequencing is complete.
	This will greatly facilitate the process of pathway discovery and homology prediction
	In contrast, the genomes of primates and humans will not be completely sequenced for several years after completion of the *C. elegans* genome.

positional cloning to isolate specific genes, and testing hypotheses about causes and effects of various treatments.

One of the most powerful features of the mouse genetic map is that it can be related quickly to the human genetic map. Large segments of mouse and human chromosomes contain the same genes in the same orders[5]. A mouse gene chromosomal location correlates fairly accurately to that in humans. As a result, one can locate positional candidate cDNA clones using the cDNA clones mapped to human chromosomes by the Human Genome Project. These cDNA clones can then be examined for their roles in mouse and human type 2 diabetes.

Genetically altered mice are useful for testing hypotheses about the role of specific genes in diabetes. Many methods are available for testing hypotheses about genes involved in the pathogenesis of diabetes. In rodent models, this includes transgenic and knockout mice. There are many variations on both of these methods. Transgenic mice can be used to: (1) overexpress genes in their normal tissues; (2) overexpress genes in specific tissues; (3) express particular mouse or human genes; (4) express genes with inducible promoters; or (5) express novel proteins designed to test specific hypotheses (for example, chimeric proteins or proteins with specific mutations). Knockout mice can also be used in a wide variety of experiments. Examples of knockout approaches include: (1) to test the effects of complete absence of a specific protein; (2) to test the effect of a specific protein that is absent in a specific tissue; and (3) to introduce specific mutations into the germline of mice[6]. Transgenic and knockout methods can be combined to eliminate expression of the normal mouse protein, which can then be replaced by the homologous human protein to 'humanize' the mouse. Alternatively, the missing protein can be replaced by transgenic constructs that are used to test specific hypotheses about in vivo structure and function.

There are a wide variety of 'normal' inbred strains as well as hundreds of spontaneously mutant mouse strains. These mutations probably existed as variant alleles in wild populations, but were not apparent because the allele frequency was low. Every person and animal carries some mutant recessive genes the phenotypes of which are not expressed. During the process of inbreeding, some rare recessive mutant genes become homozygous and then the phenotype appears. These mutant inbred strains have provided very useful resources for cloning genes for complex disease, such as the leptin gene that was cloned from the *ob* mouse.

Limitations

Although many of the limitations of rodent models are obvious, such as differences of size and life span from humans, others are more subtle. One limitation is that one cannot easily correlate traits in an animal model to cause-and-effect relationships and then extrapolate to humans. The same mutation in different mouse strains has very different effects on traits. Understanding the strain effect may alter the understanding of the usefulness of animal models and influence thinking about the roles of genes in human diabetes. For example, the *ob* and *db* mutations have very different phentoypes when they are placed on the background of C57BL/6J or C57BL/6Ks[7]. The *ob* and *db* mutations both cause type 1 diabetes on the C57BL/6Ks background and these same mutations cause a much milder type 2 diabetes when they are placed on the C57BL/6J background. Similarly, the original Zucker (*fa/fa*) rat strains are insulin resistant but not diabetic. On the other hand, in a substrain selectively inbred for hyperglycemia (ZDF), animals homozygous for the *fa* mutation develop frank diabetes[8].

Some history of the inbred rodent strains will elucidate the differences between the strains better. Virtually all mice used in research laboratories are inbred. Inbred rodents are the product of at least 20 generations of brother-to-sister matings that began from a founding pair of wild outbred mice. Inbreeding produces strains in which all animals are genetically identical. However, each inbred strain will have a different set of the alleles present in the founding outbred population. Phenotypic differences *between* inbred animals of a single strain result from environmental influences or measurement error. Phenotypic differences *among* strains are the result of genetic differences. A survey of inbred animals for any one trait almost always identifies strains with differing phenotypes.

The main reason for strain dependence of observed phenotypes is that type 2 diabetes is a complex disease influenced by many genes. Each animal model will exhibit a different set of phenotypes because each inbred animal has fixed different sets of alleles for each of the many genes that influence type 2 diabetes. Lists of correlated traits in animal models do not necessarily represent lists of cause-and-effect traits. These correlated traits in each model are so strongly influenced by the background and modifier genes that it may be impossible to draw conclusions about the cause-and-effect relationships. This may also help to explain why there are so many models – each appears to provide some novel information.

Even diseases clearly influenced by mutations in a single gene exhibit varying phenotypes in different people and animals. This is because there are many modifiers that influence the severity of the trait, e.g., this is probably true of type 1 diabetes, where the HLA effect is modified by many other genes. There is one exception – transgenic and knockout mice may be bred so that they all share the same background; one can then directly compare effects of specific mutations. In this case, all the background genes are the same, so one can compare the specific effects of the altered gene on type 2 diabetes.

One caveat that should be considered in knockout studies is that knockout animals will lack the 'knocked out' gene throughout embryogenesis and all phases of development. Therefore, a normal phenotype in a specific knockout does not in itself suggest that the missing gene is unimportant in a normal animal. Developmental compensation and redundant pathways can mask the normal role of a knockout protein. In one key example of this redundancy, the neuropeptide Y (NPY) knockout mouse is not obese or hyperphagic[9], yet, when combined with the *ob* mutation, *ob/ob* mice are less obese than those with an intact NPY gene[10], demonstrating that NPY is involved in mediating a portion of the central effects of leptin deficiency. Thus, the role of NPY as a central transducer of energy balance was likely masked by the development or recruitment of redundant pathways. This problem may be minimized with the advent of inducible knockout models in which the gene of interest is targeted in adult animals.

These lessons from animal models about the impact of background genes on observed phenotypes have important implications for human studies. They suggest that alleles of background genes present in different ethnic groups may have profound influences on the phenotypes observed with any given gene.

Recent contributions

Identification of chromosomal loci for type 2 diabetes, and the construction of knockout mice with phenotypes of polygenic type 2 diabetes, are two areas in which there have been many recent publications using mouse models. Whole genome linkage mapping methods have identified chromosomal loci (quantitative trait loci, or QTLs) that influence type 2 diabetes[11]. However, isolation of the specific underlying genes requires two more large steps – production of monogenic models for each type 2 chromosomal locus and then using these new monogenic models as tools for classic positional cloning. Each of these steps requires several years, so it is perhaps not surprising that no genes influencing type 2 diabetes have yet been isolated by positional cloning of animal model QTL genes. However, recent results suggest that QTL genes can be cloned because some groups have produced monogenic models from complex models. This is accomplished by selective breeding of two mouse strains to produce a congenic strain, in which the congenic strain is identical to a background strain except for a small, selected, donor strain region. Although no congenic strains have as yet been constructed for type 2 diabetes loci, a congenic strain has been developed for type 1 diabetes in the biobreeding BB rat[12]. Additional details on linkage mapping of type 2 diabetes loci are provided in the section on recent developments.

Analysis of mice with knockouts of two independent genes is the second major area of recent contributions of mouse models to the understanding of type 2 diabetes. As is discussed in more detail later, it has been possible to produce animals with polygenic type 2 diabetes in double knockout mice. In some cases, the phenotype of the double knockouts is quite different from either of the single-gene knockout mice. The results provide an unambiguous demonstration of gene interactions that lead to type 2 diabetes.

NONHUMAN PRIMATES

Advantages

Although they are less well studied than rodents, nonhuman primates have been studied for several decades as animal models of type 2 diabetes. Spontaneous insulin-resistant diabetes has been reported in most common species of nonhuman primates and occurs with a high prevalence in *Macaca niger*[13] and, with a lesser, but significant, prevalence, in rhesus monkeys[14]. The progression of obesity-related type 2 diabetes in the aging rhesus monkey has been well characterized in longitudinal studies, and it shares many of the features of the progression to type 2 diabetes observed in cross-sectional studies in humans[15]. An insulin-resistant form of diabetes can be induced by administering nicotinic acid to baboons with reduced β-cell mass, resulting from low-dose administration of streptozotocin[16].

The most obvious advantage of the nonhuman primate models is their genetic and physiologic similarity to humans. The presence of islet amyloidosis, characteristic of type 2 diabetes in humans, is also observed in diabetic monkeys. This suggests a similar etiology of islet lesions in monkeys and humans[17]. Maps of genetic markers have been established for baboon and rhesus monkeys[18] and some genes relevant to type 2 diabetes and obesity, such as the *ob* gene[19] and the β_3-adrenergic receptor[20], have been cloned in monkeys. Other advantages of nonhuman primates include their relatively large size, which allows for frequent serial blood sampling (e.g., minimal model assessment of insulin sensitivity and secretion by fast-sampled intravenous glucose tolerance tests or, FSIVGTT). Furthermore, one can obtain serial tissue biopsies from nonhuman primates that would likely be precluded in humans. Last, diet composition and amount can be well controlled in nonhuman primates, whereas compliance with dietary regimens is poor in free-living human subjects.

Limitations

One of the major limitations of nonhuman primates versus other animal models is the limited numbers of animals available for study. Other important limitations include: the long periods of time required for breeding, the considerable expense of maintaining nonhuman primates, and the limited number of facilities that provide support for research, e.g., regional primate research centers.

Recent Contributions

As previously discussed, the aging obese rhesus monkey develops a form of type 2 diabetes that shares a large number of features with human type 2 diabetes including, but not limited to, hyperinsulinemia, insulin resistance, impaired glucose tolerance, dyslipidemia, and hypertension[14,15]. One of the more important contributions from nonhuman primates studies is that the development of insulin resistance can be prevented in rhesus monkeys by dietary restriction[21]; the onset of type 2 diabetes can be prevented by maintaining the animals at a stable body weight[22], and prevention of obesity prevents the development of type 2 diabetes in rhesus monkeys. These results are in agreement with cross-sectional and interventional studies in humans. They also provide additional rationale for efforts to prevent obesity in people with a family history of diabetes.

CAENORHABDITIS ELEGANS

Advantages

C. elegans is the first animal model for which the genome is completely sequenced. There are many advantages to the *C. elegans* model for gene discovery efforts. *C. elegans* provides experimental advantages for reductionist gene cloning and pathway identification experiments. For instance, many of the genes involved in apoptosis were first identified in *C. elgans*. Many *C. elegans* genes are clearly homologous to human proteins – for example, *C. elegans* has a clear homolog to the insulin receptor[23]. In addition, there are many mutants of *C. elegans* available for elucidating biologic pathways. There are mutants that live longer (longevity mutants) and ones that may accumulate fat[24,25]. These mutants have identified candidate human diabetes genes and are being used to determine pathways of insulin and tissue growth factor β (TGF-β) signalling.

Limitations

There are many potential limitations to *C. elegans* as a diabetes model. For *C. elegans*, the biggest problem is that the phenotype has not been investigated. Although genome project resources have shown that *C. elegans* or other animal models have proteins with sequences homologous to those of humans, in many cases the relationship of the observed phenotype to human disease is unclear. All mammals have homologous genes – such as the fact that insulin and insulin receptors are widely distributed – but not all mammals are diabetes models. Diabetes models require the exhibition of a phenotype that is recognizable. The *C. elegans* analogy relies heavily on sequence homology, so it is unclear what will be learned[26]. There is no evidence that *C. elegans* exhibits phenotypes characteristic of type 2 diabetes, even though *C. elegans* clearly has genes that are homologous to insulin, insulin receptor, and many other proteins of the insulin-signaling pathways. The diabetes phenotypes observed are confined to the identification of Sudan black staining of intestinal particles in Dauer phase worms. These have been interpreted as 'fat,' but there has been no chemical characterization of Dauer phase worms. Nevertheless, the accumulation of 'fat' in these worms has provided the data to suggest a diabetes phenotype.

Recent Contributions

Several genes that influence *C. elegans* longevity, which are also part of the insulin-signaling pathway have been cloned. The human homologs for these genes become candidate type 2 diabetes genes, which should be examined in detail for potential roles. Many chromosomal loci for type 2 diabetes have been identified in rodent models, and several pathways for insulin-like signaling have been identified in *C. elegans*. Thus, *C. elegans* is not so much a model organism as a pathway discovery tool, packaged inside a worm. Still, especially for the rodent models, which clearly exhibit type 2 diabetes phenotypes, isolation of the underlying genes has not been carried out. In fact, frustration with gene identification progress in humans and rodents is a part of the driving force behind the experiments with the very simple animal models.

CHARACTERISTICS OF SEVERAL NOVEL MODELS OF TYPE 2 DIABETES

We discuss briefly several of the recent developments in type 2 diabetes models and some developments in older models, where recent findings have imparted a renewed interest. For example, novel polygenic models have been constructed from two or more knockout mice. Also, genes influencing type 2 diabetes have been mapped by whole genome approaches in several genetic models. As discussed in the section on *C. elegans*, novel species are being used as diabetes models, primarily because these species provide experimental advantages for reductionist gene cloning and pathway identification experiments.

DOUBLE KNOCKOUTS

One novel and interesting development is the double knockout model in which two genes that interact with one another are ablated. Double knockouts have shown that mice heterozygous for knockout of the insulin receptor and for insulin receptor substrate-1 (IRS-1) develop characteristics of type 2 diabetes[27]. Mice with double knockouts of glucokinase and IRS-1 exhibit a type 2 diabetes phenotype that is not apparent in either single knockout[28]. By studying double knockouts, one may be able to reconstruct polygenic traits and to gain insight into the underlying causes of diabetes.

NEW ZEALAND OBESE MOUSE

The New Zealand obese (NZO) mouse is an obese polygenic model exhibiting hyperphagia, mild hyperglycemia, and hyperinsulinemia with marked insulin resistance[29]. Although the NZO mouse is not a new model, it has recently been shown that it is resistant to the effects of peripherally administered leptin to reduce food intake, but that it responds normally to central leptin administration, suggesting a defect of leptin transport into the central nervous system (CNS) in these animals[30]. There is increasing evidence that leptin is an important regulator of energy balance in humans[31,32] and there are data suggesting impaired leptin transport across the blood–brain barrier in humans[33]. The NZO mouse may be a useful model for investigating the mechanism of leptin resistance resulting from a failure of leptin to gain access to its targets in the CNS. Leptin-deficient mice are hyperphagic, obese, insulin resistant, and diabetic. Although leptin-deficient and leptin receptor-mutant humans are not frankly diabetic, they might be diabetic on a different genetic background or when they get older. Increased energy intake and obesity clearly contribute to type 2 diabetes in humans. Finally, leptin appears to have central and peripheral effects on both insulin sensitivity and insulin secretion, increasing its relevance to type 2 diabetes.

OLETF RAT

The OLETF rat is a spontaneous genetic model that exhibits impaired glucose tolerance, hyperglycemia, and modest hyperinsulinemia[34]. Several studies have investigated genes underlying type 2 diabetes in the OLETF rat and identified loci on several chromosomes[35,36]. One defect defined in the OLETF model is a deficiency of the cholecystokinin A (CCK-A) receptor subtype. These animals are hyperphagic and do not reduce food consumption in response to exogenous CCK. One hypothesis is that a lack of CCK-induced satiety leads to increased meal size, obesity, and diabetes[37]. However, OLETF rats also do not secrete insulin in response to CCK[38]. In addition, CCK has an important role in maintaining pancreatic differentiation[39], which suggests that the development of diabetes in these animals may be multifactorial. Of potential relevance to human type 2 diabetes is that exercise training attenuates obesity and prevents the development of diabetes in this model[40].

GOTO–KAKIZAKI RAT

The Goto–Kakizaki (GK) rat model of type 2 diabetes was developed by selectively breeding rats with impaired glucose tolerance for more than 35 generations[11]. The rats exhibit moderate insulin resistance, which is associated with decreased numbers of hepatic insulin receptors. They also show impaired insulin secretion, which is associated with decreased ATP-sensitive channel activity in β cells and underexpression of *GLUT2* in islets[8,40]. As this is a nonobese model, one interesting aspect of the GK rat model is the ability to study insulin resistance and glucose intolerance in the absence of obesity.

DIET-INDUCED MODELS

The advantage of diet-induced models of type 2 diabetes is that the availability of high-energy and highly palatable foods may contribute to obesity and the progression to diabetes in humans. Unfortunately, most rodent models of diet-induced obesity do not develop more than mild hyperglycemia[41–43]. There is one recently described model of experimentally induced type 2 diabetes in which high fat feeding was combined with bilateral ventromedial hypothalamic (VMH) lesions in rats. These combined treatments produced rats with fasting hyperglycemia of more than 10 μmmol/l (180 μmg/dl)[44].

MATERNAL LOW-PROTEIN RAT MODEL

Associations have been found between markers of fetal and early growth retardation and the subsequent development of diabetes (the 'thrifty phenotype' hypothesis). These observations in humans have been reproduced in the offspring of pregnant rats fed a low-protein diet. The thrifty phenotype hypothesis and this animal model of diabetes are discussed at length in chapter 9.

FUTURE PROSPECTS FOR ANIMAL MODELS

Future prospects for animal models are excellent, e.g. it is almost certain that a rodent type 2 diabetes gene will be positionally cloned. Why are there so many animal models? The answer is that each is unique, and relatively easy to find. But what has been found and what is missing? Phenotype characterization is excellent for many rodent models and for rhesus monkeys, but practically non-existent for *C. elegans*. Many chromosomal loci for type 2 diabetes have been identified in rodent models and several pathways for insulin-like signaling have been identified in *C. elegans*. As mentioned earlier use of the more simple models is the result of the frustration with gene identification progress in humans and rodents.

Cloning of genes underlying QTLs has been difficult. Even criteria for success are hard to develop. It has been suggested that one needs to show that a specific candidate chromosomal region contains the underlying gene by constructing interval specific congenic strains (ISCSs) surrounding the QTL[45]. ISCSs are congenic strains in which several congenics each contain adjacent donor strain chromosomal regions. Congenic strains are derived from a cross between two strains, followed by repeated backcrosses to the major background strain and selection for a minor or donor strain chromosomal region. The resulting congenic is almost identical to the background strain, except for the selected donor strain region. One can test phenotypic effects of genes that are linked, but 1–2 cM apart, in the different ISCS mice. Once an ISCS has been identified that retains the phenotype observed in the original QTL, then one can test specific candidate genes by making transgenic or knockouts. This has been accomplished for a cancer-susceptibility gene[46]. Diabetes may be influenced by complex genetic interactions, such as epistasis and nonadditive interactions. Epistasis occurs when phenotypes are influenced by two or more genes, where each gene alone may have no effect on the trait, but where two or more together can influence the trait. Nonadditive interactions are gene-to-gene interactions in which the two genes make unequal contributions to the overall phenotype. One of the advantages of animal genetic studies is cloning genes that influence complex diseases by complex interactions. Although there is at least some possibility that these genes can be identified in animal models, genes involved in such complex interactions will be even more difficult to identify in human studies alone.

REFERENCES

1. Shafrir E. Development and consequences of insulin resistance: lessons from animals with hyperinsulinaemia. *Diabetes Metab* 1996; **22**:122–31.
2. 6th International Workshop on Lessons from Animal Diabetes. Copenhagen, Denmark, July 14–17, 1997. Abstracts. *Exp Clin Endocrinol Diabetes* 1997; **105**(suppl 3): 1–98.
3. Ahringer J. Turn to the worm! *Curr Opin Genet Dev* 1997; **7**:410–15.
4. Sonnhammer EL, Durbin R. Analysis of protein domain families in *Caenorhabditis elegans*. *Genomics* 1997; **46**:200–16.
5. Nadeau JH. Maps of linkage and synteny homologies between mouse and man. *Trends Genet* 1989; **53**: 82–6.
6. Pandolfi PP. Knocking in and out genes and trans genes: the use of the engineered mouse to study normal and aberrant hemopoiesis. *Semin Hematol* 1998; *35*:136–48.
7. Hummel KP, Coleman DL, Lane PW. The influence of genetic background on expression of mutations at the diabetes locus in the mouse. I. C57BL-KsJ and C57BL-6J strains. *Biochem Genet* 1972; **7**(1): 1–13.
8. Shafrir E. Diabetes in animals: Contributions to the understanding of diabetes by studying its etiopathology in animal models. In: Sherwin R, ed. *Diabetes Mellitus, Theory and Practice* vol 5. Stanford: Appleton Lange, 1997: 310–48.
9. Erickson JC, Clegg KE, Palmiter RD. Sensitivity to leptin and susceptibility to seizures of mice lacking neuropeptide Y. *Nature* 1996; **381**(6581): 415–21.
10. Erickson JC, Hollopeter G, Palmiter RD. Attenuation of the obesity syndrome of ob/ob mice by the loss of neuropeptide Y. *Science* 1996; **274**(5293): 1704–7.
11. Ktorza A, Bernard C, Parent V, et al. Are animal models of diabetes relevant to the study of the genetics of non-insulin-dependent diabetes in humans? *Diabetes Metab* 1997; **23**(suppl 2): 38–46.
12. Bieg S, Koike G, Jiang J et al. Genetic isolation of iddm 1 on chromosome 4 in the biobreeding (BB) rat. *Mamm Genome* 1998; **9**:324–6.

13. Howard CF Jr. Longitudinal studies on the development of diabetes in individual *Macaca Nigra*. *Diabetologia* 1986; **29**:301–6.
14. Hansen B. Primate animal models of non-insulin-dependent diabetes mellitus. In: LeRoith D, Taylor S, Olefsky J, eds. *Diabetes Mellitus*. Philadelphia: Lippincott-Raven, 1996: 595–603.
15. Hansen B. Animal models of aging-associated metabolic syndrome of obesity. In: Bouchard C, Bray G, eds. *Regulation of Body Weight: Biological and behavioral mechanisms*. Chichester: John Wiley & Sons, 1996: 45–60.
16. McCulloch DK, Kahn SE, Schwartz MW, Koerker DJ, Palmer JP. Effect of nicotinic acid-induced insulin resistance on pancreatic β-cell function in normal and streptozocin-treated baboons. *J Clin Invest* 1991; **87**:1395–401.
17. de Koning EJ, Bodkin NL, Hansen BC, Clark A. Diabetes mellitus in *Macaca mulatta* monkeys is characterized by islet amyloidosis and reduction in beta-cell population. *Diabetologia* 1993; **36**:378–84.
18. Rogers J, Hixson JE. Baboons as an animal model for genetic studies of common human disease. *Am J Hum Genet* 1997; **61**:489–93.
19. Hotta K, Gustafson TA, Ortmeyer HK, Bodkin NL, Nicolson MA, Hansen BC. Regulation of obese (ob) mRNA and plasma leptin levels in rhesus monkeys. Effects of insulin, body weight, and non-insulin-dependent diabetes mellitus. *J Biol Chem* 1996; **271**:25327–31.
20. Walston J, Lowe A, Silver K et al. The beta3-adrenergic receptor in the obesity and diabetes prone rhesus monkey is very similar to human and contains arginine at codon 64. *Gene* 1997; **188**:207–13.
21. Kemnitz JW, Roecker EB, Weindruch R, Elson DF, Baum ST, Bergman RN. Dietary restriction increases insulin sensitivity and lowers blood glucose in rhesus monkeys. *Am J Physiol* 1994; **266** (4 Pt 1): E540–7.
22. Hansen BC, Bodkin NL. Primary prevention of diabetes mellitus by prevention of obesity in monkeys. *Diabetes* 1993; **42**:1809–14.
23. Kimura KD, Tissenbaum HA, Liu Y, Ruvkun G. daf-2, an insulin receptor-like gene that regulates longevity and diapause in *Caenorhabditis elegans* [see comments]. *Science* 1997; **277**(5328): 942–6.
24. Tissenbaum HA, Ruvkun G. An insulin-like signaling pathway affects both longevity and reproduction in *Caenorhabditis elegans*. *Genetics* 1998; **148**:703–17.
25. Lin K, Dorman JB, Rodan A, Kenyon C. daf-16: An HNF-3/forkhead family member that can function to double the life-span of *Caenorhabditis elegans* [see comments]. *Science* 1997; **278**(5341): 1319–22.
26. Hekimi S, Lakowski B, Barnes TM, Ewbank JJ. Molecular genetics of life span in *C. elegans*: how much does it teach us? *Trends Genet* 1998; **14**:14–20.
27. Bruning JC, Winnay J, Bonner-Weir S, Taylor SI, Accili D, Kahn CR. Development of a novel polygenic model of NIDDM in mice heterozygous for IR and IRS-1 null alleles. *Cell* 1997; **88**:561–72.
28. Terauchi Y, Iwamoto K, Tamemoto H et al. Development of non-insulin-dependent diabetes mellitus in the double knockout mice with disruption of insulin receptor substrate-1 and beta cell glucokinase genes. Genetic reconstitution of diabetes as a polygenic disease. *J Clin Invest* 1997; **99**:861–6.
29. Proietto J, Larkins R. A Perspective on the New Zealand Obese Mouse. In: Shafrir E, ed. *Lessons from Animal Diabetes*. London: Smith-Gordon, 1992: 65–74.
30. Halaas JL, Boozer C, Blair-West J, Fidahusein N, Denton DA, Friedman JM. Physiological response to long-term peripheral and central leptin infusion in lean and obese mice. *Proc Natl Acad Sci USA* 1997; **94**:8878–83.
31. Havel PJ. Leptin production and action: relevance to energy balance in humans [editorial, comment]. *Am J Clin Nutr* 1998; **67**:355–6.

32. Keim N, Stern J, Havel P. Relationship between circulating leptin concentrations and appetite during a prolonged moderate energy deficit in women. *Am J Clin Nutr* 1998: in press.
33. Schwartz MW, Peskind E, Raskind M, Boyko EJ, Porte D Jr. Cerebrospinal fluid leptin levels: relationship to plasma levels and to adiposity in humans. *Nature Med* 1996; **2**:589–93.
34. Shafrir E. Animal models of non-insulin-dependent diabetes. *Diabetes Metab Rev* ***1992;*** **8**:179–208.
35. Kanemoto N, Hishigaki H, Miyakita A et al. Genetic dissection of 'OLETF', a rat model for non-insulin-dependent diabetes mellitus [In Process Citation]. *Mamm Genome* 1998; **9**:419–25.
36. Moralejo DH, Wei S, Wei K, Yamada T, Matsumoto K. X-linked locus is responsible for non-insulin-dependent diabetes mellitus in the OLETF rat. *J Vet Med Sci* 1998; **60**:373–5.
37. Moran TH, Katz LF, Plata-Salaman CR, Schwartz GJ. Disordered food intake and obesity in rats lacking cholecystokinin A receptors. *Am J Physiol* 1998; **274**(3 Pt 2): R618–25.
38. Tachibana I, Akiyama T, Kanagawa K et al. Defect in pancreatic exocrine and endocrine response to CCK in genetically diabetic OLETF rats. *Am J Physiol* 1996; **270**(4 Pt 1): G730–7.
39. Miyasaka K, Ohta M, Tateishi K, Jimi A, Funakoshi A. Role of cholecystokinin-A (CCK-A) receptor in pancreatic regeneration after pancreatic duct occlusion: a study in rats lacking CCK-A receptor gene expression. *Pancreas* 1998; **16**:114–23.
40. Shima K, Shi K, Mizuno A, Sano T, Ishida K, Noma Y. Exercise training has a long-lasting effect on prevention of non-insulin-dependent diabetes mellitus in Otsuka–Long–Evans–Tokushima Fatty rats. *Metabolism* 1996; **45**:475–80.
41. Ahren B, Simonsson E, Scheurink AJ, Mulder H, Myrsen U, Sundler F. Dissociated insulinotropic sensitivity to glucose and carbachol in high- fat diet-induced insulin resistance in C57BL/6J mice. *Metabolism* 1997; **46**:97–106.
42. Ahren B, Mansson S, Gingerich RL, Havel PJ. Regulation of plasma leptin in mice: influence of age, high-fat diet, and fasting. *Am J Physiol* 1997; **273**(1 Pt 2): R113–20.
43. Surwit RS, Petro AE, Parekh P, Collins S. Low plasma leptin in response to dietary fat in diabetes- and obesity-prone mice [published erratum appears in *Diabetes* 1997; **46**:1920]. *Diabetes* 1997; **46**:1516–20.
44. Axen KV, Li X, Fung K, Sclafani A. The VMH-dietary obese rat: a new model of non-insulin-dependent diabetes mellitus. *Am J Physiol* 1994; **266**(3 Pt 2): R921–8.
45. Gould KA, Luongo C, Moser AR et al. Genetic evaluation of candidate genes for the Mom1 modifier of intestinal neoplasia in mice. *Genetics* 1996; **144**:1777–85.
46. Cormier RT, Hong KH, Halberg RB et al. Secretory phospholipase Pla2g2a confers resistance to intestinal tumorigenesis. *Native Genet* 1997; **17**:88–91.

Part C

Other Factors Relevant to Prediction

8

Non-genetic Transmission

L. AERTS, K. HOLEMANS AND F.A. VAN ASSCHE
Laboratory of Obstetrics and Gynaecology, U.Z. Gasthuisberg, Herestraat 49, Leuven B-3000, Belgium

It has been well established that the development of a fetus in an abnormal intrauterine environment implies structural and functional adaptations with long-lasting consequences for the metabolism of the offspring in later life. Different experimental designs of altered maternal metabolism have demonstrated a diabetogenic effect in the offspring, including the occurrence of gestational diabetes. The fetuses of these mothers also develop in an abnormal intrauterine environment, which will once again transmit the diabetogenic effect to the next generation.

This phenomenon appears to be of crucial importance, because it induces the transmission of a diabetogenic tendency over consecutive generations, without any genetic interference. The transmission can indeed be prevented by normalizing maternal glycaemia during pregnancy.

Several epidemiological studies in the human have described similar effects of maternal diabetes or malnutrition on the metabolism of the offspring, including impaired glucose tolerance, gestational diabetes and type 2 diabetes.

This chapter deals mainly with the different experimental animal models, linking them to the human situation; the latter is described in more detail in other chapters of this book.

OFFSPRING OF MILDLY DIABETIC MOTHERS

When mild diabetes is induced in pregnant rats, with glycaemia of more than 20% above the normal, the fetuses also have to deal with this hyperglycemia. Development of the islets of Langerhans in the fetal pancreas, which occurs during the last trimester, is enhanced, leading to islet hypertrophy and β-cell

Type 2 Diabetes: Prediction and Prevention. Edited by Graham A. Hitman

hyperplasia[1,2], and increased β-cell sensitivity and responsiveness[3], which results in hyperinsulinaemia[1,3,4]. Increased glucose and amino acid utilization[5,6] results in macrosomia[1]. Plasma glucagon[7] and corticosterone[8] levels are low. At birth, when the mother's hyperglycaemic stimulus is withdrawn and the pups are fed by their mother's milk, which is poor in carbohydrates, the normal initiation of hepatic glycogenolysis is impaired[9] and the relative involution of the endocrine pancreas is even more pronounced than in the control pups[10]. Despite normal basal insulin levels, glucose-stimulated insulin secretion is deficient in these pups, and this impairment of glucose tolerance is aggravated with advancing age, eventually leading to overt diabetes in elderly animals[11].

As adults, these animals have a normal islet and β-cell mass[10,12], and normal basal glucose and insulin levels[10]; their glucose-stimulated insulin response is, however, deficient, both in vivo and in vitro[13,14]. This impairment must be induced *in utero* by the fetal hyperinsulinaemia, because a similar defect in adult animals occurs after neonatal exposure of their hypothalamus to high insulin concentrations[15,16]. Amelioration of impaired glucose tolerance in the adult offspring, through modulation of the adrenergic activation of insulin secretion, also points to a neuroendocrine involvement in the deficient insulin-response[14]. However, an increased amino acid turnover also seems to play a role, because circulating amino acid levels are still low in these animals (as they are in fetal life)[6] and restoration to normal levels normalizes the insulin secretion, at least in vitro[17].

When these youngsters become pregnant, the adaptation of their endocrine pancreas to pregnancy includes a normal doubling of the islet and β-cell mass[12]. Nevertheless, they develop mild gestational diabetes[17–19], thereby again exposing the next generation of fetuses to a mildly diabetic intrauterine environment. Indeed these fetuses display all the characteristics of fetuses from mildly diabetic mothers: islet hyperplasia, β-cell hyperactivity, hyperinsulinaemia and macrosomia[17–19]. As adults, they have an impaired glucose tolerance and, when pregnant, they develop gestational diabetes[17–19].

The effects on the offspring up to the third generation are similar, whether the first-generation mothers were made either mildly diabetic by partial destruction of their pancreatic β-cells with streptozotocin[17,18] or mildly hyperglycaemic during the last trimester by continuous glucose infusion[19]. The effect on the third generation is transmitted only via the maternal line: female offspring of diabetic mothers develop gestational diabetes and transmit the diabetogenic effect to their fetuses; male offspring have impaired glucose tolerance, but do not affect the glucose tolerance of their offspring[20]. This difference again stresses the importance of the intrauterine environment, and excludes a genetic factor in this transgeneration effect.

OFFSPRING OF SEVERELY DIABETIC MOTHERS

When severe diabetes is induced in pregnant rats, with glycaemia at the limit for survival of pregnancy and lactation without treatment, the developing fetuses also have to deal with this abundant fuel supply. The development of their islets of Langerhans is thereby enhanced and results in islet hypertrophy[1,3]. β cells do, however, get overstimulated by the continuous excessive glucose challenge. Insulin secretion occurs faster than insulin synthesis, and many β cells become degranulated, disorganized[1] and unable to secrete insulin, whether in vivo or in vitro[3,4,21,22]. Circulating insulin levels are therefore very low and insulin binding is decreased, at least in the liver and lungs[23]; the fetuses cannot profit from the abundant food and they display intrauterine growth retardation[1,3,22].

In these pups, the involution of the endocrine pancreas during lactation is also more pronounced than that in the controls[10], but at adulthood they have largely recovered. The total mass of endocrine tissue and of β cells exceeds even the control values, mainly as a result of an abundance of very small iselts[12], and ultrastructural examination of the β cells reveals an increased β-cell recruitment[24]. These youngsters are still smaller than normal, but they display normal basal glucose and insulin levels[10]. During glucose infusion, glycaemia remains within the normal range, but associated with very high insulin levels. Insulin output on glucose stimulation appears to be excessive, both in vivo and in vitro, whereas insulin uptake is deficient[13,14,25]. Euglycaemic/hyperinsulinaemic clamps on these adult youngsters demonstrate normal glucose use in basal conditions, but clear-cut insulin resistance in the presence of hyperinsulinaemia. This resistance is characterized by a decreased sensitivity and responsiveness of the liver and a decreased sensitivity of the peripheral tissues[26,27], mainly the skeletal muscles[28]. In fact, these animals, in many ways, display the characteristics of pregnant animals. At the level of the pancreas, there is islet hypertrophy and β-cell hyperplasia, β-cell hyperactivity and enhanced recruitment, increased sensitivity and responsiveness. At the level of insulin action, there is a similar insulin resistance as that seen during normal pregnancy, in both the peripheral tissues and the liver. All these parameters do not in fact increase further when these adult youngsters become pregnant[12,29]. Despite their adequate condition, they develop gestational diabetes, and their fetuses display the typical characteristics of fetuses from mildly diabetic mothers, thus transmitting once again the diabetogenic effect to the next generation[17].

The primary factor inducing all these events is evidently the extreme maternal and fetal hyperglycaemia in the first generation. Indeed the effects in fetal and adult offspring are prevented by normalizing the maternal glycaemia during the last trimester by transplantation of an adequate number of healthy islets[30]. The occurrence of insulin resistance at adulthood is similar, whether the pups were fed by their own diabetic mothers[17] or by healthy controls[25]. The low circulating insulin levels, resulting from β-cell exhaustion in these hyperglycaemic fetuses, might prevent the normal development of the peripheral insulin receptor system, which may lead to insulin resistance at adulthood, and to increased β-cell mass and responsiveness. The overstimulation of the fetal β-cells might, however, have directly induced a deficiency in the control of β-cell mass and responsiveness in later life, resulting in an increased insulin output by the pancreas and a decreased insulin sensitivity in the peripheral tissues.

OFFSPRING OF SEMISTARVED MOTHERS

When rats are semistarved (50% of normal food intake) throughout the second half of pregnancy and lactation, levels of maternal and fetal glycaemia are very low[31] and result in intrauterine growth retardation[31,32]. The poor nutrient supply fails to stimulate the development of the fetal pancreas, the β-cell mass and insulin content are significantly reduced[32], and the circulating insulin reaches only half of the normal value at term gestation[31]. Continuing the food restriction of the mother during lactation further aggravates the growth retardation and reduces the β-cell mass to about 30% of the normal value[31,33]. Weaning on a normal laboratory diet partially restores the body weight[31].

At adulthood, circulating insulin levels in these youngsters are low, and basal glycaemia is increased[31]. Glucose uptake is normal in basal conditions and during an euglycaemic/hyperinsulinaemic clamp. In contrast, hyperinsulinaemia induces hepatic insulin resistance, characterized by a decreased responsiveness of the liver[31,34]. When these newborns of semistarved mothers are fed normally, they recover very quickly from their growth retardation[35], but at weaning β-cell mass and insulin content are still deficient[32], and at adulthood they show the same decreased insulin responsiveness of the liver[31]. The altered glucose metabolism in these youngsters must thereby be induced by the intrauterine rather than the postnatal environment.

In this experimental model, fetal plasma insulin levels are also very low and do not present a stimulus for the development of the insulin receptor system; nevertheless insulin resistance at adulthood occurs only in the liver, whereas peripheral insulin sensitivity and responsiveness are normal.

OFFSPRING OF PROTEIN-DEFICIENT MOTHERS

When pregnant rats are fed a protein-deficient (8% vs 20% protein content) but isocaloric diet, keeping their levels of glycemia within the normal range, their fetuses are born growth retarded, with a decreased islet size and β-cell proliferation capacity, and with a deficient insulin content and vascularization of the islets of Langerhans[36]. Insulin secretion from these islets after in vitro stimulation with amino acids is impaired[37].

If the mothers, during lactation, and the pups, after weaning, are further kept on this low-protein diet, the adult offspring remain smaller than normal, with low circulating insulin levels and impaired glucose tolerance[37,38]. The vascularization of the pancreas and its blood flow are impaired in these animals[39] and gluconeogenesis from the liver is increased, with hepatic resistance to both glucagon and insulin[38,40].

The damage in these cases must have been induced by the intrauterine environment because recovery on normal feeding after birth restores adult body weight, but does not improve glucose tolerance[41].

From the previously described experimental models, it is clear that alterations, even mild, in maternal metabolism during the last part of gestation induce disturbances in the development of the fetus with lasting consequences for the glucose handling of this offspring throughout life. Alterations in food intake postnatally obviously influence the growth rate of the pups, but do not seem to affect their later glucose tolerance.

The exact mechanisms for this non-genetic transmission of disturbed glucose tolerance are not yet clear, and they are not necessarily the same for each of the described models. The maternally derived changes in fetal plasma composition (glucose, amino acids, fatty acids) certainly influence the development and function of the fetal pancreas, but they might affect other organs and functions as well, in either a direct or an indirect way. High glucose concentrations are known to promote β-cell replication, but the typical β-cell hyperplasia in fetuses of diabetic mothers occur only if the fetus has a functioning hypothalamo-hypophyseal system[42], stressing the involvement of the derived hormones. Moreover, fetal hyperglycaemia induces fetal hyperinsulinaemia, which is known to damage the ventromedial part of the hypothalamus, controlling insulin secretion by modulating the tone on the vagus nerve[15,16]; other body functions might also be affected by similar mechanisms. Fetal hypoinsulinaemia, resulting from β-cell exhaustion or malnutrition, might have an opposite effect; moreover it presents a lack of stimulus for the development of the insulin-receptor system and this effect might differ in the various insulin-sensitive organs depending on whether it is associated with hyper- or hypoglycaemia. It is also evident that the mother's metabolic condition influences the maturation of the fetal gastrointestinal tract[43] and the extent of vascularization, not only in the pancreas but also in other organs, including the brain.

From all this, it must be concluded that the development of the organs and functions associated with fetal glucose metabolism are determined by the intrauterine metabolic environment, and that the nature of this influence is very complex, involving many different aspects and interactions. This applies even more to the long-lasting effects on the offspring in adulthood, and might explain the differences between the various experimental models. Insulin response to glucose stimulation could be deficient or excessive and, insulin-dependent glucose uptake could be normal or decreased. This insulin resistance can be present only in the liver, associated with alterations in glucose handling by the liver, or it can be located principally in the peripheral glucose-consuming tissues, such as the skeletal muscles. The turnover of amino acids can also be involved. The deficiency in vascularization in the different organs could persist into adulthood, and even the blood pressure and heart rate might be affected.

Although, in each of the models described here, glucose tolerance is in some way disturbed, and insulin secretion and/or action altered, not all of the animals spontaneously develop diabetes in normal conditions. In most models, only a diabetologenic tendency is transmitted, which becomes apparent in stimulated situations, such as a glucose tolerance test, glucose infusions, clamps or pregnancy. It should be stressed, however, that laboratory animals are raised in very standardized conditions, and are fed on standard laboratory chow that has a very balanced composition. Their glucose tolerance is hardly challenged throughout their life span.

Several epidemiological studies in humans confirm a similar non-genetic transmission of a diabetogenic tendency, leading to type 2 diabetes in the offspring. In the Pima Indians, a population with a very high incidence of type 2 diabetes, the influence of the intrauterine environment appears to be more important than genetic transmission of the disease. The occurrence of impaired glucose tolerance, gestational diabetes and type 2 diabetes in this population is much higher in the children of mothers who had diabetes during that particular pregnancy, than in children from mothers who developed diabetes only after that pregnancy[44]. A higher incidence of type 2 diabetes is reported in children from diabetic mothers than in those from diabetic fathers[45], and a higher incidence of diabetes is present in offspring from diabetic great-grandmothers via the maternal than via the paternal line[46]. Systematic treatment of diabetic pregnant women drastically decreases the occurrence of diabetes in the offspring[47]. Excessive insulin secretion in fetuses of diabetic mothers, as assessed by amniotic fluid insulin concentrations, can be used as a strong predictor of impaired glucose tolerance in these children[48,49].

In addition, microsomia of the newborn, whether resulting from maternal malnutrition or from a gestational pathology, is strongly associated with metabolic disorders in adulthood. From extensive epidemiological studies that relate birthweight to health condition in adulthood[50–54], small babies appear to be predisposed to the development of impaired glucose tolerance, insulin resistance and increased blood pressure in adult life. The correlation applies, however, only to babies who were small for gestational age and thin for their length – two conditions that are related to poor fetal nutrition. The symptoms at adulthood are worse in those individuals who gain more weight than in those who remain slim. In developing countries, where maternal malnutrition and low birthweight are common, disturbed glucose tolerance and type 2 diabetes often become apparent only when the society becomes Westernized and switches from traditional to high-calorie food[55–58].

The conclusions are that, in the human as in the laboratory animal, an abnormal intrauterine environment during the later part of pregnancy induces alterations in the fetal metabolism, which may lead to lasting consequences for the health of the offspring in later life. The primary symptoms are impaired glucose tolerance and insulin resistance, eventually leading to type 2 diabetes, especially when food intake is excessive.

REFERENCES

1. Aerts L, Van Assche FA. Rat foetal endocrine pancreas in experimental diabetes. *J Endocrinol* 1977; **73**:339–46.
2. Reusens-Billen B, Remacle C, Daniline J, Hoet JJ. Cell proliferation in pancreatic islets of rat fetuses and neonates from normal and diabetic mothers. An in vitro and in vivo study. *Hormone Metab Res* 1984; **16**:565–71.
3. Kervran A, Guillaume M, Jost A. The endocrine pancreas of the fetus from diabetic pregnant rat. *Diabetologia* 1978; **15**:387–93.
4. Bihoreau MT, Ktorza A, Kervran A, Picon L. Effect of gestational hyperglycemia on insulin secretion in vivo and in vitro by fetal rat pancreas. *Am J Physiol* 1986, **251**:E86–91.
5. Leturque A, Revelli JP, Hauguel S, Kande J, Girard J. Hyperglycemia and hyperinsulinemia increase glucose utilisation in fetal rat tissues. *Am J Physiol* 1987; **253**:E616–20.
6. Aerts L, Van Bree R, Feytons V, Rombauts W, Van Assche FA. Plasma amino acids in diabetic pregnant rats and their fetal and adult offspring. *Biol Neonate* 1989; **56**:31–9.
7. Ktorza A, Girard J, Kinebanyan MF, Picon L. Hyperglycaemia induced by glucose infusion in the unrestrained pregnant rat during the last three days of gestation: metabolic and hormonal changes in the mother and the fetuses. *Diabetologia* 1981; **21**:569–74.
8. Mulay S, Solomon S. Influence of streptozotocin-induced diabetes in pregnant rats on plasma corticosterone and progesterone levels and on cytoplasmic glucocorticoid receptors in fetal tissues. *J Endocrinol* 1983; **96**:335–45.
9. Jame P, Ktorza A, Bihoreau MT et al. Impaired hepatic glycogenolysis related to hyperinsulinemia in newborns from hyperglycemic pregnant rats. *Pediatr Res* 1990; **28**:646–651.
10. Aerts L, Van Assche FA. Endocrine pancreas in the offspring of rats with experimentally induced diabetes. *J Endocrinol* 1981; **88**:81–8.
11. Bihoreau MT, Ktorza A, Kinebanyan MF, Picon L. Impaired glucose homeostasis in adult rats from hyperglycemic mothers. *Diabetes* 1986; **35**:979–84.
12. Aerts L, Vercruysse L, Van Assche FA. Morphometric evaluation of the islets of Langerhans in an experimental model of impaired glucose tolerance and gestational diabetes. *Diabetes Res* 1997; in press.
13. Aerts L, Sodoyez-Goffaux F, Sodoyez JC, Malaisse WJ, Van Assche FA. The diabetic intrauterine milieu has a long-lasting effect on insulin secretion by β-

cells and on insulin uptake by target tissues. *Am J Obstet Gynecol* 1988; **159**:1287–92.

14. Gauguier D, Bihoreau MT, Picon L, Ktorza A. Insulin secretion in adult rats after intrauterine exposure to mild hyperglycemia during late gestation. *Diabetes* 1991; **40** (suppl 2): 109–14.
15. Plagemann A, Heidrich I, Gotz F, Rohde W, Dorner G. Lifelong enhanced diabetes susceptibility and obesity after temporary intrahypothalamic hyperinsulinism during brain organisation. *Exp Clin Endocrinol* 1992; **99**:91–5.
16. Plagemann A, Heidrich I, Rohde W, Gotz F, Dorner G. Hyperinsulism during differentiation of the hypothalamus is a diabetogenic and obesity risk factor in rats. *Neuroendocrinol Lett* 1992; **5**:373–8.
17. Aerts L, Holemans K, Van Assche FA. Maternal diabetes during pregnancy: consequences for the offspring. *Diabetes Metab Rev* 1990; **6**:147–67.
18. Aerts L, Van Assche FA. Is gestational diabetes an acquired condition? *J Dev Physiol* 1979; **1**:219–25.
19. Gauguier D, Bihoreau MT, Ktorza A, Berthault MF, Picon L. Inheritance of diabetes mellitus as consequence of gestational hyperglycemia in rats. *Diabetes* 1990; **39**:734–9.
20. Aerts L. Transmission of experimentally induced diabetes in pregnant rats to their offspring in subsequent generations. A morphometric study of maternal and fetal endocrine pancreases at histological and ultrastructural level. In: Shafrir E, Renold AE, eds. *Frontiers in Diabetes Research. Lessons from animal diabetes*. London: John Libbey; 1984: 705–10.
21. Bihoreau MT, Ktorza A, Picon L. Gestational hyperglycaemia and insulin release by the fetal rat pancreas in vitro: effect of amino acids and glyceraldehyde. *Diabetologia* 1986; **29**:434–9.
22. Eriksson U, Andersson A, Efendic S, Elde R, Hellerstrom C. Diabetes in pregnancy: effects on the foetal and newborn rat with particular regard to body weight, serum insulim concentration and pancreatic contents of insulin, glucagen and somatostatin. *Acta Endocrinol* (Copenh) 1980; **94**:354–64.
23. Mulay S, Philip A, Solomon S. Influence of maternal diabetes on fetal rat development: alteration of insulin receptors in fetal liver and lung. *J Endocrinol* 1983; **98**:401–10.
24. Aerts L, Van Assche FA. Morphometric evaluation β-cell function during glucose infusion in control and hyperresponsive rats. *Diabetes Res* 1991; **18**:1–10.
25. Grill V, Johansson B, Jalkanan P, Eriksson UJ. Influence of severe diabetes mellitus early in pregnancy in the rat: effects on insulin sensitivity and insulin secretion in the offspring. *Diabetologia* 1991; **34**:373–8.
26. Holemans K, Aerts L, Van Assche FA. Evidence for an insulin resistance in the adult offspring of pregnant streptozotocin-diabetic rats. *Diabetologia* 1991; **34**:81–5.
27. Ryan EA, Liu D, Bell RC, Finegood DT, Crawford J. Long-term consequences in offspring of diabetes in pregnancy: studies with syngeneic islet-transplanted streptozotocin-diabetic rats. *Endocrinology* 1995; **136**:5587–92.
28. Holemans K, Van Bree R, Verhaeghe J, Aerts L, Van Assche FA. In vivo glucose utilisation by individual tissues in virgin and pregnant offspring of severely diabetic rats. *Diabetes* 1993; **42**:530–6.
29. Holemans K, Aerts L, Van Assche FA. Absence of pregnancy-induced alterations in tissue insulin sensitivity in the offspring of diabetic rats. *J Endocrinol* 1991; **131**:387–93.
30. Aerts L, Van Assche FA. Islet transplantation in diabetic pregnant rats normalises glucose homeostasis in their offspring. *J Dev Physiol* 1992; **17**:283–7.

31. Holemans K, Verhaeghe J, Dequeker J, Van Assche FA. Insulin sensitivity in adult female offspring of rats subjected to malnutrition during the perinatal period. *J Soc Gynecol Invest* 1996; **3**:71–7.
32. Garafano A, Czernikow P, Breant B. *In utero* undernutrition impairs rat beta cell development. *Diabetologia* 1997; **40**:in press.
33. Bréant B, Garafano A, Czernichow P. Late fetal and early post-natal malnutrition impairs rat β-cell development. *Diabetologia* 1997; **40**:A121.
34. Holemans K, Van Bree R, Verhaeghe J, Meurrens K, Van Assche FA. Maternal semistarvation and streptozotocin-diabetes in rats have different effects on the in vivo glucose uptake by peripheral tissues in their female adult offspring. *J Nutr* 1997; **127**:1371–6.
35. Holemans K, Spiessens C, Meurrens K, Van Assche FA. Growth patterns after growth retardation in the rat: effect of pregnancy and lactation. *Am J Obstet Gynecol* 1997; **176**:S128.
36. Snoeck A, Remacle C, Reusens B, Hoet JJ. Effect of a low protein diet during pregnancy on the fetal rat endocrine pancreas. *Biol Neonate* 1990; *57*:107–18.
37. Dahri S, Snoeck A, Reusens-Billen B, Remacle C, Hoet JJ. Islet function in offspring of mothers on low-protein diet during gestation. *Diabetes* 1991; **40** (suppl 2): 115–20.
38. Hales CN. Fetal growth retardation and consequences for insulin secretion and resistance in adult life. *Exp Clin Endocrinol Diabetes* 1997; **105**:A15–16.
39. Iglesias-Barreira V, Ahn MT, Reusens B, Dahri S, Hoet JJ, Remacle C. (1996) Pre- and postnatal low protein diet affect pancreatic islet blood flow and insulin release in adult rats. *Endocrinology* 1996; **137**:3797–801.
40. Hales CN. Fetal nutrition and adult diabetes. *Sci Am Sci Med* 1994; **1**:54–63.
41. Dahri S, Reusens B, Remacle C, Hoet JJ. Nutritional influences on pancreatic development and potential links with non-insulin-dependent diabetes. *Proc Nutr Soc* 1995; **54**:345–56.
42. Van Assche FA. Histological, histochemical and biochemical study of the endocrine pancreas in anencephalics. *Excerpta Medica* 1969; 191.
43. Reusens-Billen B, Remacle C, Hoet JJ. The development of the fetal rat intestine and its reaction to maternal diabetes II. Effect of mild and severe maternal diabetes. *Diabetes Res Clin Pract* 1989; **6**:213–219.
44. Pettitt DJ. Diabetes in subsequent generations. In: Dornhorst A, Hadden DR, eds. *Diabetes and Pregnancy. An international approach to diagnosis and management*, vol. 22. Chichester: John Wiley & Sons, 1996: 367–76.
45. Martin AO, Simpson JL, Ober C, Freinkel N. Frequency of diabetes mellitus in mothers of probands with gestational diabetes: possible maternal influence on the predisposition to gestational diabetes. *Am J Obstet Gynecol* 1985; **151**:471–5.
46. Dorner G, Plagemann A, Reinagel H. Familial diabetes aggregation in type I diabetics: gestational diabetes an apparent risk factor for increased diabetes susceptibility in the offspring. *Exp Clin Endocrinol* 1987; **89**:84–90.
47. Dorner G, Steindel E, Thoelke H. Evidence for decreasing prevalence of diabetes mellitus in childhood apparently produced by prevention of hyperinsulinism in the foetus and newborn. *Exp Clin Endocrinol* 1984; **84**:134–42.
48. Silverman BL, Metzger BE, Cho NH, Loeb C. Impaired glucose tolerance in adolescent offspring of diabetic mothers. Relationship to fetal hyperinsulinism. *Diabetes Care* 1995; **18**:611–17.
49. Zimmet PZ, Collins VR, Dowse GK, Knigh LT. Hyperinsulinemia in youth is a predictor of type 2 (non insulin dependent) diabetes mellitus. *Diabetologia* 1992; **35**:534–91.

50. Baird J, Phillips DIW. Birth weight and adult disease. In: Dornhorst A, Hadden DR, eds. *Diabetes and Pregnancy. An international approach to diagnosis and management*. Chichester: John Wiley & Sons, 1996: **23**:377–89.
51. Lithel HO, McKeigue PM, Berglund L, Mohsen R, Lithell UB, Leon DA. Relation of size at birth to non-insulin dependent diabetes and insulin concentrations in men aged 50–60 years. *BMJ* 1996; **312**:406–10.
52. Phillips DIW, Barker DJ. Low birthweight and glucose intolerance: a role for the sympathetic nervous system? *Diabetologia* 1997; **40**:A43.
53. Wahl MA, Straub SG, Ammon HP. Vasoactive intestinal polypeptide-augmented insulin release: actions on ionic fluxes and electrical activity of mouse islets. *Diabetologia* 1993; **36**:920–5.
54. Shaw JTE. Association of low birth weight with reduced beta-cell function. *Diabetologia* 1997; **40**:A44.
55. Yajnik CF, Fall CHD, Vaidya U. Fetal growth and glucose and insulin metabolism in four-year-old Indian children. *Diabetic Med* 1995; **12**:330–6.
56. Oliveira JE, Milech A, Franco LJ. The prevalence of diabetes in Rio de Janeiro, Brazil. *Diabetes Care* 1992; **15**:1509–16.
57. Gault A, O'Dea K, Rowley KG, McLeay T, Traianedes K. Abnormal glucose tolerance and other coronary heart disease risk factors in an isolated aboriginal community in central Australia. *Diabetes Care* 1996; **19**:1269–73.
58. O'Dea K. Westernization and non-insulin dependent diabetes in Australian Aborigines. *Ethn Dis* 1991; **1**:171–87.

9

Intrauterine Development and its Relationship to Type 2 Diabetes Mellitus

C.J. PETRY AND C.N. HALES

Department of Clinical Biochemistry, Box 232, Addenbrooke's Hospital, Hills Road, Cambridge CB2 2QR, UK

Any hypothesis generated to explain the aetiology of type 2 diabetes mellitus has to be able to address a number of irrefutable facts. The first of these is the tendency for type 2 diabetes to cluster in families[1]. There is also evidence of high concordance rates among identical twins. Although early studies showed concordance rates of 70–85% for type 2 diabetes among twins, these studies have recently been criticized for selection biases[2]. More recent studies, designed to be less affected by such biases, have shown lower rates of concordance (e.g. 16% for dizygotic twins and almost 34% for monozygotic twins in a Finnish study[3]), although the values are still higher than those from the general populations in which these studies were performed[4]. The next factor that has to be addressed is the association of type 2 diabetes with lower socioeconomic status, at least in some 'Westernized' populations[5,6]. An explanation is also required for the finding that there is a higher prevalence of type 2 diabetes in urban rather than rural locations. Thus, in a large multinational study by King and Rewers[4] on behalf of the World Health Organization Ad Hoc Diabetes Reporting Group, this not only applied to migrants who relocated to countries in which they were racial minorities, but was also apparent among Chinese and Indian migrants relocated to Singapore and Mauritius, respectively. Much of this migration would have been from rural to urban locations.

Finally, one of the strongest factors that has to be addressed in any theory regarding the aetiology of type 2 diabetes is the rapid rise in its incidence

Type 2 Diabetes: Prediction and Prevention. Edited by Graham A. Hitman

and prevalence that have taken place this century. Both the lowest and the highest prevalences of type 2 diabetes in the world are in people who have traditionally lived hunter–gatherer or early agricultural lifestyles[4]. Those groups that have continued to live in such circumstances in the 'least developed' communities, such as the indigenous populations of Tanzania and Chile, have a prevalence of diabetes that is less than 3%. In contrast, the highest prevalence of diabetes is found in those people who have switched from traditional ways of life to more sedate 'Westernized' lifestyles. Thus, in Micronesian Nauruans the prevalence of diabetes is around 40%, and in Pima and Papago Indians in Arizona it is closer to 50%[4]. The rapid change in the prevalence of type 2 diabetes in Pima Indians has been dramatic, because it was rare 80 years ago, relatively uncommon 40 years ago and, by the late 1960s, had reached around 40% in subjects aged over 35 years old[7,8]. Further demonstration that the Westernization of people who switch from a more traditional lifestyle leads to an increase in the prevalence of diabetes comes from young Ethiopian Jews who were airlifted to Israel during a time of severe famine[9]. After residing in Israel for 4 years or less, 8.9% of those studied had type 2 diabetes and a further 89% had impaired glucose tolerance (IGT) These rates are likely to be much higher than those in age-matched controls still residing in Ethiopia. Remarkably all the subjects were less than 30 years of age and were lean (at least by Western standards) with body mass indices (BMIs) at the time of the study of less than 27.

The clustering of type 2 diabetes in families and the bimodal distribution of plasma glucose in oral glucose tolerance tests[10] (at least in some populations with a high prevalence of diabetes) have largely been interpreted as suggesting that this form of diabetes is genetic in origin. Fervent searching for 'diabetogenes' resulted in the discovery that defects in the pancreatic glucokinase gene were responsible for the development of maturity-onset diabetes of the young (MODY) in some people[11] – an important but numerically minor subset of people with type 2 diabetes. More recently mutations in genes encoding hepatic nuclear factor-1α (HNF-1α)[12] and hepatic nuclear factor-4α (HNF-4α)[13] have also been shown to cause MODY. Given that this appears to be the only form of diabetes that follows classic Mendelian inheritance (in this case being autosomal dominant) (reviewed by Fajans et al.[14]), and that, even after extensive searching, no single gene responsible for causing diabetes in most people has been discovered to date[15], the genetic mode of inheritance for type 2 diabetes is largely assumed to be polygenic.

In 1962, Neel proposed the 'thrifty genotype hypothesis'[16] in an attempt to explain the rapid changes that have occurred in the prevalence of diabetes this century (these changes have taken place over a time span that is too short for a major change in 'diabetogenes' to occur in the worldwide gene pool). He proposed that, in the early stages of human evolution, a series of genes could have been selected that gave a survival advantage to individuals who underwent cyclic changes in food availability associated with the hunter–gatherer or early agricultural lifestyle. Expression of these genes would result in a 'quick insulin trigger' in response to hyperglycaemia, which would reduce urinary energy loss in times of food scarcity. This would therefore be a survival advantage through the more efficient use of dietary energy. At times when food was readily available, this would allow the efficient storage of dietary energy as fat, and this would be available as an energy store for times when food was more scarce. Neel further proposed that, with the availability of a more constant food supply, these genes, which produced a survival advantage when there was a cyclic availability of food, would become detrimental to health because this quick insulin response would become overstimulated in many people. Ultimately β-cell decompensation would result with the associated development of diabetes. Neel modified his hypothesis 2 decades later to take into account increases in knowledge about the distinction between the major subtypes of diabetes[17]. Neel has now applied it specifically to type 2 diabetes and updated the possible mechanisms behind the detrimental effects of a thrifty genotype to ones that occur as possible consequences of insulin resistance.

INTRAUTERINE GROWTH AND ADULT DISEASE

An alternative explanation for the aetiology of type 2 diabetes and the insulin resistance syndrome, from the genetic-by-environment view of the thrifty genotype hypothesis, is the 'thrifty phenotype hypothesis' suggested by Hales and Barker in 1992[18]. This hypothesis arose to account for the factors described earlier and those from a series of epidemiological studies by Barker, Hales and colleagues, which found associations between markers of fetal and early growth retardation and the subsequent development of adult degenerative diseases. An early observation was made by Forsdahl[19], showing that geographical variations in current death rates from arteriosclerotic heart disease in Norway showed a significant positive relationship with geographical variations in past infant mortality rates (but not with current infant mortality rates). A similar study was performed by Williams et al.[20] who found that, in England and Wales, geographical variations in death rates from ischaemic heart disease (IHD) showed positive correlations with geographical variations in both current and past infant mortality rates. Barker and Osmond[21] then showed that the geographical pattern of mortality from cardiovascular disease in England and Wales resembled the pattern of maternal and neonatal mortality earlier in the century. They found that the distribution was more closely related to neonatal and maternal death rates in the past than to more recent postneonatal death rates[22].

An association was therefore established between poor maternal and neonatal health and subsequent disease many years later. Forsdahl[19] proposed that the link was the result of poverty during adolescence. In contrast, Barker and Osmond[21] suggested that the association was the result of poor nutrition in fetal and early life. To clarify the reason for the association, a population in whom early weight data were available was studied. Barker et al.[23] observed that there were increased death rates from IHD in men with low weights at birth and one year of age, favouring their initial hypothesis. The link between low weights at birth and one year of age and the subsequent development of IHD raised the possibility that early growth retardation could also be associated with the various risk factors for IHD. Other populations in whom both weight and early weight data were available were then studied, especially with regard to these risk factors.

One such factor known to increase the risk of developing IHD is hypertension. Barker et al.[24] found an inverse link in males and females at both 10 and 36 years of age between birthweight and systolic blood pressure. Current weight showed a positive association with systolic blood pressure in both age groups, but the risk was independent from that associated with low birthweight. Thus the highest mean systolic blood pressures in both sexes and in both age groups were found in the groups with the lowest birthweights and the highest current weights. In a follow-up study of 50 year olds born in Preston, England, hypertension was predicted by a combination of low birthweight and high placental weight[25]. It was speculated that discordance between placental and fetal size may lead to circulatory adaptation in the fetus, altered arterial structure in the the child and hypertension in the adult. A number of other studies have now also found links between fetal growth restriction and the subsequent development of hypertension (reviewed by Law[26]).

INTRAUTERINE GROWTH AND TYPE 2 DIABETES

Type 2 diabetes is associated with both IHD and hypertension and insulin deficiency is thought to play a part in its pathogenesis[27]. Fetal and early life are critical periods for pancreatic β-cell development, because about half the adult mass of β-cells is present by one year of age[28]. Studies were therefore performed to investigate whether fetal and early growth are connected to subsequent glucose tolerance. Oral glucose tolerance tests were performed on 64-year-old men from Hertfordshire, England, in whom birthweight details were available[29]. The plasma glucose values 2 hours after the 75 g glucose load were used to categorize the men into those with normal glucose tolerance (<7.8 mmol/l), impaired glucose tolerance (7.8–11.0 mmol/l) or diabetes (>11.0 mmol/l). The proportion of men with either impaired glucose tolerance or diabetes fell progressively as their birthweights increased. This meant that those born the lightest (<2.5 kg or 5.5 lb) were almost seven times more likely to have either impaired glucose tolerance or diabetes at age 64 than those born heaviest (>4.3 kg or 9.5 lb), when odds ratios were adjusted for current BMIs. Similar trends were found when comparing the post-load glucose levels with the men's weights at one year of age. These relationships were independent of social class and held for each level of the BMI.

The mean plasma glucose levels 2 hours after the 75 g glucose load are shown in Table 9.1, with the men categorized into tertiles for both weight at one year of age and current BMI. For each tertile of BMI, the plasma glucose levels fell as the weight at one year of age increased. Also for each tertile of weight at one year of age, there was a rise in plasma glucose as the current BMI of the 64-year-old men increased. The highest glucose values were therefore found in the men who were lightest at one year of age, but who had the highest BMIs when they were 64. This suggests that factors associated with low birthweight at 1 year of age and with high BMI in adult life contribute towards an individual's glucose tolerance.

A similar study was then performed on 50-year-old men and women from Preston, England, for whom more extensive data on measurements at birth were available[30]. As in Hertfordshire, people with either impaired glucose tolerance or diabetes were found to have significantly lower birthweights than those with normal glucose tolerance. They also had smaller head circumferences and were thinner at birth. Their placental to birthweight ratios were higher, which suggests possible maternal undernutrition. The inverse association found in this population between the plasma glucose concentration 2 hours after the glucose load and the birthweights was independent of the duration of gestation. This implies that the low birthweights resulted from reduced fetal growth rather than from any effects of prematurity. However, as the numbers were too small, it was not possible to determine whether prematurity itself might play a role in some individuals.

In both the Hertfordshire[29] and Preston[25,30] cohorts, low birthweight was associated with the development of both glucose intolerance and hypertension, key features of the insulin resistance syndrome[31]. These populations

Table 9.1. Mean plasma glucose 2 hours after 75 g oral glucose load, according to weight at 1 year and adult body mass index (BMI) in Hertfordshire men aged 64

	Weight at 1 year (kg)			
Adult BMI (kg/m^2)	≤9.75	−10.66	>10.66	All
≤25.4	6.6 (45)	6.1 (39)	5.8 (36)	6.2 (120)
−28	6.7 (47)	6.9 (44)	5.9 (36)	6.5 (127)
>28	7.7 (39)	7.4 (43)	6.6 (41)	7.2 (123)
All	7.0 (131	6.8 (126)	6.1 (113)	6.6 (370)

Numbers of men in parentheses.
Reproduced, with permission of the BMJ Publishing Group, from Hales et al.[29]

were therefore studied to investigate whether the insulin resistance syndrome might in some way be associated with fetal growth restriction[32]. Subjects were defined as having the insulin resistance syndrome if they had a 2-hour post-load plasma glucose of more than 7.8 mmol/l, a systolic blood pressure of 160 mmHg or more in Hertfordshire or 150 mmHg or more in the younger population in Preston, and a fasting triglyceride concentration that was equal to or above the median value for that population. In both Hertfordshire and Preston, the prevalence of the insulin resistance syndrome fell progressively from those with the lowest to those with the highest birthweights. When adjusted for the current BMI, the odds ratio for the insulin resistance syndrome in the Hertfordshire men whose birthweights were 2.50 kg or less, in comparison to those born weighing more than 4.31 kg, was 18. In Preston, where women were included in the study and the highest birthweight category was more than 3.41 kg, the equivalent odds ratio was almost 14. The association with low birthweight was found to be independent of duration of gestation, smoking history, alcohol consumption and social class, either currently or at birth.

Since these initial studies, at least 13 other studies have shown links between poor fetal and early growth and either loss of glucose tolerance or markers of insulin resistance (Table 9.2). In Pima Indians the prevalence of type 2 diabetes was greatest in those subjects with the lowest and those with the highest birthweights[35]. The link between high birthweight and the

Table 9.2. Studies showing a link between fetal and early growth restriction and either subsequent loss of glucose tolerance or markers of insulin resistance

Population	Country	Reference
Hertfordshire men	UK	Hales et al.[29]
Salisbury young men	UK	Robinson et al.[33]
Preston men and women	UK	Phipps et al.[30]
		Barker et al.[32]
		Phillips et al.[34]
Pima Indian men and women	USA	McCance et al.[35]
Mexican–Americans and non-Hispanic whites	USA	Valdez et al.[36]
Salisbury children	UK	Law et al.[37]
Pune young children	India	Yajnik et al.[38]
Swedish men		Lithell et al.[39]
Jamaican school children		Forrester et al.[40]
Pregnant women	UK	Olah[41]
American men		Curham et al.[42]
Australian Aboriginies		Hoy et al.[43]
British children		Whincup et al.[44]
Danish twins		Pousen et al.[45]

development of type 2 diabetes has not been found in other populations studied to date and is presumably the result of macrosomic babies of mothers with gestational diabetes (a common condition in Pima Indians[35]) who subsequently develop type 2 diabetes. In the San Antonio Heart Study[36], 562 subjects were split into tertiles for both birthweight and current BMI. The prevalence of the insulin resistance syndrome fell with increasing birthweight in each of the BMI tertiles and with rising current BMIs in each of the birthweight tertiles. None of the 61 subjects with the highest birthweights and the lowest BMIs was classified as having the insulin resistance syndrome. This contrasts with 25 of 64 subjects having the insulin resistance syndrome in the category containing those people with the lowest birthweights and the highest current BMIs. The authors stated that for each tertile decrease in birthweight (a decrease of 535 g on average) the odds of developing conditions related to insulin resistance increased by 72%[36].

Poulsen et al[45] studied mono- and dizygotic twins in Denmark who were disconcordant for type 2 diabetes. They found that, in both mono- and dizygotic twins, birthweights were considerably lower in the diabetic twins in comparison to their non-diabetic siblings. As monozygotic twins share the same genetic make-up, the mechanism of the link between low birthweights and the development of type 2 diabetes was purely environmental. Although this study does not disprove any role that genetics may play in changing the susceptibility of an individual to type 2 diabetes it does show that the link with birthweight can occur independently of a genetic influence.

It is important to consider, but hard to calculate, what proportion of type 2 diabetes might be the result of early growth retardation. One view[35] is that, as only a small proportion of birthweights in Western populations are low, the amount of type 2 diabetes for which it accounts will also be low. We believe that this is a misinterpretation of data. Birthweight alone is a very crude index of successful fetal growth and development. It is also clear that there is a continuous relationship rather than a threshold between birthweight and risk thus 3.2-kg babies are at a greater risk than 4.0-kg babies in the Hertfordshire studies[29,32]. In populations in which the data are adequate for making the calculation, thinness at birth provides a better estimate of risk than weight alone[34]. Another way to look at what proportion of type 2 diabetes or the insulin resistance syndrome could be the result of poor early growth is to examine the prevalence of these conditions in those infants with the best early growth. Put another way, what would their occurrence be if all infants could be induced to undergo optimal early growth. Examined in this way one can see the potential for a very large reduction in type 2 diabetes or insulin resistance[29,32,36], suggesting that whatever explains the link between early growth retardation and adult glucose intolerance is a major factor.

THE THRIFTY PHENOTYPE HYPOTHESIS

An attempt to explain these various associations has been made with the thrifty phenotype hypothesis, described by Hales and Barker in 1992[18] (shown schematically in Figure 9.1). Central to this hypothesis is that the predisposition to type 2 diabetes and the other conditions that cluster as the insulin resistance syndrome occurs through adaptations to malnutrition by a developing fetus. Low birthweight is a proxy for a variety of intrauterine influences (Figure 9.1), but worldwide it is probably predominantly caused by maternal malnutrition. Maternal malnutrition may be (or may have been) especially prevalent in the populations that have undergone rapid transitions during the twentieth century from traditional to more Western lifestyles and in which prevalences of type 2 diabetes are now extremely high[4].

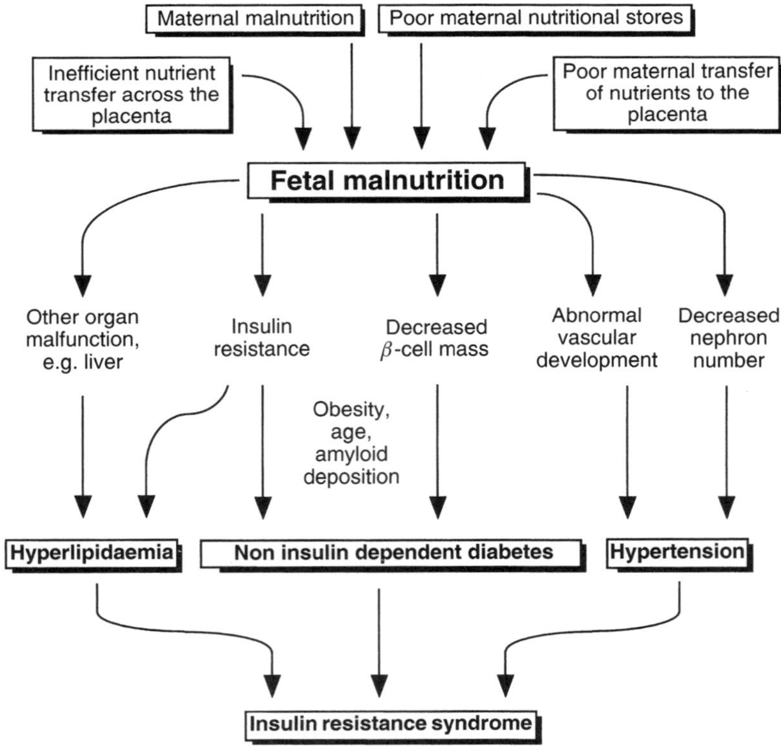

Figure 9.1. Diagrammatic representation of key features of the thrifty phenotype hypothesis: *shown* is the central role of fetal malnutrition in the development of type 2 diabetes and the insulin resistance syndrome. (Adapted with permission of Springer-Verlag GmbH & Co. KG, from Hales and Barker[18].)

Thus, the fetus would adapt its growth and metabolism to the expectation of poor availability of nutrition postnatally. This could have survival advantages both for the present, in terms of targeting available nutrients to more essential organs such as the brain, and for the future, in terms of being more able to store energy as fat to provide energy reserves for use when food is scarce. These adaptations would provide survival advantages whenever there was a constant, relatively poor nutrition or cyclic availability of adequate nutrition. If there was a constant supply of good nutrition, however, the adaptations could become detrimental to health with the possible development of type 2 diabetes and the insulin resistance syndrome.

The factors that change the adaptations made by the malnourished fetus from those conferring survival advantages to those detrimental to health are perceived as being the development of obesity, ageing and a sedentary lifestyle[18]. Clearly the development of type 2 diabetes occurs most commonly in obese individuals who are in their 40s and 50s or older[4]. In the Hertfordshire cohort, those men with newly diagnosed type 2 diabetes or impaired glucose tolerance, in addition to having lower birthweights and higher blood pressure, had higher current BMIs[29]. Also analysis of the men from the cohorts in both Preston and Hertfordshire showed that the current waist:hip ratios fell progressively with increasing birthweights (independently of current BMIs), suggesting that fetally malnourished babies have a greater tendency to store abdominal fat in later life[46]. This would be consistent with the idea that one of the adaptations made by the malnourished fetus allows metabolism to be altered such that fat storage is favoured. The thrifty phenotype hypothesis suggests that the occurrence and timing of onset of the different conditions associated with the insulin resistance syndrome would depend on the exact timing of growth impairment during fetal or possibly during infant life[18]. Clearly the development of obesity, whether or not it arose as a result of having a 'thrifty' metabolism, could interact with the effects of fetal growth restriction to hasten the occurrence of such conditions.

A number of possible mechanisms through which a thrifty phenotype could operate have been suggested. The first of these is a deficiency of pancreatic β-cell function. In the study of Hertfordshire men, plasma concentrations of 32,33-split-proinsulin fell sharply with an increase in weight at one year (and showed a tendency to fall with an increase in birthweight)[29], possibly reflecting a deficit of β-cells. A deficit of insulin production may be associated with fetal growth restriction because insulin is essential for early growth and development[47] and small-for-dates babies have reduced numbers of pancreatic β-cells[48]. A deficit of insulin production in individuals who were growth restricted *in utero* has not currently been demonstrated[48], presumably as a result of difficulties in controlling adequately for degrees of insulin resistance. However, any deficit of β-cell function, perhaps combined with an associated insulin resistance, would obviously render an individual more susceptible in later life to the development of type 2 diabetes.

Effects of the thrifty phenotype could also be mediated through insulin resistance[18], especially with regard to the development of the insulin resistance syndrome. Phillips et al.[34] tested some of the Preston cohort with either normal or impaired glucose tolerance for their insulin sensitivity. They found that babies who were thinner at birth became more insulin resistant in adult life. These results were strengthened by results from a study in which 50-year-old men in Sweden were given intravenous glucose tolerance tests[39]. After adjustment for current BMIs, birthweight was shown to be inversely related to both fasting and 60-minute plasma insulin concentrations post-glucose load. These results suggest that adult insulin sensitivity, at least in part, may be determined *in utero*.

Other effects of thrifty phenotype may be mediated through alterations in vasculature[18]. Animal studies have shown that maternal protein restriction during pregnancy can dramatically reduce pancreatic islet vascularization in the offspring[50]. If these changes reflect more widespread reductions, insulin resistance could result given that it has been shown to be associated with a lower density of capillaries in skeletal muscle[51]. A less compliant vasculature could be more resistant to blood flow and therefore contribute towards the development of hypertension[52]. The advantage to the developing fetus of such an altered vasculature could be the targeting of blood flow to essential organs such as the brain, at the expense of other organs. Indeed blood flow to the brain has been shown to be increased in small-for-dates fetuses[53].

Alterations in organ structure and function may also cause some of the effects associated with a thrifty phenotype. Changes in kidney structure, with low birthweight being associated with a reduced nephron endowment, has been suggested as a cause of the hypertension seen in individuals with early growth retardation[54]. Further, it has been suggested that, when kidney growth lags behind somatic growth, sodium retention is favoured, predisposing an individual to hypertension[55].

MATERNAL LOW-PROTEIN RAT MODEL

In the thrifty phenotype hypothesis[18] and in a recent review describing progress in this area since the hypothesis was put forward[15], attention was drawn to how poor maternal protein intake may be a possible factor in the development of a thrifty phenotype in the offspring. Protein restriction was chosen because of the many previous studies in humans and animals that have shown that it lends to detrimental effects on insulin secretion and glucose homeostasis[18]. Also, protein is generally a relatively scarce and expensive foodstuff for many populations and for deprived communities within affluent societies[15]. Although other nutritional deficiencies in pregnancy are in no way excluded as mediators of the establishment of a thrifty phenotype in the offspring, our studies to test and model the thrifty phenotype in the rat have focused on feeding rats a diet that contains a reduced amount of protein throughout pregnancy and lactation.

Snoeck et al.[50] noted that feeding a rat a low-protein diet during pregnancy caused growth restriction in the pups. These pups had reduced pancreatic β-cell proliferation, islet size and islet vascularization. In our studies, we used the same low-protein diet (containing 8% protein) and fed it to rats during pregnancy and lactation. Offspring from these rats were compared with offspring from rats fed an isocaloric diet containing 20% protein, after both groups of offspring were weaned onto a standard laboratory chow. By 3 months of age, the low-protein offspring had a reduced insulin-inhibitory effect on glucagon-stimulated gluconeogenesis, increased numbers of hepatic insulin receptors (and decreased glucagon receptors) and increased levels of the glucose transporter GLUT2 in the liver[56]. In skeletal muscle, low-protein offspring had raised levels of GLUT4 in plasma membranes, which appeared not to rise with insulin stimulation[57]. They also had double the number of insulin receptors in the muscle membranes compared with controls. Adipocytes from low-protein offspring had significantly higher basal and insulin-stimulated glucose uptakes than controls, along with increased numbers of insulin receptors[58]. They also showed changes in expression of insulin-signalling components. All these results are consistent with an adaptation of metabolism caused by the maternal protein restriction. At 3 months of age and less, the low-protein offspring were more glucose tolerant than controls[59,60]. However, the glucose tolerance of the low-protein offspring deteriorated more rapidly than that of the controls, so that by 15 months of age they were more glucose intolerant.

More recently, the effect of obesity on previously protein-restricted rats has been investigated. Rats were severely growth retarded by extending the protein restriction from purely maternal to include the time from when the pups were weaned to when they were 70 days old. They then became obese by eating a highly palatable cafeteria-style diet. By one year of age the maternal and early protein restrictions were shown to be associated with the development of hypertension[61] (Figure 9.2a) (an effect that was previously shown using a similar low-protein diet during pregnancy alone[62]). The obese cafeteria-fed rats were also hypertensive, and the effects of early protein restriction and obesity were shown to be independent and additive, so that the highest blood pressures were seen in rats that were obese and had been protein restricted in early life. This reflects the human situation where low birthweight and high current weight have been shown to be associated independently with raised blood pressures[24]. At this age the obese rats had worse glucose tolerances than non-obese, chow-fed rats independent of whether they had been previously protein restricted[61] (Figure 9.2b). The maternal and early protein restrictions were not associated with a detectable alteration in glucose tolerance. By 16 months of age, however, there was a relative deterioration in the glucose tolerance of the low-protein rats

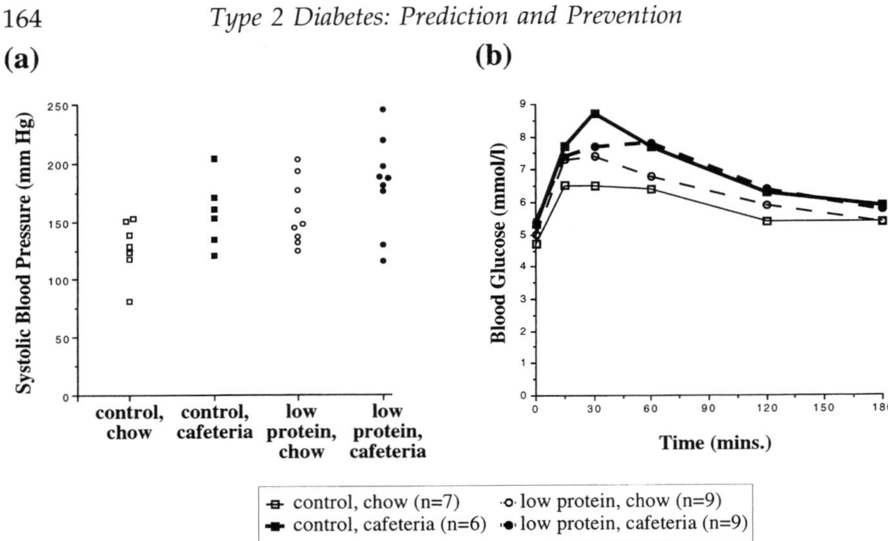

Figure 9.2. (a) Systolic blood pressures and (b) intraperitoneal glucose tolerance tests of 1-year-old female rats[61]. The mothers of low protein rats had been fed a diet containing 8% protein throughout pregnancy and lactation. The low-protein rats were weaned onto this diet and fed until they were 70 days old. Equivalent control rats were fed a 20% protein diet. From 70 days of age, the rats were fed either a standard chow or a highly palatable cafeteria-style diet to make them obese. (Reproduced with permission of the Biochemical Society and the Medical Research Society, from Petry et al.[61].)

(Table 9.3). The obese rats still had worse glucose tolerances overall than those that were non-obese, independent of whether or not they had previously been protein restricted. In contrast, in the non-obese rats, although there was an improvement in glucose tolerance in the controls, the previously protein-restricted rats showed a deterioration such that in comparison they were glucose intolerant. Thus, in this study both the early growth restriction and the subsequent obesity were shown to have detrimental effects on both

Table 9.3. The deterioration in glucose tolerance of rats between 12 and 16 months of age.

	Adult diet	
	Chow	Cafeteria
Control	−468 (616)	−216 (600)
Low protein	82 (469)	−18 (522)

Results are shown as mean (SD) of area under the glucose tolerance curve units. Note: a negative value denotes an improvement in glucose tolerance. Two-way analysis of variance: relative deterioration in early protein-restricted rats ($p = 0.014$), relative deterioration in cafeteria-fed rats ($p = 0.603$), interaction ($p = 0.236$).

glucose tolerance and blood pressure. These results are entirely consistent with the thrifty phenotype hypothesis[18] and suggest that the maternal low-protein rat is a suitable model for investigating the mechanisms involved in its evolution.

CONCLUSIONS

There is now substantial evidence that growth restriction *in utero* and possibly in early infancy, is associated with an increased risk of developing type 2 diabetes and other features of the insulin resistance syndrome. This risk can occur independently of any genetic influence. Animal studies suggest that fetal nutrition plays a causative role in this process and that influences in adult life can modify that risk. At a recent symposium addressing this subject[63] a call was made to an international audience to start a study in a developing country in which pregnant women could be freely given adequate nutrition to see whether the burden of type 2 diabetes could be reduced in their offspring. Although this has immense cost implications, faced with a future type 2 diabetes edpidemic[64] the benefits to health are likely to be enormous.

REFERENCES

1. Pierce M, Keen H, Bradley C. Risk of diabetes in offspring of parents with non-insulin-dependent diabetes. *Diabetic Med* 1993; **12**:6–13.
2. Hawkes CH. Twin studies in diabetes mellitus. *Diabetic Med* 1997; **14**:347–52.
3. Kaprio J, Tuomilehto J, Koskenvuo M et al. Concordance for type 1 (insulin dependent) and type 2 (non insulin dependent) diabetes in a population-based cohort of twins in Finland. *Diabetologia* 1992; **35**:1060–7.
4. King H, Rewers M, World Health Organisation Ad Hoc Diabetes Reporting Group. Global estimates for prevalence of diabetes mellitus and impaired glucose tolerance in adults. *Diabetes Care* 1993; **16**:157–77.
5. Barker DJP, Gardner MJ, Power C. Incidence of diabetes amongst people aged 18–50 years in nine British towns: a collaborative study. *Diabetologia* 1982; **22**:421–5.
6. Stern MP, Rosenthal M, Haffner SM, Hazuda HP, Franco LJ. Sex difference in the effects of sociocultural status on diabetes and cardiovascular risk factors in Mexican Americans. The San Antonio Heart Study. *Am J Epidemiol* 1984; **120**:834–51.
7. Bennett PH, Burch TA, Miller M. Diabetes mellitus in American (Pima) Indians. *Lancet* 1971; **ii**:125–8.
8. West KM. Diabetes in American Indians and other native populations of the new world. *Diabetes* 1974; **23**:841–55.
9. Cohen MP, Stern E, Rusecki Y, Zeidler A. High prevalence of diabetes in young Ethiopian immigrants to Israel. *Diabetes* 1988; **37**:824–8.

10. Zimmet P, Whitehouse S. Bimodality of fasting and two-hour glucose tolerance distributions in a Micronesian population. *Diabetes* 1978; **27**:793–800.
11. Vionnet N, Stoffel M, Takeda J et al. Nonsense mutation in the glucokinase gene causes early-onset non-insulin-dependent diabetes mellitus. *Nature* 1992; **356**:721–2.
12. Yamagata K, Oda N, Kaisaki PJ et al. Mutations in the hepatocyte nuclear factor-1 alpha gene in maturity-onset diabetes of the young (MODY3). *Nature* 1996; **384**:455–8.
13. Yamagata K, Furuta H, Oda N et al. Mutations in the hepatocyte nuclear factor-4 alpha gene in maturity-onset diabetes of the young (MODY1). *Nature* 1996; **384**:458–60.
14. Fajans SS, Bell GI, Bowden DW, Halter JB, Polonsky KS. Maturity-onset diabetes of the young. *Life Sci* 1994; **55**:413–22.
15. Hales CN, Desai M, Ozanne SE. The thrifty phenotype hypothesis: how does it look after 5 years? *Diabetic Med* 1997; **14**:189–95.
16. Neel JV. Diabetes mellitus: a 'thrifty' genotype rendered detrimental by 'progress'? *Am J Hum Genet* 1962; **14**:353–62.
17. Neel JV. The thrifty genotype revisited. In: Köbberling J, Tattersall R, eds. *The Genetics of Diabetes Mellitus*, Serono Symposium No 47. London: Academic Press, 1982: 283–93.
18. Hales CN, Barker DJP. Type 2 (non-insulin-dependent) diabetes mellitus: the thrifty phenotype hypothesis. *Diabetologia* 1992; **35**:595–601.
19. Forsdahl A. Are poor living conditions in childhood and adolescence an important risk factor for arteriosclerotic heart disease? *Br J Prev Soc Med* 1977; **31**:91–5.
20. Wiliams DRR, Roberts SJ, Davies TW. Deaths from ischaemic heart disease and infant mortality in England and Wales. *J Epidemiol Community Health* 1979; **33**:199–202.
21. Barker DJ, Osmond C. Infant mortality, childhood nutrition, and ischaemic heart disease in England and Wales. *Lancet* 1986; **i**:1077–81.
22. Barker DJP, Osmond C. Death rates from stroke in England and Wales predicted from past maternal mortality. *BMJ* 1987; **295**:83–6.
23. Barker DJ, Winter PD, Osmond C, Margetts B, Simmonds SJ. Weight in infancy and death from ischaemic heart disease. *Lancet* 1989; **ii**:577–80.
24. Barker DJP, Osmond C, Golding J, Kuh D, Wadsworth MEJ. Growth in utero, blood pressure in childhood and adult life, and mortality from cardiovascular disease. *BMJ* 1989; **298**:654–7.
25. Barker DJP, Bull AR, Osmond C, Simmonds SJ. Fetal and placental size and risk of hypertension in adult life. *BMJ* 1990; **301**:259–62.
26. Law, C. Fetal origins of adult hypertension. *J Hum Hypertens* 1995; **9**:649–51.
27. Cerasi E, Kaiser N, Gross DJ. From sand rats to diabetic patients: is non-insulin-dependent diabetes mellitus a disease of the beta cell? *Diabetes Metab.* 1997; **23** (Suppl 2): 47–51.
28. Rahier J, Wallon J, Henquin JC. Cell populations in the endocrine pancreas of human neonates and infants. *Diabetologia* 1981: **20**:540–6.
29. Hales CN, Barker DJP, Clark PMS et al. Fetal and infant growth and impaired glucose tolerance at age 64. *BMJ* 1991; **303**:1019–22.
30. Phipps K, Barker DJP, Hales CN, Fall CHD, Osmond C, Clark PMS. Fetal growth and impaired glucose tolerance in men and women. *Diabetologia* 1993; **36**:225–8.
31. Reaven G. Role of insulin resistance in human disease. *Diabetes* 1988; **37**: 1595–607.

32. Barker DJP, Hales CN, Fall CHD, Osmond C, Phipps K, Clark PMS. Type 2 (non-insulin-dependent) diabetes mellitus, hypertension and hyperlipidaemia (syndrome x): relation to reduced fetal growth. *Diabetologia* 1993; **36**:62–7.
33. Robinson S, Walton RJ, Clark PMS, Barker DJP, Hales CN, Osmond C. The relation of fetal growth to plasma glucose in young men. *Diabetologia* 1992; **35**:444–6.
34. Phillips DIW, Barker DJP, Hales CN, Hirst S, Osmond C. Thinness at birth and insulin resistance in adult life. *Diabetologia* 1994; **37**:150–4.
35. McCance DR, Pettitt D, Hanson RL, Jacobsson LTH, Knowler WC, Bennett PH. Birth weight and non-insulin dependent diabetes: thrifty genotype, thrifty phenotype, or surviving small baby genotype? *BMJ* 1994; **308**:942–5.
36. Valdez R, Athens MA, Thompson GH, Bradshaw BS, Stern MP. Birthweight and adult health outcomes in a biethnic population in the USA. *Diabetologia* 1994; **37**:624–31.
37. Law CM, Gordon GS, Shiell AW, Barker DJP, Hales CN. Thinness at birth and glucose tolerance in seven-year-old children. *Diabetic Med* 1995; **12**:24–9.
38. Yajnik CS, Fall CHD, Vaidya U et al. Fetal growth and glucose and insulin metabolism in four-year-old Indian children. *Diabetic Med* 1995; **12**:330–6.
39. Lithell HO, McKeigue PM, Berglund L, Mohsen R, Lithell U-B, Leon DA. Relation of size at birth to non-insulin dependent diabetes and insulin concentrations in men aged 50–60 years. 1996; **312**:406–10.
40. Forrester TE, Wilks RJ, Bennett FI et al. Fetal growth and cardiovascular risk factors in Jamaican school children. *BMJ* 1996; **312**:156–60.
41. Olah KS. Low maternal birth weight – an association with impaired glucose tolerance in pregnancy. *J Obstet Gynaecol* 1996; **16**:5–8.
42. Curhan GC, Willett WC, Rimm EB, Spiegelman D, Ascherio AL, Stampfer MJ. Birth weight and adult hypertension, diabetes mellitus, and obesity in US men. *Circulation* 1996; **94**:3246–50.
43. Hoy W, Kyle E, Rees M et al. Birth weight, adult weight and insulin levels: associations in an Australian Aboriginal (AA) community. *Communication to the First World Congress on Prevention of Diabetes and its Complications*. Lejngby, Denmark April 1996.
44. Whincup PH, Cook DG, Adshead F et al. Childhood size is more strongly related than size at birth to glucose and insulin levels in 10–11-year-old children. *Diabetologia* 1997; **40**:319–26.
45. Poulsen P, Vaag AA, Kyvik KO, Møller Jensen D, Beck-Nielsen H. Low birth weight is associated with NIDDM in disconcordant monozygotic and dizygotic twin pairs *Diabetologia* 1997: **40**:439–46.
46. Law CM, Barker DJ, Osmond C, Fall CH, Simmonds SJ. Early growth and abdominal fatness in adult life. *J Epidemiol Community Health* 1992; **46**:184–6.
47. Fowden AL. The role of insulin in prenatal growth. *J Dev Physiol* 1989; **12**: 173–82.
48. Van Assche FA, Aerts L. The fetal endocrine pancreas. *Contrib Gynecol Obstet* 1979; **5**:44–57.
49. Phillips DIW, Hirst S, Clark PMS, Hales CN, Osmond C. Fetal growth and insulin secretion in adult life. *Diabetologia* 1994: **37**:592–6.
50. Snoeck A, Remacle C, Reusens B, Hoet JJ. Effect of a low protein diet during pregnancy on the fetal rat endocrine pancreas. *Biol Neonate* 1990; **57**:107–18.
51. Lillioja S, Young AA, Culter CL et al. Skeletal muscle capillary density and fiber type are possible determinants of in vivo insulin resistance in man. *J Clin Invest* 1987; **80**:415–24.

52. Martyn CN, Barker DJ, Jespersen S, Greenwald S, Osmond C, Berry C. Growth in utero, adult blood pressure and arterial compliance. *Br Heart J* 1995; **72**: 116–21.
53. Al-Ghazali W, Chita S, Chapman MG, Allan LD. Evidence of redistribution of cardiac output in asymmetrical growth retardation. *Br J Obstet Gynaecol* 1989; **96**:697–704.
54. MacKenzie HS, Brenner BM. Fewer nephrons at birth: a missing link in the etiology of essential hypertension? *Am J Kidney Dis* 1995: **26**:91–8.
55. Weder AB, Schork NJ. Adaptation, allometry, and hypertension. *Hypertension* 1994: **24**:145–56.
56. Ozanne SE, Smith GD, Tikerpae J, Hales CN. Altered regulation of hepatic glucose output in the male offspring of protein-malnourished rat dams *Am J Physiol* 1996; **270** (Endocrinol Metab 33):E559–64.
57. Ozanne SE, Wang CL, Coleman N, Smith GD. Altered muscle insulin sensitivity in the male offspring of protein-malnourished rats. *Am J Physiol* 1996; **271** (Endocrinol Metal 34): E1128–34.
58. Ozanne SE, Nave BT, Wang CL, Shephard PR, Prins J, Smith GD. Poor fetal nutrition causes long-term changes in expression of insulin signaling components in adipocytes. *Am J Physiol* 1997; **273** (Endocrinol Metab 36):E46–51.
59. Hales CN, Desai M, Ozanne SE, Crowther NJ. Fishing in the stream of diabetes: from measuring insulin to the control of fetal organogenesis. *Biochem Soc Trans* 1996; **24**:341–50.
60. Shepherd PR, Crowther NJ, Desai M, Hales CN, Ozanne SE. Altered adipocyte properties in the offspring of protein malnourished rats. *Br J Nutr* 1997; **78**:121–9.
61. Petry CJ, Ozanne SE, Wang CL, Hales CN. Early protein restriction and obesity independently induce hypertension in 1-year-old rats. *Clin Sci* 1997; **93**:147–52.
62. Langley SC, Jackson AA. Increased systolic blood pressure in adult rats induced by fetal exposure to low protein diets. *Clin Sci* 1994; **86**:217–22.
63. Hales CN. The thrifty phenotype hypothesis. 16th International Diabetes Federation Congress, 20–25 July 1997, Helsinki. Abstracts for the state-of-the-art lectures and symposia: 47.
64. Zimmet P, McCarty D. The NIDDM epidemic: global estimates and projections – a look into the crystal ball. *IDF Bull* 1995; **40**:8–16.

10

Lessons from Gestational Diabetes

M.R. DRUCE AND A. DORNHORST

Department of Metabolic Medicine, Imperial College School of Medicine, Hammersmith Hospital, London W12 0NN, UK

This chapter addresses the lessons that can be learned from the study of gestational diabetes mellitus (GDM) that are relevant to the prediction and prevention of type 2 diabetes. To be able to undertake this exercise one needs to be able to define GDM and to describe its metabolic phenotype.

Gestational diabetes mellitus is currently defined as glucose intolerance first recognized in pregnancy[1]. This definition includes mothers with previously undiagnosed diabetes or impaired glucose tolerance (IGT) that was first recognized in pregnancy. Post partum it is inevitable that glucose intolerance that pre-dates pregnancy persists, although it is usual for it to abate when it has arisen *de novo* in pregnancy.

The World Health Organization (WHO) have attempted to subclassify glucose intolerance recognized in pregnancy into two categories, namely, true GDM for pregnant women who fulfil the non-pregnant WHO criteria for diabetes, and a lesser category of gestational impaired glucose tolerance (GIGT) for women who fulfil the non-pregnant criteria for impaired glucose tolerance[2]. The underlying assumption is that GDM represents unrecognized pre-existing IGT or diabetes, whereas GIGT is temporally related to the pregnancy. This subclassification of glucose intolerance in pregnancy has not been widely accepted because of the ambiguity surrounding the validity of the WHO diagnostic criteria, as discussed below.

Type 2 Diabetes: Prediction and Prevention. Edited by Graham A. Hitman

THE HETEROGENEITY OF GDM

The first lesson to be learned from the study of GDM, as with diabetes outside pregnancy, is that it is a heterogeneous group of disorders[3]. Women with GDM include those with unrecognized type 2 diabetes, IGT and early type 1 diabetes, in addition to those with pregnancy-induced glucose intolerance[4]. After pregnancy this last group is itself heterogeneous[5–7]. Although most women have metabolic abnormalities that predict type 2 diabetes, a minority (about 5%) have immunological markers that predict type 1 diabetes[7–9] and some have genetic conditions (<2%) associated with maturity-onset diabetes of the young (MODY)[10] or other monogenetic forms of diabetes[11].

ESTABLISHING DIAGNOSTIC CRITERIA

Universally accepted diagnostic criteria for GDM are required if comparisons are to be made between and within different populations. They also need to define the population at clinical risk. Established diabetes is associated with an increased pregnancy risk, including congenital abnormalities, abortions, accelerated fetal growth and unexplained stillbirth, in addition to obesity and diabetes in the child[12–16]. At what level of maternal hyperglycaemia these adverse outcomes are increased is unknown. The controversy surrounding the diagnosis of GDM is focused on precise definition of the level of maternal hyperglycaemia that is associated with no added risk to pregnancy outcome, whether to the fetus or the mother[17,18].

The original WHO diagnosis of diabetes was based on the plasma glucose after fasting and 120 minutes after 75 g oral glucose tolerance test (OGTT), which is associated with microvascular disease, namely retinopathy and nephropathy[19]. However, these outcomes are pathognomonic for diabetes. In contrast, the pregnancy outcomes associated with GDM are non-specific. In addition, the fetal outcomes studied are influenced by external factors, including the availability and provision of obstetric health care.

To date, the criteria for GDM have used adverse pregnancy outcome measures (either maternal or fetal) or have been statistically derived[12]. Original studies in Boston in the late 1950s by O'Sullivan led to the present-day American criteria for GDM[20]. These were established using a 3-hour 100-g OGTT with the outcome measure being the future risk of maternal diabetes. It was recommended that this diagnostic test be performed on women after an initial positive screening test. Other diagnostic criteria have used different glucose loads and different pregnancy outcome measures. In the 1960s, criteria based on the 50-g OGTT were validated using neonatal hypoglycaemia and hyperinsulinaemia[21]. These criteria are no longer used, but remain the only criteria derived using a specific glycaemia-related fetal endpoint.

In the late 1970s a European study group applied a purely statistical approach to the diagnosis of GDM[22]. In 11 European cities over 1000 unselected pregnant women underwent a 75-g OGTT. By the second trimester, about 10% of the women had IGT by WHO non-pregnant criteria. As this figure was considered to be too high, the diagnostic limits were set at the 95th percentile values of plasma glucose for 0, 60 and 120 minutes. This ensured that around 5% of a European population would have a diagnosis of GDM. The statistically derived glucose values were all higher than others in use for the diagnosis of GDM (Table 10.1).

The application of the WHO non-pregnant criteria for the diagnosis of glucose intolerance in pregnancy remains a pragmatic solution. The use of the 75-g OGTT ensures a universal diagnostic test that is applicable both during and after pregnancy. However, this ignores the normal metabolic adaptation of pregnancy[23] (Table 10.2). The exact fasting and post-prandial plasma glucose levels used to define glucose intolerance in pregnancy can, if necessary, be adjusted up or down in the future, in the light of epidemiological data[24]. For example, the recent diagnostic criteria for diabetes and IGT recommended by the American Diabetic Association have been amended in this way, placing greater emphasis on the fasting values[3]. These new recommendation are expected to be endorsed in the near future by the WHO.

SIMILARITIES BETWEEN GDM AND IGT

The next lesson to be learned from the study of GDM is from its similarities with IGT. Both represent the grey area between normal and frankly diabetic. The term 'impaired glucose tolerances' was introduced by the WHO in recognition of the distribution frequency of the 120-minute OGTT plasma glucose within the normal population, which was invariably skewed to the right. Only later was this population shown to be at increased risk of future diabetes and macrovascular disease[25,26]. Neither the diagnosis for IGT nor that for GDM on a standardized OGTT is reproducible. Up to 50% of non-gravid subjects diagnosed as having IGT have a normal glucose tolerance test on subsequent testing[27,28]. The progression of IGT to diabetes is a function of the degree of hyperglycaemia and the relative degree of insulinopenia.

The above scenario is similar to GDM, where the recurrence rate for GDM in subsequent pregnancies is between 30% and 50%[29]. The likelihood of a recurrence increases with the degree of glucose intolerance. Gestational diabetes in one, but not a subsequent pregnancy has a significantly lower risk of future diabetes than if it does recur – 3% vs 30% over 16 years in one

Table 10.1. Different diagnostic criteria for gestational diabetes based on the oral glucose tolerance test

Diagnostic criteria	Glucose load (g)	Fasting plasma glucose (mmol/l)	60-min plasma glucose (mmol/l)	120-min plasma glucose (mmol/l)	180-min plasma glucose (mmol/l)
American Diabetic Association[a]	100	≥ 5.8	≥ 10.6	≥ 9.2	≥ 8.1
World Health Organization GDM[b]	75	≥ 7.8	–	≥ 11.1	–
World Health Organization Gestational IGT[c]	75	≤ 7.8	–	≥ 7.8 < 11.0	–
Diabetic Pregnancy Study Group–European Association for the Study of Diabetes[d]	75	–	≥ 10.5	≥ 9.0	–

[a]Diagnosis of gestational diabetes dependent on two or more values being exceeded[1].
[b]Diagnosis of gestational diabetes reserved for those women fulfilling the criteria for diabetes in the non-pregnant population[3].
[c]Diagnosis of IGT in pregnancy having similar criteria as IGT in the non-pregnant population[3].
[d]Diagnosis of gestational diabetes dependent on both values being exceeded[22].

Table 10.2. Changes in maternal carbohydrate metabolism associated with normal pregnancy

Fall in fasting plasma glucose values
Rise in postprandial glucose values
Increased hepatic glucose output
Rise in fasting and postprandial insulin concentrations
Decreased insulin sensitivity
Increased circulating proinsulin concentrations
Decreased hepatic insulin extraction
Increased circulating amylin polypeptide
β-cell hypertrophy
Enhanced lipolysis

Australian series[30]. However, even a 3% risk puts these women above the background prevalence rate for diabetes; this is again similar to the IGT population who revert to normal glucose tolerance while retaining a higher lifetime prevalence than the background population[28].

As well as highlighting the similarities, there is also a lesson to be drawn regarding the value of the OGTT as a 'diagnostic' test. The inconsistency in the reproducibility of the OGTT in diagnosing IGT[31] and GDM[32] is probably a reflection of the poor predictive value of the OGTT for diagnosing abnormality close to, or within, the normal range. At this point, in a bimodal population the upper tail of the normal distribution curve will overlap with the lower tail of the abnormal distribution curve. This is confounded by an inherent variability in post-prandial glucose values, which are influenced by dietary factors, levels of physical activity and anxiety[31].

PREGNANCY AS A METABOLIC MODEL FOR TYPE 2 DIABETES

GDM pregnancy acts as a β-cell stress test[33–35]. Women with GDM pregnancy are a selected group identified by their inability to maintain glucose tolerance at levels of insulin resistance that most women can. Although the majority of pregnant women have sufficient β-cell capacity to cope with the sudden and extreme increases in insulin resistance seen in normal pregnancy, a minority of women do not, and it is these women who become glucose intolerant.

Understanding why some insulin-resistance subjects remain glucose tolerant whereas others do not is central to understanding the pathogenesis of type 2 diabetes[36]. Insulin resistance is a universal feature of type 2 diabetes; however, as with pregnancy and other insulin-resistant conditions, only a minority of subjects actually develop diabetes[37].

In pregnancy, insulin resistance increases as a result of circulating placental hormones[38,39]. A 30–85% increase in insulin resistance occurs by the third trimester which requires postprandial insulin secretion to increase two- to threefold[23,33,34,40,41]. Normal pregnancy is associated with marked β-cell hypertrophy and hyperplasia[42], indicative of an increase in insulin synthesis and release. Not only is insulin secretion increased, so too is IAPP (islet amyloid polypeptide), which is synthesized and co-secreted with insulin from the β-cell[43]. The exact physiological role of IAPP remains to be defined[44]. The small reduction in hepatic insulin clearance that occurs in normal pregnancies also contributes to peripheral hyperinsulinaemia[34]. The insulin response in women with GDM to both oral and intravenous glucose is consistently lower than that of glucose-tolerant women[33]. Post partum, abnormalities in the early insulin response to glucose persist, even when insulin resistance improves sufficiently to restore glucose tolerance[45,46]. The extent of this relative insulinopenia both in pregnancy and post partum is predictive of future type 2 diabetes[47,48]. From these observations, it can be seen that an individual's β-cell function is central in determining whether GDM will develop, and the likelihood of future diabetes.

In GDM, insulin resistance as a result of pregnancy can be viewed as the precipitating factor, and insulin secretory capacity the variable factor that determines who will and who will not, develop diabetes. The insulin resistance of obesity rather than that of pregnancy may be viewed as a similar precipitant, and insulin-secretory capacity is also the variable in determining IGT and type 2 diabetes. Obesity, like pregnancy, is associated with an increase in β-cell secretory function with 24-hour insulin secretory profiles three- to fourfold higher than those of non-obese controls[41,49]. Obesity, like pregnancy, is also associated with morphological changes in the pancreas with an approximately 20% increase in overall β-cell mass compared with non-obese controls[50]. In contrast, type 2 diabetic subjects have a 20–30% decrease in β-cell mass[51].

The maintenance of normoglycaemia is likely to depend on the individuals' ability to increase their β-cell mass in response to demand, whether it is increased demand as a result of pregnancy, obesity or another cause of insulin resistance. Future work needs to examine why individuals with GDM or type 2 diabetes are unable to increase their β-cell function and possibly mass in response to increased demand.

UNDERSTANDING INSULIN PROCESSING AND PACKAGING

Pregnancy is a time of β-cell hypersecretion, and this provides an opportunity to examine insulin processing, by measuring proinsulin secretion and its conversion intermediates. Rodent models of diabetes have shown that increased insulin demand in the presence of pre-existing β-cell defects leads to an increased release of insulin precursors from immature islet cell granules[52]. Type 2 diabetes is characterized by an increase in the secretion of proinsulin and its cleaved product 32,33-split-proinsulin[53]. The proportion of 32,33-split-proinsulin to proinsulin-like molecules is increased in conditions associated with insulin resistance[54], including normal and GDM pregnancies[55], and non-pregnant IGT and type 2 diabetic subjects[56]. As with type 2 diabetes, total proinsulin-like molecules are increased in women with GDM[55] and remain increased postpartum[43]. During pregnancy the proportion of proinsulin-like molecules to true insulin has been reported to be predictive of GDM[55] and to be highest in those pregnancies requiring insulin therapy[57].

This might be hoped to act as a predictor of GDM/type 2 diabetes, but to date, increased proinsulin-like molecules either during or after a GDM pregnancy have not been shown to predict type 2 diabetes[58].

THE ROLE OF INSULIN RESISTANCE IN DIABETES

Important lessons about insulin resistance can be learned from the study of normal and GDM pregnancies. The insulin resistance syndrome is sometimes regarded as the 'metabolic scourge' of the twentieth century, held responsible for premature cardiovascular disease and the current global epidemic of diabetes[37]. Pregnancy provides an unique opportunity to see insulin resistance in a favourable light.

Normal pregnancy is associated with increased resistance to insulin[23,33]. Insulin sensitivity falls by 45–75% by the third trimester, achieving values similar to those of type 2 diabetes[34,59]. This fall in insulin sensitivity facilitates the diversion of glucose in the postprandial state to the fetus, while optimizing maternal fat deposition, and thus ensuring maternal fuel for later in pregnancy and lactation. Theoretically, decreased maternal insulin sensitivity may also improve metabolic efficiency by reducing postprandial thermogenesis, thereby maximizing anabolic usage of undigested calories[60]. However, when maternal β-cell function is unable to increase sufficiently to maintain normal glucose tolerance, these theoretical advantages are jeopardized.

Various techniques have been used to assess insulin resistance in pregnancy, including the euglycaemic clamp[40,61], short insulin tolerance test[35], and the use of mathematical modelling for both intravenous and oral glucose tolerance tests[33,34,62]. All studies confirm that both normal pregnancies and those identified as having GDM are associated with marked increases in insulin resistance which improves post partum. However, there is inconsistency in the literature in the degree to which women with GDM are more insulin resistant than controls either during or after pregnancy[34,63]. This may reflect differences in methodologies employed to assess insulin resistance. Not all techniques used may be sufficiently sensitive to detect differences in insulin resistance at the levels encountered in pregnancy. The other possibility is that the contribution of insulin resistance to the insulin secretory defect in the pathogenesis of GDM differs according to the population.

It is important to realize that the insulin resistance associated with pregnancy differs from that of type 2 diabetes. It is of short duration with a common aetiology, namely placental hormones[38,39]. By contrast, the increased insulin resistance that precedes the development of IGT and type 2 diabetes occurs over years, if not decades. The insulin resistance associated with IGT and type 2 diabetes is multifactorial, involving an admixture of genetic and environmental factors, which include obesity, lack of physical activity and ethnicity[64,65].

Many of the risk factors for developing GDM are also risk factors for type 2 diabetes and increased insulin resistance. The prevalence of GDM increases with age, obesity and parity having the highest prevalence among ethnic groups known to be insulin resistant[66–69]. From this, one would expect many GDM women to be insulin resistant both before and after pregnancy. However, there are no prospective studies examining the cause, extent and duration of any insulin resistance in women predating a GDM pregnancy.

Both in pregnancy and post partum, obese women with GDM are more insulin resistant than lean controls[34,40]. Whether these obese women with GDM are more insulin resistant than obese non-diabetic women either during or after pregnancy is unclear[45]. In contrast, non-obese GDM women are clearly more insulin resistant when compared with non-obese controls[34]. It is likely that these non-obese GDM women come from the upper levels of the normal insulin resistance distribution curve seen in the non-obese, non-pregnant, non-diabetic population.

Overall the literature suggests that, both in pregnancy and post partum, women with GDM are more insulin resistant as a group than women who remain glucose tolerant. However, what distinguishes women who develop GDM from those who do not is the coexisting insulin secretory defect, which is proportionally greater than that seen in other prediabetic groups with similar levels of insulin resistance. However, the degree of insulin resistance may play a more important role in certain populations. In the highly insulin-resistant Pima-Indian women, those with GDM have a slower progression to diabetes than non-pregnant women with IGT[70]. This is probably explained by insulin resistance in GDM women correcting itself sufficiently post partum to maintain normoglycaemia for longer than it takes for highly insulin-resistant, non-pregnant IGT women to become diabetic. These observations suggest that GDM women may not be wholly metabolically representative of the future female type 2 diabetic population. It is possible that non-obese GDM women have a more marked β-cell defect than the more typical obese GDM women.

Insulin resistance, however, is known to be multifactorial, and can and does occur among the non-obese general population[71]. Regardless of the aetiology of the insulin resistance, if present before pregnancy it would be expected to have a similar cumulative effect on the β cells, with an initial increase in β-cell mass[51] and changes in insulin processing[54], resulting finally in a loss in first-phase insulin release and responsiveness to glucose[65,72]. In some non-obese women, genetic factors may be contributing more than environmental factors to the insulin resistance. In others, the secretory defect may be the result of slowly evolving autoimmune type 1 diabetes[4]. With either scenario, the model of GDM emphasizes the balance between insulin resistance and β-cell function. The diagnosis of GDM tells the physician that this equilibrium is threatened. Over time, the insulin resistance increases and β-cell capacity falls, as a natural consequence of ageing. The study of GDM emphasizes that the primacy of insulin resistance and insulin secretion in the pathogenesis of type 2 diabetes should not be viewed in terms of 'either, or'.

LESSONS FROM EPIDEMIOLOGY

There are important lessons to be learned from the epidemiology of GDM and type 2 diabetes which should prove informative for the prediction and prevention of type 2 diabetes. However, epidemiology remains a purely observational science and the information derived depends on interpretation and extrapolation of observational data in the light of clinical and scientific knowledge. The translation from epidemiological facts on prediction to the prevention of diabetes remains one of the greatest challenges to the clinical diabetologist[73].

There are striking similarities in the demographic characteristics of the population with GDM and those of the female population with type 2 diabetes. Both conditions are strongly influenced by genetic susceptibility as seen by the effects of ethnicity[66,68] and family history. This commonality of genetic susceptibility to both GDM and type 2 diabetes is suggested by the fact that the prevalence of GDM for any one ethnic group is similar to that for type 2 diabetic women who are 10–20 years older[74,75]. This susceptibility appears to be influenced by environmental factors, which include diet, and levels of obesity and physical activity.

An important epidemiological problem is the extent to which women with GDM are the future female population with type 2 diabetes. Harris argued that, as the prevalence of GDM within a population was similar to that of the background prevalence of IGT for women of similar age, it was these two conditions that were synonymous rather than future type 2 diabetes[76]. The prevalence rate for GDM obtained from large population studies in the USA is around 3%[69]; this is, however, likely to be higher if universal antenatal screening for GDM occurs. It will also be considerably higher in certain ethnic groups[68]. The prevalence of GDM is similar to type 2 diabetes in ethnically matched middle-aged women, and lower than that for older women[77]. However, follow-up studies have shown that only 30–40% of GDM women actually become diabetic by late middle age[78]. Overall, therefore, at face value only a minority of parous type 2 diabetic women aged under 60 years would be expected to have had previous GDM.

There are two plausible explanations for this apparent mismatch of GDM with future diabetes. One is that many future diabetic women may have completed their families during their 20s at a time when they were not obese and at low risk of GDM. The second important possibility is that GDM identifies only a subfraction of potentially diabetic women – those characterized by poor β-cell function – and the development of future diabetes in this group is highly dependent on the increase of insulin resistance to levels that approach those seen in pregnancy. This later explanation is compatible with the known risk factors associated with progression to type 2 diabetes after a GDM pregnancy, as discussed below[47,48].

GDM RISK FACTORS FOR PREDICTING TYPE 2 DIABETES

The prediction of type 2 diabetes can be helped by the study of which risk factors are associated with the progression to type 2 diabetes after an index GDM pregnancy[79]. Several well-recognized risk factors have been identified; some are modifiable and others are not (Table 10.3). Some can be used to predict a woman's risk of future diabetes whereas others are potentially amenable to modification, which could delay or prevent type 2 diabetes. Many of these factors are associated either directly or indirectly with increased insulin resistance.

Table 10.3. Risk factors associated with type 2 diabetes after a GDM pregnancy

Unmodifiable risk factors at time of index pregnancy
Age
Ethnicity
Parity
Family history
Degree of glucose intolerance and insulinopenia
Obesity
Modifiable risk factors after index pregnancy
Level of obesity and weight gain
Further pregnancies, especially associated with recurrence of GDM
Potentially modified risk factors after index pregnancy
Level of physical activity
Dietary fat
Drugs that increase insulin sensitivity, including smoking

The prevalence of subsequent diabetes depends on the length of follow-up and the age at follow-up. The background prevalence of type 2 diabetes increases throughout life[73]. The excess of diabetes among previous GDM women is likely to be greatest in middle age, but to remain above background throughout life[30]. As life expectancy increases, so too will the cumulative lifetime risk of diabetes after GDM.

One of the most important unmodifiable risk factors for future type 2 diabetes after a GDM pregnancy is ethnicity. Ethnicity also influences cultural and behavioural patterns that impinge on other diabetic risk factors[73]. Within certain populations, up to half of the women are diabetic within 5 years[48,80]. This contrasts with less than 10% for non-Hispanic white populations by 10 years, and 30–40% by 30 years[78]. Early detection and treatment of diabetes can be targeted to the very-high-risk ethnic groups (secondary prevention).

In large population studies, parity itself has little or no effect on the risk of type 2 diabetes, when all the other causally related risk factors have been accounted for, namely, increasing obesity and age[81,82]. The first pregnancy is associated with significant changes in weight and abdominal fat distribution[83], however, it would appear that subsequent pregnancies are not associated with any further changes that cannot be accounted for by age. It is possible that, if adipocytes undergo differentiation during the first pregnancy which promotes abdominal fat disposition, the age of first pregnancy rather than the number of pregnancies may also influence the lifetime risk of abdominal obesity and diabetes. A threefold increase in the annual incidence of type 2 diabetes postpartum was reported in Hispanic women who developed GDM after an additional pregnancy[84], in contrast to a lack of increasing parity on future type 2 diabetes seen in the large American Nurse's Study[81].

Obesity is a major risk factor for both GDM[68] and type 2 diabetes[85], and increased pregnancy weight during a GDM pregnancy has long been recognized as a risk factor for future type 2 diabetes[47,86]. A recent study shows a synergistic effect of obesity at the time of pregnancy and poor insulin secretory function on the subsequent risk of diabetes[47]. Women who previously developed GDM in the highest tertiles for obesity in pregnancy, but the lowest for insulin area under the OGTT curve, had an eightfold increased 5-year risk of diabetes, compared with women in the more favourable tertiles for both[47]. Women who were just in the highest tertile for obesity had a twofold increase. The degree of obesity post partum, especially abdominal obesity[85], will be a major determinant of postpartum insulin sensitivity; a previous history of obesity will be an indication of how long the woman's β-cells have been subjected to an excessive secretory demand. Of O'Sullivan's original cohort followed up for 16 years, 47% of the obese women or those who had gained weight had become glucose intolerant, compared with 28% for those who remained non-obese or who had lost weight since pregnancy[86]. The contribution of obesity to diabetes after a GDM pregnancy is in keeping with the epidemiological studies in large non-diabetic cohorts[87]. Epidemiological and clinical studies therefore confirm a high percentage of obesity in newly diagnosed type 2 diabetic women[73,88,89]. Abdominal obesity is a more permissive risk factor than BMI alone[90]. Up to 80% of the variability of insulin sensitivity in non-diabetic subjects has been attributed to abdominal obesity[85,91,92].

A family history of type 2 diabetes in a first-degree relative of a woman with GDM further increases her risk of diabetes[5,30,47] with 35% of Australian women who had developed GDM being diabetic by 16 years compared with 22% for those with no family history[30]. An interesting finding in a 5-year follow-up study in Chicago was that it was only a maternal family history that was associated with the progression to type 2 diabetes[47], highlighting the importance of the maternal transmission of diabetes[93].

The degree of metabolic disturbance both in pregnancy and immediately post partum, as assessed by fasting plasma glucose, glucose area under the OGTT curve, the need for insulin therapy or early diagnosis in pregnancy, is predictive of future type 2 diabetes[5,47]. About three-quarters of women with GDM from Chicago were diabetic within 6 months when their fasting pregnancy plasma glucose exceeded 7.2 mmol/l. This dropped to 10% when fasting values were below 5.8 mmol/l[94]. In a 5-year follow-up study of over 600 Latino women with GDM, Kjos and colleagues[48] found that 84% of the women in the highest glucose area quartile during an OGTT were diabetic, compared with 12% in the lowest quartile. In less high-risk populations, the degree of glycaemia post partum is equally predictive of type 2 diabetes, although the progression rate is slower[6]. Diabetes at 5 and 10 years postpartum is also shown to increase with the extent of β-cell dysfunction[47], as assessed by a low insulin response during an OGTT, at 30–60 min or 1–3 h.

MODIFIABLE GDM RISK FACTORS

Women with GDM provide an ideal population to identify modifiable risk factors for the development of type 2 diabetes[79]. To date, the risk factors shown to be associated with type 2 diabetes or recurrence of GDM after an index GDM pregnancy include further pregnancy[84], increasing weight[86] and high dietary fat intake[95] (see Table 10.3). Other potential risk factors that have not been proved are level of physical activity[96] and smoking[97]. Although, the influence of risk factors is known, however, the effect of intervention on those factors is less clear cut.

One could argue that parity is a modifiable risk factor. This has been discussed previously. It is likely that, although most women have sufficient β-cell reserves to sustain consecutive pregnancies, women with previous GDM, with their already compromised β-cell reserves, do not. These women may be legitimate targets for counselling about potential risks of further pregnancies, but there is still conflicting evidence.

Obesity and further weight gain are important modifiable risk factors for future diabetes and again these have already been addressed. Although obesity is clearly an important risk factor in GDM women for future diabetes[47], and remains a potentially modifiable one through dietary invention, it is unknown whether the benefit of weight reduction would be as protective against future type 2 diabetes in women with previous GDM as in those without. In the background female population, it has been estimated that a weight loss of 10 kg could lessen the reduction in life expectancy associated with type 2 diabetes by as much as 35%[87,98].

Dietary content is another important contributor to the epidemic of type 2 diabetes[99–101]. The prevalence of type 2 diabetes is highest in those countries with a high fat consumption[73], and increases when the percentage of the diet derived from fat exceeds 40%[99,102]. Recently, a study on women with a history of GDM reported that the dietary fat intake between the index pregnancy and a subsequent pregnancy influences the recurrence rate of GDM, being greater in those women who consumed more fat between pregnancies[95]. What is currently not known is whether a low-fat diet reduces the risk of future diabetes in those women with a previous history of GDM[103].

Physical activity represents an important, but as yet unproven, potential modifiable risk factor for the prevention of type 2 diabetes after a GDM pregnancy. Lifestyle changes in the industrialized world have brought about a radical fall in physical activity, which has not been matched by a sufficient compensatory fall in calorie intake[104]. These changes are particularly apparent in young women[105]. Newly diagnosed women with type 2 diabetes report lower levels of physical activity than non-diabetic controls; this is especially true among certain ethnic groups[106]. Exercise has known metabolic benefits, which include reducing insulin resistance, decreasing abdominal fat mass, and ameliorating the detrimental effect of dietary fat on insulin sensitivity[107,108]. Longitudinal studies in both men and women[96,109] suggest that regular moderate and vigorous exercise can reduce the risk of developing type 2 diabetes by 30–50%[110,111]. Exercise has also been shown to delay the progression of IGT to type 2 diabetes[112]. We await the results of ongoing interventional studies to see whether exercise programmes introduced after an index GDM pregnancy can delay the progression to diabetes[113].

PRACTICAL LESSONS FOR PREVENTION

At present, primary prevention of diabetes is not widely practised. Instead, the treatment of diabetes is centred on preventing the development of diabetic complications (secondary prevention) and minimizing the morbidity from established complications (tertiary prevention). The proven benefits of secondary and tertiary prevention have formed the basis of our clinical practice.

The persuasive theoretical argument for the primary prevention of diabetes has resulted in the European section of the World Health Organization (WHO) and the International Diabetic Federation (IDF) endorsing primary preventive strategies[114], which are summarized in the 1995 Acropolis Affirmation[115]. Targeting high-risk groups for primary prevention, to include previous gestational diabetic women and those with IGT, are advocated. However, it is at present unknown whether primary prevention of diabetes is either practical or effective. We advise culinary restraint and exercise over gluttony and sloth to all our newly diagnosed diabetic patients, appreciating that this advice is given too little too late. It is not known at what stage in the natural history of type 2 diabetes behavioural modification can delay or prevent its development. Interventional studies have shown a benefit, over 6 years, from diet and exercise, either alone or together, in delaying the progression from IGT to diabetes[112]. However, other studies suggest that, when the fasting blood glucose is above 6 mmol/l, diet and exercise are for the most part ineffectual in preventing further deterioration of glucose tolerance, despite improving physical fitness[116].

Gestational diabetic women are an ideal study group for interventional lifestyle studies on the prevention of diabetes[79]. As most women become pregnant in their lifetime, the screening for GDM provides an opportunity to identify a large proportion of women at risk of diabetes, at an age when lifestyle modification may reduce or delay not only diabetes but also cardiovascular disease. These women will have received basic diabetic eduction during pregnancy, when their motivation would have been high; extending this beyond the pregnancy may prove easier than attempting lifestyle modification in other less motivated groups.

Although it is likely that weight control and physical exercise may prolong the period of normal glucose tolerance after a GDM pregnancy, the development of IGT and later type 2 diabetes is still to be expected. Evidence suggests that the progression of IGT to type 2 diabetes in previous GDM women occurs over a shorter period of time than for the background population in most[48], but not all, populations studied[70]. All women with gestational diabetes should be made aware of the early symptoms of diabetes. Public awareness of the symptoms is generally poor; even in the presence of symptoms, the diagnosis of type 2 diabetes is often delayed by 10 years[117,118]. In ethnic minority groups, especially when literacy and language difficulties are present, the delay in diagnosis is even greater. It is this long period of undiagnosed and untreated diabetes that accounts for the high prevalence of micro- and macrovascular complications at diagnosis. Appropriate education and follow-up of women with gestational diabetes should make it possible to achieve earlier diagnosis and treatment.

LESSONS FROM THE FETUS

One of the most interesting observations arising from the study of maternal hyperglycaemia has been the observation that there is an increased prevalence of early diabetes and obesity in the children[14,15,93,119]. Numerous studies have reported higher rates of diabetes in the offspring of men and women who have diabetes than in the offspring of those who do not[120]. There is a clear genetic component in the inheritance of type 2 diabetes marking out offspring of diabetic parents as at risk and therefore legitimate targets for primary prevention.

Perhaps less well known is the effect of the diabetic intrauterine environment. The effects of this on glucose metabolism may lead to the development of type 2 diabetes. The influence of the intrauterine environment in GDM is likely to explain why more individuals with type 2 diabetes/IGT have a maternal, as opposed to a paternal, history of diabetes[93,121,112].

The Pima Indians of Arizona have the world's highest rate of type 2 diabetes, which often develops at a young age[123]. This population has been intensively screened and monitored. Prospective family data are available for this population before and after pregnancy. Overall, there are few cases of diabetes before the age of 15, but when present it is almost always in the offspring of diabetic women. At all ages, there are more cases of diabetes in the offspring of diabetic than of non-diabetic or prediabetic women; the rates for the last two groups are in fact similar[93]. This suggests that genetic predisposition, acting on offspring of both diabetic and prediabetic women, is less important than the effect of the diabetic intrauterine environment[93,119]. The higher rate of diabetes may, in part, be mediated by the earlier development of obesity in the offspring of the diabetic women, but this does not appear to account for the magnitude of the effect. One possibility is the effect of the diabetic intrauterine environment on the development of adipocytes and pancreatic β cells[124–126].

Animal studies also help to demonstrate the lasting effects of the diabetic intrauterine environment in the absence of genetically inherited diabetes. The developing fetal pups of genetically non-diabetic rats, which are made hyperglycaemic during pregnancy, either by destruction of the pancreas with streptozotocin[127,128] or by glucose infusion[129], suffer problems that are typical of diabetic pregnancy. As adults, the second-generation rats have abnormal glucose tolerance tests[127], together with abnormalities of insulin resistance[130]. In addition, the females have gestational diabetes so that the third generation is also affected[127]. As these animals are not genetically predisposed to diabetes, the effects may be attributed to the diabetic intrauterine environment.

From the fetal outcomes, we learn a number of valuable lessons. With regard to prediction of type 2 diabetes, diabetic pregnancy appears to be a risk factor for type 2 diabetes in the offspring regardless of genetic propensity. In addition, the intrauterine environment is highlighted, providing a window on its potential importance as an aetiological agent. Thus, good control of hyperglycaemia during a diabetic pregnancy may be important, not just for the health of the mother or to reduce peripartum complications in the fetus (such as macrosomy, hypoglycaemia, etc.), but also because it is in itself a contributor to primary prevention of type 2 diabetes in the offspring.

CONCLUSIONS

Gestational diabetes is an opportunity to identify some, if not all, women at risk of type 2 diabetes. These women provide an opportunity to examine the metabolic events in the evolution of type 2 diabetes. These women also represent a potential group for interventional studies for both the prevention of type 2 diabetes and diabetic macrovascular disease. Diabetes is a familial disease, with an increased maternal transmission. Young parents are ideally placed in the home setting to have a favourable influence on the diets and eating habits of today's children. By targeting women who have previous gestational diabetes with advice on healthy eating and living, one has the potential for modifying their risk of future diabetes in two generations at increased risk. The study of diabetes in pregnancy will bring a greater understanding to the influence of the intrauterine environment on the susceptibility of the child to future obesity and diabetes. We believe that many more lessons on the prediction and prevention of type 2 diabetes will emerge from further studies on gestational diabetes. If lifestyle modification or therapeutic interventions are shown to delay the onset of type 2 diabetes significantly, the screening for GDM in pregnancy will provide an ideal opportunity to reach a high proportion of the female population at risk.

REFERENCES

1. Metzger BE. Summary and recommendations of the Third International Workshop – Conference on Gestational Diabetes Mellitus. *Diabetes* 1991; **40**(suppl 2): 197–201.
2. WHO. Diabetes mellitus. *Tech Report Series* 1985; **729**:9–17.
3. The Expert Committee on the Diagnosis and Classification of Diabetes Mellitus. Report on the expert committee on the diagnosis and classification of diabetes mellitus. *Diabetes Care* 1997; **20**:1183–1197.
4. Buschard K, Buch I, Mølsted-Pedersen L, Hougaard P, Kurl C. Increased incidence of true type I diabetes acquired during pregnancy. *BMJ* 1987; **294**:275–279.
5. Dornhorst A, Bailey PC, Anyaoku V, Elkeles RS, Johnson DG, Beard RW. Abnormalities of glucose tolerance following gestational diabetes. *Q J Med* 1990; **284** (New Series 7): 1219–1228.

6. Damm P, Kühl C, Bertelsen A, Mølsted-Pedersen L. Predictive factors for the development of diabetes in women with previous gestational diabetes mellitus. *Am J Obsted Gynecol* 1992; **167**:607–616.
7. Damm P, Kuhl C. Buschard K et al. Prevalence and predictive value of islet cell antibodies in women with gestational diabetes. *Diabetic Med* 1994; **11**:558–563.
8. Beischer NA, Wein P, Sheedy MT, Mackay IR, Rowley MJ, Zimmet P. Prevalence of antibodies to glutamic acid decarboxalase in women who have had gestational diabetes. *Am J Obsted Gynecol* 1996; **173**:1563–1569.
9. Fuchtebbusch M, Ferber K, Standl E, Ziegler AG. Prediction of type 1 diabetes postpartum in patients with gestational diabetes mellitus by combined islet cell autoantibody: a prospective multicenter study. *Diabetes* 1997; **46**:1459–1467.
10. Saker PJ, Hattersley AT, Barrow B et al. High prevalence of a missense mutation of the glucokinase gene in gestational diabetic patients due to a founder-effect in a local population. *Diabetologia* 1996; **39**:1325–1328.
11. Alan CJ, Agryopoulos G, Bowker M et al. Gestational diabetes and gene mutations which affect insulin secretion. *Diabetes Res Clin Pract* 1997; **36**:135–141.
12. Reece EA. The history of diabetes mellitus. In: Reece EA, Coustan DR, eds. *Diabetes Mellitus in Pregnancy*. New York: Churchill Livingstone, 1988: 3–15.
13. Casson IF, Clarke CA, Howard CV et al. Outcomes of pregnancy in insulin dependent diabetic women: results of a five year population cohort study. *BMJ* 1997; **315**:275–278.
14. Pettitt DJ, Bennett PH, Knowler WC, Baird HR, Aleck KA. Gestational diabetes mellitus and impaired glucose tolerance during pregnancy. Long-term effects on obesity and glucose tolerance in the offspring. *Diabetes* 1985; **34**(suppl 2): 119–122.
15. Silverman BL, Metzger BE, Cho NH, Leob CA. Impaired glucose tolerance in adolescent offspring of diabetic mothers. *Diabetes Care* 1995; **18**:611–617.
16. Girling JC, Dornhorst A. Pregnancy and diabetes mellitus. In: Pickup JC, Williams G, eds. *Textbood of Diabetes*. Oxford: Blackwell Science, 1997: 72.1–72.34.
17. Jarrett RJ. Gestational diabetes: a non-entity? *BMJ* 1993; **306**:37–38.
18. Dornhorst A, Chan S. The elusive diagnosis of gestational diabetes. *Diabetes Med* 1998; **15**:7–10.
19. World Health Organization. *WHO Expert Committee on Diabetes Mellitus, Second Report*. Geneva: WHO, 1980.
20. O'Sullivan JB, Mahan CM. Criteria for oral glucose tolerance test in pregnancy. *Diabetes* 1964; **13**:278–285.
21. Gillmer MDG, Oakley NW, Beard RW, Niththyananthan R, Cawston M. Screening for diabetes during pregnancy. *Br J Obstet Gynaecol* 1980; **87**:377–382.
22. Lind T. A prospective multicentre study to determine the influence of pregnancy upon the 75 g oral glucose tolerance test: The Diabetic Pregnancy Study Group of the European Association for the Study of Diabetes. In: Sutherland HW, Stowers JM, Pearson DWM, eds. *Carbohydrate Metabolism in Pregnancy and the Newborn IV*. London: Springer-Verlag, 1989: 209–226.
23. Catalano PM, Tyzbir ED, Wolfe RR et al. Carbohydrate metabolism during pregnancy in control subjects and women with gestational diabetes. *Am J Physiol* 1993; **264**(Endocrinol Metab): E60–E67.
24. McCance DR, Hanson RL, Pettitt DJ, Bennett PH, Hadden DR, Knowler WC. Diagnosing diabetes mellitus-do we need new criteria? *Diabetologia* 1997; **40**:247–255.
25. Jarrett RJ, Keen H, Fuller JH, McCartney M. Worsening to diabetes in men with impaired glucose tolerance ('borderline diabetes'). *Diabetologia* 1979; **16**:25–30.

26. Jarrett RJ. Risk factors of macrovascular disease in diabetes mellitus. *Hormone Metab Res* 1985; **15**(suppl): 1–3.
27. Keen H, Jarrett RJ, McCartney P. The 10 year follow-up of the Bedford survey (1962–1972). *Diabetologia* 1982; **22**:73–78.
28. Saad MF, Knowler WC, Pettitt DJ, Nelson RJ, Bennett PH. The natural history of impaired glucose tolerance in the Pima Indians. *N Engl J Med* 1988; **319**: 1500–1506.
29. Moses RG. The recurrence rate of gestational diabetes in subsequent pregnancies *Diabetes Care* 1996; 19:1349–1356.
30. Henry OA, Beisher NA. Long-term implication of gestational diabetes for the mother. *Baillières Clin Obstet Gynaecol* 1991; **5**:461–483.
31. Mooy JM, Gootenhuis PA, de Vries HPJK, Popp-Snijders C, Bouter LM, Heine RJ, Intra-individual variation of glucose, specific insulin and proinsulin concentrations measured by two oral glucose tolerance tests in general Caucasian population: the Hoorn Study. *Diabetologia* 1996; **39**:298–305.
32. Catalano PM, Avallone DA, Drago NM, Amini SB. Reproducibility of the oral glucose tolerance test in pregnant women. *Am J. Obstet Gynecol* 1993; **169**: 874–881.
33. Buchanan TA, Dornhorst A. The metabolic stress of pregnancy. In: Dornhorst A, Hadden D eds. *Diabetes and Pregnancy: An international approach to management*. Chichester: John Wiley & Sons, 1996: 45–62.
34. Kautzky-Willer A, Prager R, Waldhäusl W et al. Pronounced insulin resistance and inadequate β-cell secretion characterizes lean gestational diabetes during and after pregnancy. *Diabetes Care* 1997; **20**:1717–1723.
35. Nicholls JSD, Chan SP, Ali K, Beard RW, Dornhorst A. Insulin secretion and sensitivity in women fulfilling WHO criteria for gestational diabetes. *Diabetic Med* 1995; **12**:56–50.
36. Polonsky KS, Sturis J, Graeme I. Non-insulin-dependent diabetes mellitus – A genetically programmed failure of the β-cell to compensate for insulin resistance. *N Engl J Med* 1996; **334**:777–783.
37. DeFronzo RA, Ferrannini E. Insulin resistance. A multifaceted syndrome responsible for NIDDM, obesity, hypertension, dyslipidemia and atherosclerotic cardiovascular disease. *Diabetes Care* 1991; **14**:173–194.
38. Langhoff-Roos J, Wibell L, Gebre-Medhin M, Lindmark G. Placental hormones and maternal glucose tolerance: a study of fetal growth in normal pregnancy. *Br J Obstet Gynaecol* 1989; **96**:320–326.
39. Handwerger S. Clinical counterpoint: the physiology of placental lactogen in human pregnancy. *Endocrine Rev* 1991: **12**:329–336.
40. Ryan EA, O'Sullivan MJ, Skyler JS. Insulin action during pregnancy: studies with the euglycemic glucose clamp technique. *Diabetes* 1985; **34**:380–389.
41. Spellacy WN, Goetz FC. Plasma insulin in normal late pregnancy. *N Engl J Med* 1963; **268**:988–991.
42. Van Assche FA, Aerts L, De Prins F. A morphological study of the endocrine pancreas in human pregnancy. *Br J Obsted Gynaecol* 1978; **85**:818–820.
43. Kautzky-Willer A, Thomaseth K, Ludvik B et al. Elevated islet amyloid pancreatic polypeptide and proinsulin in lean gestational diabetes. *Diabetes* 1997; **46**:607–614.
44. Ludvik B, Kautzky-Willer A, Prager R, Thomaseth K, Pacini G. Amylin: history and overview. *Diabetic Med* 1997; **14**(suppl 2): S9–13.
45. Ryan EA, Imes S. Liu D et al. Defects in insulin secretion and action in women with a history of gestational diabetes. *Diabetes* 1995; **44**:506–512.

46. Dornhorst A, Chan SP, Gelding SV et al. Ethnic differences in insulin secretion in women at risk of future diabetes. *Diabetic Med* 1992; **9**:258–262.
47. Metzger BE, Cho NH, Roston SM, Radvany R. Prepregnancy weight and antepartum insulin secretion predict glucose tolerance five years after gestational diabetes mellitus. *Diabetes Care* 1993; **16**:1598–1605.
48. Kjos Sl, Peters RK, Xiang A, Henry OA, Montoro M, Buchanan TA. Predicting future diabetes in Latino women with gestational diabetes. *Diabetes* 1995; **44**:586–591.
49. Polonsky KS, Given BD, Van Cauter E. Twenty-four-hour profiles and pulsatile patterns of insulin secretion in normal and obese subjects. *J. Clin Invest* 1988; **81**:442–448.
50. Kloppel G, Lohr M, Habich K, Oberholzer M, Heitz PU. Islet pathology and the pathogenesis of type 1 and type 2 diabetes revisted. *Surv Synth Pathol Res* 1985; **4**:110–125.
51. Rahier J, Goebgels RM, Henquin JC. Cellular composition of the human diabetic pancreas. *Diabetologia* 1988; **24**:366–371.
52. Gadot M, Ariav Y, Cerasi E, Kaiser N, Gross DJ. Hyperproinsulinemia in the diabetic *Pasmmomys obesus* is a result of increased secretory demand on the beta-cell. *Endocrinology* 1995; **136**:4218–4223.
53. Ward WK, LaCava EC, Paquette TL, Beard JC, Wallum BJ, Porte D. Disproportionate elevation of immunoreactive proinsulin in Type 2 diabetes (non-insulin dependent) diabetes mellitus. *Diabetologia* 1987; **31**:698–702.
54. Nagi DK, Hindra JJ, Ryle AJ et al. Relationship of concentrations of insulin, proinsulin and 32,33 split proinsulin and future cardiovascular risk in type II diabetes. *Diabetologia* 1990; **33**:532–537.
55. Swinn RA, Wareham NJ, Gregory R et al. Excessive secretion of insulin precursors characterizes and predicts gestational diabetes. *Diabetes* 1995; **44**: 911–915.
56. Davies MJ, Metcalf J, Day JL, Gray IP, Hales CN. Insulin deficiency rather than hyperinsulinaemia in newly diagnosed type 2 diabetes mellitus. *Diabetes Med* 1993; 10:305–312.
57. Nicholls JSD, Ali K, Gray IP et al. Increased maternal fasting proinsulin as a predictor of insulin requirement in women with gestational diabetes. *Diabetes Med* 1994; 11:57–61.
58. Hanson U, Persson B, Harling SG, Binder C. Increased molar proinsulin-to-insulin ratio in women with previous gestational diabetes does not predict later impairment of glucose tolerance. *Diabetes Care* 1996; **19**:17–20.
59. Bergman RN, Phillips LS, Cobelli C. Physiological evaluation of factors controlling glucose tolerance in man. Measurement of insulin sensitivity and beta-cell sensitivity from the response to intravenous glucose. *J Clin Invest* 1981; **68**:1456–1467.
60. Robinson SR, Johnson DJ. Advantage of diabetes? (letter) *Nature* 1995; **375**:640.
61. Catalano PM, Tyzbir ED, Wolfe RR, Roman NM, Amini SB, Sims EA. Longitudinal changes in basal hepatic glucose production and suppression during insulin infusion in normal pregnant women. *Am J Obstet Gynecol* 1992; **167**:913–919.
62. Buchanan TA, Metzger BE, Freinkel N, Bergman RN. Insulin sensitivity and β-cell responsiveness to glucose during late pregnancy in lean and moderately obese women with normal glucose tolerance or mild gestational diabetes. *Am. J Obstet Gynecol* 1990; **162**:1008–1114.

63. Dornhorst A, Edwards SMG, Nicholls JSD et al. A defect in insulin release in women at risk of future non-insulin dependent diabetes. *Clin Sci* 1991; **81**: 195–199.
64. Rich SS. Mapping genes in diabetes. Genetic epidemiogical perspective. *Diabetes* 1990; **39**:1315–1319.
65. DeFronzo RA, Bonadonna RC, Ferrannina E. Pathogenesis of NIDDM: a balanced overview. *Diabetes Care* 1992; **15**:318–368.
66. Dooley SL, Metzger BE, Cho NH. Gestational diabetes mellitus. Influence of race on disease and perinatal outcome in a U.S. population. *Diabetes* 1991; **40**(suppl 2): 25–29.
67. Berkowitz GS, Lapinski RH, Wein R, Lee D. Race/ethnicity and other risk factors for gestational diabetes. *Am J Epidemiol* 1991; **135**:965–973.
68. Dornhorst A, Paterson CM, Nicholls JSD et al. High prevalence of gestational diabetes in women from ethnic minority groups. *Diabetic Med* 1992; **9**:820–825.
69. Engelgau MM, Herman WH, Smith PJ, German RR, Aubert RE. The epidemiology of diabetes and pregnancy in the USA 1988. *Diabetes Care* 1995; **18**: 1029–1033.
70. Pettitt DJ, Narayan KM, Hanson RL, Knowler WC. Incidence of diabetes mellitus in women following impaired glucose tolerance in pregnancy is lower than following impaired glucose tolerance in the non-pregnant state. *Diabetologia* 1996; **39**:1334–1337.
71. Hollenbeck CB, Reaven GM. Variations in insulin-stimulated glucose uptake in healthy individuals with normal glucose tolerance. *J Clin Endocrinol Metab* 1987; **64**:1169–1173.
72. Yki-Järvinen H. Glucose toxicity. *Endocrinol Rev* 1992; **13**:415–431.
73. Zimmet P. Challenges in diabetes epidemiology–from West to the rest. *Diabetes Care* 1992; **15**:232–252.
74. Beischer NA, Oats JN, Henry OA, Sheedy MT, Walstab JE. Incidence and severity of gestational diabetes mellitus according to country of birth in women living in Australia. *Diabetes* 1991; **40**(suppl 2): 35–38.
75. Hadden DR. Geographic, ethnic and racial variation in the incidence of gestational diabetes mellitus. *Diabetes* 1985; **34**(suppl 2): 8–12.
76. Harris MI. Gestational diabetes may represent discovery of preexisting glucose intolerance. *Diabetes Care* 1988; **11**:402–411.
77. WHO Ad Hoc Diabetic Reporting Group. Diabetes and impaired glucose tolerance in women aged between 20 and 39 years. *World Health Stats Q* 1992; **45**:321–327.
78. Henry OA, Beischer NA, Sheedy MT, Walstab JE. Gestational diabetes and follow-up among immigrant Vietnam-born women. *Aust NZ J Obstet Gynaecol* 1993; **33**:109–114.
79. Dornhorst A, Rossi M. Risk and prevention of type 2 diabetes in women with gestational diabetes. *Diabetes Care* 1998; **21**(suppl 2): 43–49.
80. Benjamin E, Winters D, Mayfield J, Gohdes D. Diabetes in pregnancy in Zuni Indian women. Prevalence and subsequent development of clinical diabetes after gestational diabetes. *Diabetes Care* 193; **16**:1231–1235.
81. Manson JE, Rimm EB, Colditz GA et al. Parity and incidence of non-insulin dependent diabetes. *Am J Med* 1992; **93**:13–18.
82. Kritz-Silverstein D, Barrett-Connor E, Wingard DL. The effect of parity on the later development of non-insulin dependent diabetes mellitus or impaired glucose tolerance. *N Engl J Med* 1989; **321**:1214–1219.
83. Smith DE, Lewis CE, Caveny JL, Perkins LL, Burke GL, Bild DE. Longitudinal changes in adiposity associated with pregnancy. *JAMA* 1994; **271**:1747–1751.

84. Peters Rk, Kjos SL, Xiang A, Buchanan TA. Long-term diabetogenic effect of single pregnancy in women with previous gestational diabetes mellitus. *Lancet* 1996; **347**; 227–230.
85. Carey DG, Jenkins AB, Campbell JF, Chisholm DJ. Abdominal fat and insulin resistance in normal and overweight women: direct measurements reveal a strong relationship in subjects at both low and high risk of NIDDM. *Diabetes* 1996; **45**:633–638.
86. O'Sullivan JB. Body weight and subsequent diabetes mellitus. *JAMA* 1982; **248**:949–952.
87. Manson JE, Willett WC, Stamfer MJ et al. Body weight and mortality among women. *N Engl J Med* 1995; **333**:677–685.
88. United Kingdom Prospective Diabetes Study Group UK. UK Prospective Diabetes Study (UKDPS) VIII. Study design, progress and performance. *Diabetologia* 1991; **34**:877–890.
89. Colditz GA, Willett WC, Stampfer MJ. Weight as a risk for the clinical diabetes in women. *Am J. Epidemiol* 1990; **132**: 501–513.
90. Kaye SA, Folsom AR, Sprafka JM, Prineas RJ, Wallace RB. Increased incidence of diabetes mellitus in relationship to abdominal adiposity in older women. *J Clin Epidemiol* 1991; **44**: 329–34.
91. Kissebah AH, Vydelingum N, Murray R et al. Relationship of body fat distribution to metabolic complications of obesity. *J Clin Endocrinol Metal* 1982; **54**:254–260.
92. Lemieux S, Prud'Homme D, Nadeau A, Tremblay A, Bouchard C, Després J-P. Seven-year changes in body fat and visceral adipose tissue in women. *Diabetes Care* 1996; **19**:983–991.
93. Pettitt D, Aleck K, Baird H, Carraher M, Bennett B, Knowler W. Congenital susceptibility to NIDDM: Role of intrauterine environment. *Diabetes* 1988; **37**:622–628.
94. Metzger BE, Bybee DE, Freinkel N, Phelps RL, Radvany RM, Vaisrub N. Gestational diabetes mellitus. Correlations between the phenotypic and genotypic characteristics of the mother and abnormal glucose tolerance during the first year postpartum. *Diabetes* 1985; **34**(suppl 2): 111–115.
95. Moses RG, Shand JL, Tapsell LC. The recurrence of gestational diabetes: could dietary differences in fat intake be an explanation? *Diabetes Care* 1997; **20**: 1647–1650.
96. Manson JE, Rimm EB, Stampfer MJ et al. Physical activity and incidence of NIDDM women. *Lancet* 1991; **338**:774–778.
97. Ronnemaa T, Ronnemaa EM, Puukka P, Pyorala K, Laakso M. Smoking is independently associated with plasma insulin levels in nondiabetic men. *Diabetes Care* 1996; **19**:1229–1232.
98. Goldstein DJ. Beneficial health effects of modest weight loss. *Int J Obesity* 1992; **16**:397–415.
99. Marshall JA, Hamman RF, Baxter J. High-fat, low carbohydrate diet and the etiology of non-insulin-dependent diabetes: the San Louis Valley Diabetes Study. *Am J Epidemiol* 1991; **134**:590–603.
100. Marshall JA, Hoag S, Shetterly S, Hamman RF. Dietary fat predicts conversation from impaired tolerance to NIDDM. The San Louis Valley Diabetes Study. *Diabetes Care* 1994; **17**:50–56.
101. Feskens EJM, Stengärd J, Virtanen SM et al. Dietary factors determining diabetes and impaired glucose tolerance. *Diabetes Care* 1995; **18**:1104–1112.
102. O'Dea K. Westernisation, insulin resistance and diabetes in Australian Aborigines. *Med J Aust* 1991; **155**:258–264.

103. Dornhorst A, Frost G. The potential for dietary intervention postpartum in women with gestational diabetes. *Diabetes Care* 1997; **20**:1635–1637.
104. Taylor R, Ram P, Zimmet P, Raper LR, Ringrose H. Physical activity and prevalence of diabetes in Melanesian and Indian men in Fiji. *Ann Nutr Metab* 1984; **27**:578–582.
105. Burke GL, Bild DE, Hilner JE. Differences in weight gain in relation to race, gender, age and education in young adults: the CARDIA Study. *Ethn Health* 1996; **1**: 327–35.
106. UK Prospective Diabetes Study Group. UK Prospective Diabetes Study XII: differences between Asian, Afro-Caribbean and White Caucasian Type 2 diabetic patients at diagnosis of diabetes. *Diabetic Med* 1994; **11**:670–677.
107. Eriksson J, Taimela S, Koivisto VA. Exercise and the metabolic syndrome. *Diabetologia* 1997; **40**:125–135.
108. Mayer EJ, Newman BJ, Sleby JV. Usual dietary fat intake and insulin concentrations in healthy women twins. *Diabetes Care* 1993; **16**:1459–1469.
109. Helmrich SP, Ragland DR, Leung RW, Paffenbarger RSJ. Physical activity and reduced occurrence of non-insulin-dependent diabetes mellitus. *N Engl J Med* 1991; **325**:147–152.
110. Lynch J, Helmrich SP, Lakka TA et al. Moderate intense physical activities and high levels of cardiorespiratory fitness reduce the risk of non-insulin-dependent diabetes mellitus in middle-age men. *Arch Intern Med* 1996; **156**:1307–1314.
111. Manson JE, Spelsberg A. Primary prevention of non-insulin dependent diabetes mellitus. *Am J Prev Med* 1994; **10**:172–184.
112. Pan X-R, Li G-W, Hu Y-H et al. Effects of diet and exercise in preventing NIDDM in people with impaired glucose tolerance. *Diabetes Care* 1997; **20**:537–544.
113. Diabetes Prevention Program Research Group. The Diabetes Prevention Program (DDP). *Diabetes* 1977; **46**(suppl 1): 138A.
114. WHO Study Group. *Prevention of Diabetes Mellitus*. Geneva: World Health Organization, 1994.
115. IDF (Europe). The Acropolis Affirmation. *IDF Bulletin* 1995; **40** (2): 44.
116. Dyson PA, Hammersley MS, Morris RJ, Holman RR, Turner RC. Randomised controlled trial of reinforced healthy living advice in subjects with increased but not diabetic fasting glucose levels. *Matabolism* 1997; **4** (Supp. 1): 50–55.
117. Jackson DMA, Wills R, Davies J, Meadows K, Singh B, Wise PH. Public awareness of the symptoms of diabetes mellitus. *Diabetic Med* 1991; **8**:971–972.
118. Singh B, Jackson DMA, Wills R, Davies J. Wise PH. Delayed diagnosis in non-insulin-dependent diabetes. *Diabetic Med* 1992; **304**:1154–1155.
119. Pettit DJ. Diabetes in subsequent generations. In: Dornhorst A, Hadden D eds, *Diabetes and Pregnancy: An international approach to management*. Chichester: John Wiley & Sons, 1996; 361–375.
120. Harris MI. Epidemiology, correlates of NIDDM in Hispanics, whites, and blacks in the US population. *Diabetes Care* 1991; **14**:639–648.
121. Alcolado JC, Alcolado R. Importance of maternal history of non-insulin-dependent diabetic patients. *BMJ* 1991; **302**:1178–1180.
122. Cederholm J, Wbell L. Familial influence of type 1 (insulin-dependent) diabetes mellitus by relatives with either insulin-treated or type 2 (non-insulin-dependent) diabetes mellitus. *Diabetes Res* 1991; **18**:109–113.
123. Knowler WC, Pettitt DJ, Saad MF. Diabetes mellitus in the Pima Indians: incidence risk factors and pathogenesis. *Diabetes Metab Rev* 1990; **6**:1–27.
124. Grasso S, Distefano G, Messina A. Effect of glucose priming on insulin response in the premature infant. *Diabetes* 1975; **4**:291–294.

125. Sodoyez-Goffaux F, Sodoyez JC. Effects of intermittent hyperglycaemia in pregnant rats on the functional development of the beta cells of their offspring. *Diabetologia* 1976; **12**:73–76.
126. Aerts L, Vercruysse L, Van Assche FA. The endocrine pancreas in virgin and pregnant offspring of diabetic rats. *Diabests Res Clin Pract* 1997; **38**:9–19.
127. Aerts L, Sodoyez-Goffaux F, Sodoyez JC, Malaisse WJ, Van Assche FA. The diabetic intrauterine milieu has a long lasting effect on insulin secretion by β cells and on insulin uptake by target tissues. *Am J Obstet Gynecol* 1988; **159**:1287–1292.
128. Aerts L, Holemans K, Van Assche FA. Maternal diabetes during pregnancy: consequences for the offspring. *Diabetes Metab Rev* 1990; **6**:147–67.
129. Bihoreau MT, Ktorza A, Kineanyan MF, Picon L. Impaired glucose homeostatis in adult rats from hyperglycaemic mothers. *Diabetes* 1986; **35**:979–984.
130. Holemans K, Aerts L. Van Assche FA. Evidence for an insulin resistance in the adults offspring of pregnant streptozocin-diabetic rats. *Diabetologia* 1990; **34**: 81–85.

11

Obesity

P.G. KOPELMAN

Medical Unit, St Bartholomew's and the Royal London School of Medicine and Dentistry, London E1 2AD, UK

EPIDEMIOLOGICAL EVIDENCE FOR A RELATIONSHIP BETWEEN OBESITY AND TYPE 2 DIABETES

An association between obesity and type 2 diabetes has been observed in both cross-sectional and prospective epidemiological studies[1-4]. The consistency of the association across different populations, despite different measures of fatness and criteria for the diagnosis of type 2 diabetes, reflects the strength of the relationship. The additional risk of developing type 2 diabetes in obese women aged 30–55 years who were monitored for 14 years was over 40 times that for women who remained slim (BMI < 22 kg/m^2)[5]. Colditz and colleagues[6] have estimated from their data that 64% of men and 77% of women with type 2 diabetes could theoretically have had their diabetes prevented if none had had a BMI of more than 25 kg/m^2. Although there is a continuous increase in the risk of type 2 diabetes associated with increasing body mass, the relationship is complicated by other factors – the duration of the obesity, the distribution of body fat, physical activity, ethnicity, family history of type 2 diabetes and obesity, weight loss caused by diabetes and, possibly, fetal and early infant growth rate. All of these factors may contribute to the risk of type 2 diabetes or modify the effect of fatness.

In 1985, the WHO study group on diabetes named obesity as the single most important risk factor in the development of type 2 diabetes. A number of prospective studies demonstrate that obesity is related to an increased incidence of type 2 diabetes, and prevalence studies also confirm the association. Estimates of obesity, in an analysis of six different population-based

---

Type 2 Diabetes: Prediction and Prevention. Edited by Graham A. Hitman

longitudinal studies in subjects with impaired glucose tolerance, were consistently positively associated with the incidence of type 2 diabetes[7].

ASSOCIATION BETWEEN BODY FAT DISTRIBUTION AND TYPE 2 DIABETES

Cross-sectional and longitudinal studies indicate that body fat distribution is a risk factor for type 2 diabetes independent of general obesity and, in many cases, fat distribution may be more important[2,3,8–10]. However, the measurement and definition of fat distribution is not standardized and many of the terms used to describe fat distribution patterns in these studies are not well defined. In cross-sectional epidemiological studies, which have used the waist : hip ratio (WHR) as the measurement of fat distribution, a greater importance of WHR than overall fatness to the prevalence of glucose intolerance has been reported[4,8]. Data from longitudinal studies are less consistent with the relationship with type 2 diabetes between both BMI and WHR being attenuated with age. The tendency for markers of fat distribution to be more strongly associated with prevalence of type 2 diabetes than BMI could be explained by the weight loss associated with the onset of diabetes being reflected in a fall in BMI, but not by indices of central fat distribution such as WHR. This hypothesis is supported by data from Mauritius where a decrease in BMI was observed over 5 years in a population with type 2 diabetes, whereas the WHR remained unchanged[11].

Several studies additionally suggest that a moderately high level of overall obesity is required to facilitate the effects of central obesity. These may continue to rise as body fat content increases, thereby weakening the association between fat distribution and type 2 diabetes. This explains the situation found in Pima Indians and in Western Samoa where obesity itself is the greater risk[4,12]. The comparison of prevalence of type 2 diabetes among different ethnic groups points towards residual differences after adjusting for BMI and other risk factors. Such differences may be attributed to a number of factors, including regional fat distribution, increased genetic susceptibility, increased levels of other risk factors not adjusted for and methodological difficulties.

ETHNICITY, OBESITY AND TYPE 2 DIABETES

South Indians living in the UK have a higher mortality from heart disease than Caucasians. Studies have demonstrated higher mean WHRs and trunk skinfold thickness (indicative of upper body obesity) in south Asians compared with Caucasians of similar body weight[12]. The south Asian group are also characterized by higher blood pressures, higher fasting and post-oral glucose insulin levels, and higher triglyceride but lower HDL cholesterol. These results suggest that south Asians are particularly prone to the development of upper body obesity and the associated derangement of metabolic function. In contrast, subjects of Afro-Caribbean origin have a low mortality rate from coronary heart disease in spite of a high prevalence of diabetes[14]. Glucose intolerance in Afro-Caribbean subjects is twice as common compared to that in Caucasians, whereas the prevalence of probable heart disease in Afro-Caribbean men is approximately half that seen in Caucasian men. Interestingly, Afro-Caribbean men generally have less abdominal adiposity compared with Caucasians and this seems to confer an advantageous lipid profile. It is speculated than the favourable lipoprotein profile, which persists despite glucose intolerance, is related to body fat distribution in Afro-Caribbeans and explains the lower levels of cardiac mortality.

MECHANISMS LINKING OBESITY AND TYPE 2 DIABETES

ADIPOCYTE FUNCTION IN OBESITY

Fat tissue mass is dependent on the number and size of adipocytes, which have the unique characteristic of being dominated by their contents of storage fats, the triglycerides. The mass of triglycerides in an adipocyte is dependent on the balance between triglyceride influx and mobilization; the mobilized form is as free fatty acids (FFAs) and glycerol is regulated by metabolic processes under hormonal and nervous system control. Formation of new adiopocytes seems to occur when cells reach a certain size, apparently it is dependent on various factors such as age, sex and nutrition[15]. The body fat's stores are almost entirely in the form of triacylglycerol (TAG) in adipocytes. The process of fat mobilization consists of hydrolysis of the stored TAG to release non-esterified fatty acids (NEFAs) into the circulation. The key enzyme is the intracellular TAG lipase, hormone-sensitive lipase (HSL). The major form of regulation of HSL is reversible phosphorylation by an AMP-dependent protein kinase. Lipolysis is therefore stimulated by effectors that increase the activity of adenylyl cyclase in adipocytes, leading to the formation of AMP (adenosine 3′:5′-monophosphate) from ATP. The main hormonal regulator of lipolysis is insulin, which lowers adipocyte cAMP concentrations[16].

The suppression of fat mobilization occurs in normal circumstances at very low insulin concentrations. Catecholamines acting on α_2-adrenoceptors will also inhibit lipolysis[17,18] so they have dual effects on the lipolysis rates, both accelerating through β-adrenoceptors and retarding through α_2-adrenoceptors. Activity of HSL is suppressed after meals when the physiological drive is towards fat storage rather than mobilization. In the postprandial state, the enzyme lipoprotein lipase (LPL) in adipose tissue is activated by insulin, and possibly also by some gastrointestinal peptide hormone[19]. This enzyme is synthesized within adipocytes but exported to the capillary endothelial cells, where it is attached to the luminal side of the capillary wall and acts on circulating TAG in the TAG-rich lipoproteins (chylomicrons and very-low-density lipoproteins or VLDLs). LPL releases fatty acids which may be taken up into the tissue for esterification and storage as TAG. The fatty acids released by LPL action are not all taken up by adipose tissue for storage, with approximately 50% entering the systemic circulation[20]. This release of LPL-derived fatty acids is dependent upon the insulin response to the meal and the sensitivity of LPL activation to insulin and other hormones.

The potential differences in FFA metabolism seen between lean and obese subjects may reflect a combination of factors: the antilipolytic effectiveness of insulin in obesity; the relationship of FFA release to the amount of body fat, and the lipolytic responsiveness of obese individuals to catecholamines. Adipocytes from various body regions differ from one another in many respects, in particular fat cell size, and basal lipolysis varies in adipocytes from omental, abdominal, subcutaneous and gluteal thigh depots[21]. The basal release of FFAs from adipose tissue to meet lean body mass energy needs is greater in women who are obese in the upper body than in obese women with lower body fat distribution and non-obese women. Differences in the ability of insulin to suppress and of catecholamines to stimulate lipolysis also varies according to fat distribution irrespective of the overall degree of adiposity[22].

In both men and women, the lipolytic response to noradrenaline, which acts via α_2- and β-adrenoceptors, is more marked in abdominal than in gluteal or femoral tissues[23]. An analysis of the usual pattern of male fat distribution (greater abdominal fat accumulation) suggests that this results from a greater α_2 activity in the abdominal tissue of men. Radioligand binding studies of β-adrenergic antagonists uniformly show twice as many β-adrenergic-binding sites in abdominal adipocytes as in femoral adipocytes. The pathogenic role of visceral β_3-adrenoceptors in obesity has recently been elucidated. Lonnqvist and colleagues[24] studied the responsiveness of isolated omental fat cells from obese and non-obese subjects to adrenergic-subtype receptor antagonists by measuring the rate of FFA and glycerol response. They found that the visceral fat cells from the obese subjects were highly responsive to noradrenaline stimulation. This appeared to result mainly from an enhanced lipolytic response and not from FFA re-utilization. The main finding was the markedly augmented sensitivity and coupling efficiency of the β_3-adrenoceptors; the authors suggested that this enhanced β_3-adrenoreceptor activity was caused by an increased receptor number in obese subjects. In contrast, the net lipolytic response to adrenaline is reduced in upper-obese women compared with lower-obese and non-obese women.

For lower-obese women to maintain appropriate FFA availability despite increasing fatness, there must be downregulation of lipolysis to prevent FFA release[22]. Martin and colleagues[25] measured FFA release from leg, non-leg and splanchnic adipose tissue in obese women of differing body fat distribution. Contrasting differences were observed in lipolytic activity of splanchnic fat between these obese women with predominantly upper body fat and those with lower body fat. This difference was emphasized by the finding of similar FFA release from leg fat in the two groups.

There is little published work addressing possible differences in adipocyte function between subjects from different ethnic backgrounds. An investigation of the ability of insulin to stimulate glucose transport and suppress lipolysis suggests that ethnicity is important[26]. In this study, abdominal and gluteal adipocytes from white women with upper body obesity were less sensitive, in vitro, to insulin-stimulated glucose transport and lipolytic suppression compared with adipocytes from black women of similar body weight and fat distribution. The findings support the epidemiological evidence that black women, with upper body obesity, fare better in terms of insulin resistance and dyslipidaemia than their white counterparts, and confirm the need for additional studies examining men and women from other ethnic groups.

The important metabolic interpretation of these data is the apparently elevated rate of lipolysis in visceral fat cells resulting largely from increased β_3 activity and partly from α_2-adrenoceptor activity. As a consequence, more FFAs are released into the portal system, with a detrimental action on hepatic glucose uptake and peripheral insulin sensitivity. This is discussed further in the next section.

INSULIN SECRETION IN OBESITY

Obesity is characterized by an elevated fasting plasma insulin and an exaggerated insulin response to an oral glucose load[27]. However, obesity and the regional distribution of body fat influence glucose metabolism through independent, but additive, mechanisms. Kissebah and colleagues[28] have demonstrated that increasing upper-body obesity is accompanied by a progressive increase in the glucose and insulin response to an oral glucose challenge. The in vivo insulin sensitivity in individuals was assessed further by determining the steady-state plasma glucose (SSPG) and insulin (SSPI) attained during a simultaneous intravenous infusion of somatostatin, insulin and dextrose. As endogenous insulin production was suppressed by somatostatin, and the SSPI was comparable in each situation, SSPG directly measured the subjects' ability to dispose of an intravenous glucose load under the same insulin stimulus; SSPG can be taken as an index of insulin resistance. The results showed a positive correlation between increasing upper-body obesity and SSPG. After adjustment for the effects of overall fatness (percentage ideal body weight), upper-body obesity remained independently correlated with SSPG, suggesting that the location of body fat is an independent factor that influences the degree of insulin sensitivity and, in turn, metabolic profile.

Measurement of portal plasma insulin levels (as an index of insulin secretion) shows similar levels in upper-body and lower-body obesity, although hepatic insulin extraction, both as a base level and during stimulation by intravenous or oral glucose, is reduced in upper-body obesity[29]. As a consequence, post-hepatic insulin delivery is increased in upper-body obesity, leading to more marked peripheral insulin concentrations. Studies of insulin sensitivity and responsiveness of skeletal muscle, and the relationship to overall glucose disposal in premenopausal women, with varying body fat distribution, have revealed a significant decline as upper-body fatness increases[30]. Insulin-stimulated activity of the glucose-6-phosphate-independent form of glycogen synthase (GSI) has been measured in quadricep muscle biopsies taken during an infusion of somatostatin–insulin–dextrose. Despite comparable degrees of SSPI in all women, significant reductions in percentage GSI were seen as the degree of upper-body fatness increased, and this was accompanied by decreased efficiency in insulin-stimulated glucose disposal (reflected by increasing SSPG at similar SSPI levels). Furthermore, a significant trend was reported for a decreased number of cellular insulin receptors associated with increasing upper-body fatness, which was in turn associated in some subjects with reduced glucose disposal during supramaximal insulin stimulation. Such findings suggest a defect both at the level of the insulin receptor and in post-receptor events.

Abdominal visceral adipose tissue is more sensitive to lipolytic stimuli than subcutaneous fat, although it is less sensitive to the inhibitory action of insulin; this appears to be associated with a low density of insulin receptors. Hyperinsulinaemia of obesity inhibits mainly lipolysis of insulin-sensitive subcutaneous adipocytes and may accentuate the fraction of systemic FFAs originating from visceral fat[31,32]. In addition, elevated portal concentrations of FFAs, produced by active visceral adipocytes, result in the liver being exposed to excessive FFA concentrations. The excessive visceral fat lipolysis may create a vicious chain of events with insulin resistance in liver and skeletal muscle, resulting in additional systemic insulin resistance and a further release of insulin to overcome this resistance. Leptin may be a contributory factor to the insulin resistance of obesity[33]. In obese patients, plasma leptin levels rise in parallel with body fat mass and insulin resistance. Recent reports have shown that plasma leptin levels correlate with insulin resistance independently of obesity, and leptin has been shown to inhibit aspects of insulin action on heptocytes in vitro, resulting in enhanced gluconeogenesis[34].

INSULIN SECRETION IN TYPE 2 DIABETES

The development of impaired glucose tolerance will, with time, further impair insulin action in relation to carbohydrate and lipid metabolism with resulting hyperglycaemia and raised NEFA concentration. This adds on to the effect of obesity as previously described. The further blunting of insulin's normal ability to suppress hepatic gluconeogenesis and glycogenolysis results in a sustained rise in hepatic glucose output, which contributes to an increase in basal blood glucose levels, and diminished glycogen synthesis and glucose oxidation. These defects in glucose handling lead to the exaggerated postprandial hyperglycaemia observed in type 2 diabetes. The loss of insulin's antilipolytic action results in an even greater breakdown of triglycerides in adipocytes, liberating glycerol and FFAs. The high blood NEFA levels accentuate hyperinsulinaemia which, in turn, will further decrease hepatic clearance of insulin. Chronically elevated blood glucose and NEFA levels eventually impair, rather than stimulate, β-cell function and contribute to the eventual decline in insulin secretion seen in type 2 diabetes (see below).

Insulin resistance in type 2 diabetes primarily affects post-receptor mechanisms rather than the insulin receptor itself[35]. The overall insulin receptors numbers may be reduced on target tissues, possibly through downregulation in response to hyperinsulinaemia. A variety of post-receptor defects has been identified in type 2 diabetes but most appear to be secondary to the metabolic disturbance caused by this diabetes.

β-CELL DYSFUNCTION IN TYPE 2 DIABETES

Longitudinal studies confirm that insulin resistance precedes β-cell failure by several years and that insulin levels fall at the transition from impaired glucose tolerance to overt type 2 diabetes. The rise and subsequent decline in function of the β cell can be represented by a 'bell-shaped' curve, with increased insulin production in the early stages being succeeded by a functional plateau with the development of impaired glucose tolerance, before a decline into failure and the onset of diabetes[36]. The causes of β-cell failure are presently uncertain and likely to be various. Amylin (islet amyloid polypeptide or IAPP), which is co-released by the β cell with insulin, can polymerize to form insoluble amyloid fibrils that may accumulate within the islets; these may contribute to β-cell failure in patients with type 2 diabetes[37]. Another possible mechanism is a genetic basis. The normal pulsatile pattern of basal insulin secretion is disturbed in non-diabetic, first-order relatives of some patients with type 2 diabetes[38]. Malnutrition in early life has, in addition, been suggested to impair both insulin secretion and insulin action[39].

INFLUENCE OF STEROID HORMONES

The circulating cortisol level is an important influence on insulin sensitivity and may be of particular importance in subjects with upper-body obesity. Obesity may be characterized by an increase in cortisol production rate and increased peripheral clearance, which occurs via binding to glucoreceptors present in gluococorticoid-responding tissue. Cortisol has effects on both lipid accumulation and mobilization. It inhibits the antilipolytic effect of insulin in human adipocytes, and this may be particularly pronounced in visceral abdominal fat[40]. It also has a permissive effect on lipid mobilization stimulated by catecholamine. Enlarged visceral adipocytes, as found in abdominal obesity, could be the site where this occurs because such tissue appears to have a higher density of glucocorticoid receptors compared with adipose tissue[41,42]. Abdominal subcutaneous adipose tissue demonstrates a higher expression of cortisol-induced LPL as well as a higher density of glucocorticoid receptors than femoral subcutaneous adipose tissue. Furthermore, there is a higher LPL activity in visceral compared with subcutaneous adipose tissue in both men and women[43]. This could be an explanation for the functional hypercortisolism associated with abdominal obesity in subjects who are only moderately overweight. There is a close analogy between upper body obesity and Cushing's syndrome, because both conditions are characterized by hypercortisolism and excessive visceral fat accumulation[44]. Moreover, both have similar consequences – an increase in plasma cortisol leading to insulin insensitivity and glucose intolerance, and increase in hepatic gluconeogenesis, reduced hepatic insulin uptake and insulin resistance in skeletal muscle.

DYSLIPIDAEMIA OF OBESITY AND TYPE 2 DIABETES

Hyperinsulinaemia and insulin resistance are both significant correlates of a dyslipoproteinaemic state which is characteristic of both upper-body obesity and type 2 diabetes. The lipolysis of insulin-resistant visceral adipocytes results in predictable and characteristic changes. These are reflected by an elevated fasting plasma triglyceride concentration, reduced high-density lipoprotein (HDL)-cholesterol, marginal elevations of cholesterol and low-density lipoprotein (LDL)-cholesterol concentrations and increased numbers of apo-B-carrying lipoproteins[45,46]. Measurement of the volume of visceral fat, using computed tomography (CT), confirms a close interrelationship of the volume of visceral adipose tissue, elevation of plasma triglycerides and deceased concentrations of HDL_1- and HDL_2-cholesterol in both men and women[47]. Moreover, these levels are comparable in men and women when matched for similar degrees of visceral adiposity[48].

The elevated plasma NEFA concentrations have a number of deleterious actions: plasma NEFAs are the major substrate for hepatic TAG synthesis and there is a close correlation between NEFA and VLDL-TAG concentrations or turnover rates[49]. This increased turnover appears to alter the balance between intracellular degradation of newly synthesized hepatic lipoprotein-B (apo-B) and its secretion as VLDL. The increased availability of NEFAs not only increases VLDL-TAG secretion but also the number of VLDL particles secreted[50]. This may be particularly important in the postprandial period. Insulin has an acute suppressive action on both NEFA supply to the liver and hepatic VLDL secretion in the postprandial period. In cultured hepatocytes, insulin inhibits VLDL secretion[51]. This action reduces both the competition for clearance and the postprandial rise in TAG concentration. A failure of normal suppression of the NEFA supply, seen in subjects with increased intra-abdominal fat tissue and particular with type 2 diabetes, leads to a sustained production of VLDL and an impaired clearance of TAG-rich lipoproteins in the postprandial period[15].

Plasma NEFAs arise in the postprandial period from both intracellular lipolysis and the action of LPL in capillaries. A failure of the entrapment of fatty acids in adipose tissue during the action of LPL on chylomicron-TAG may be an important mechanism leading to increased VLDL secretion[50]. A further consequence is an increase in LDL particles – VLDL is a precursor of LDL – but not necessarily an increase in LDL-cholesterol concentration because, in the presence of high VLDL-TAG concentrations, LDL particles are lipid depleted and therefore more dense. An elevation of total plasma apo-B concentration is a frequent association with upper-body obesity and type 2 diabetes which, by itself, heightens the risk of coronary heart disease[52]. Small, dense, LDL particles may be oxidized and/or glycated; such processes enhance their atherogenic potential.

Other factors that contribute to the dyslipoproteinaemia in upper-body obesity include glucocorticoids, which stimulate VLDL and apo-B production, decrease the activity of the LDL receptor and contribute to the insulin-resistant state[53].

FROM OBESITY TO TYPE 2 DIABETES

DIABETOGENIC EFFECTS OF OBESITY

Worsening of obesity is accompanied by a decline in whole-body insulin sensitivity, with abdominal fat deposition being particular associated with impaired glucose tolerance. Moreover, the deleterious metabolic effects of altered regulation of adipocyte function, observed particularly in visceral obesity, will also lead to the development of impaired glucose tolerance and type 2 diabetes (Figure 11.1).

In obesity the rate of NEFA turnover/unit lean body mass is increased[54]. The ability of insulin to suppress NEFA release in vivo is diminished in

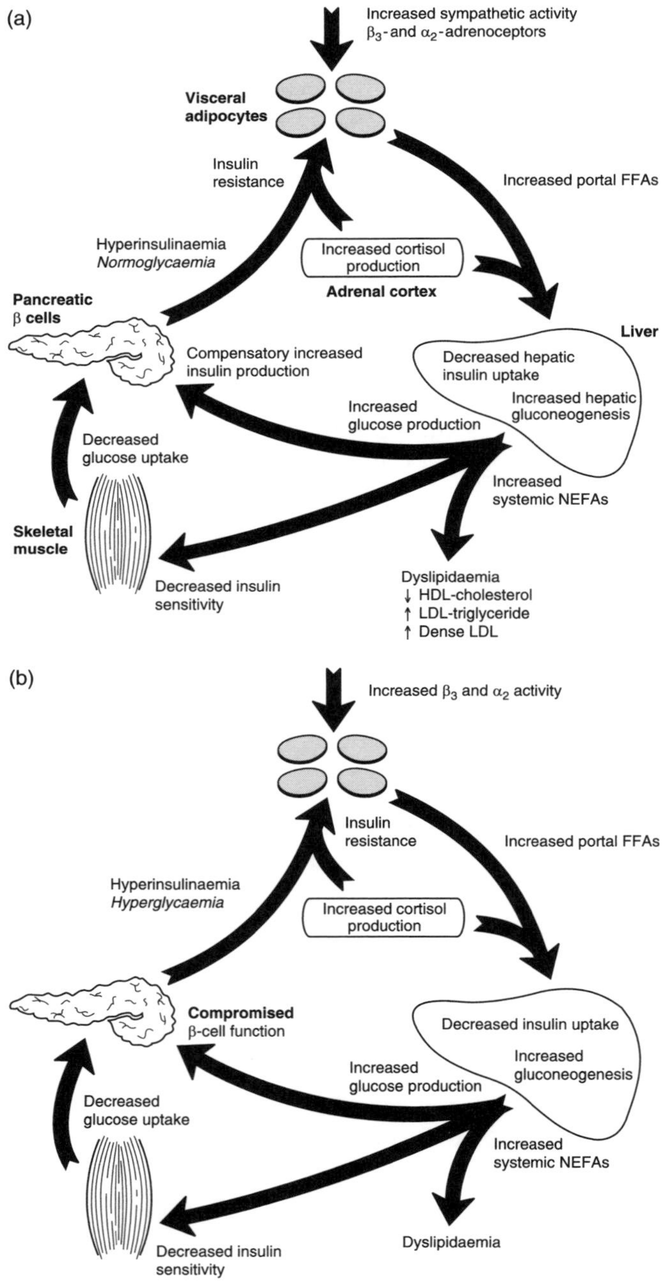
(a)
Increased sympathetic activity
β_3- and α_2-adrenoceptors
Visceral adipocytes
Insulin resistance
Increased portal FFAs
Hyperinsulinaemia
Normoglycaemia
Increased cortisol production
Adrenal cortex
Pancreatic β cells
Liver
Compensatory increased insulin production
Decreased hepatic insulin uptake
Increased hepatic gluconeogenesis
Increased glucose production
Decreased glucose uptake
Increased systemic NEFAs
Skeletal muscle
Decreased insulin sensitivity
Dyslipidaemia
↓ HDL-cholesterol
↑ LDL-triglyceride
↑ Dense LDL
(b)
Increased β_3 and α_2 activity
Insulin resistance
Increased portal FFAs
Hyperinsulinaemia
Hyperglycaemia
Increased cortisol production
Compromised β-cell function
Decreased insulin uptake
Increased gluconeogenesis
Increased glucose production
Decreased glucose uptake
Increased systemic NEFAs
Decreased insulin sensitivity
Dyslipidaemia

obese subjects as a result of insulin insensitivity of both lipolytic processes and fatty acid re-esterification. Therefore, the plasma NEFA concentration increases as insulin action becomes more and more deficient[55]. A cycle of events is thereby entered, with increasing insulin resistance resulting in increasing NEFA plasma concentration which, in turn, contributes to diminishing insulin sensitivity. The defect in insulin sensitivity observed in skeletal muscle may accentuate the defects in the regulation of lipolysis.

A number of mechanisms also link NEFA supply and impairment of glucose utilization with the supply of NEFA to the liver, this is an important determinant of the rate of hepatic glucose production. The elevation in plasma NEFA concentration, particularly postprandially when they are usually suppressed, will lead to an inappropriate maintenance of glucose production and an impairment of glucose utilization (impaired glucose tolerance). These mechanisms may be the critical links leading from obesity to the development of type 2 diabetes. The progression to type 2 diabetes may be enhanced by the suppressive effects of high NEFA concentrations on insulin secretion, or even by potentially 'toxic' effects of NEFA and sustained hyperglycaemia on pancreatic β cells[56]. A further mechanism linking increased plasma NEFA concentrations to insulin resistance is the reduced hepatic clearance of insulin – increasing delivery of NEFA to the liver reduces insulin binding to the hepatocytes. In normal circumstances, the liver removes 40% of insulin secreted from the pancreas; an impairment of this process will have a significant effect on peripheral (systemic) insulin concentrations, which contributes to hyperinsulinaemia, and leads to further downregulation of insulin receptors and increasing insulin resistance[57].

As has been described, in the initial phases of this process, the pancreas can respond by maintaining a state of compensatory hyperinsulinaemia which prevents gross decompensation of glucose tolerance. With ever-increasing plasma concentrations of NEFA, the insulin-resistant individual cannot continue to maintain this state of compensatory hyperinsulinaemia,

---

Figure 11.1. (a) Elevated rates of lipolysis in visceral adipocytes, resulting from increased β_3- and α_2-adrenoceptor activity, and insulin insensitivity (enhanced by increased cortisol production), lead to elevated free fatty acids (FFAs) being released into the portal system. This has a detrimental action on hepatic insulin uptake with an enhancement of gluconeogenesis. This, in turn, results in increased hepatic glucose production, increased systemic concentrations of non-esterified fatty acids (NEFAs) and alterations in plasma lipid profile (decreased HDL-cholesterol, increased LDL-triglyceride and increased small density LDL-cholesterol). All of these factors contribute to the prevailing systemic hyperinsulinaemia and decreased skeletal muscle insulin sensitivity. Initially, the pancreatic β cells respond with a compensatory increase in insulin production to maintain normoglycaemia but thereby creating a vicious cycle of events. Eventually (b) the insulin-resistant individual cannot maintain this state of compensatory hyperinsulinaemia and hyperglycaemia prevails.

and in time hyperglycaemia prevails. Thus, increasing NEFA concentrations, associated with a small decline in insulin secretion, will further decrease glucose uptake by muscle, increase hepatic NEFA oxidation and stimulate gluconeogenesis. This has an additive effect on plasma elevations of NEFA and glucose which, in turn, further compromise β-cell function[58].

THE EFFECT OF WEIGHT REDUCTION

The beneficial action of weight reduction suggests that many, if not all, of the deleterious events associated with upper-body obesity are a consequence, rather than a cause, of excessive visceral adipose tissue. Calorie restriction and resulting weight loss in obese diabetic patients markedly improves metabolic control, by leading to improved insulin action in both liver and muscle and, if initiated early enough, improved β-cell response to stimulation of insulin secretion.

Weight reduction in women with upper-body obesity has a marked effect on the regulation of lipolysis. There is an approximately fivefold increase in the sensitivity to noradrenaline with a specific effect on adrenoreceptor subtype – there is increased sensitivity to β_2-receptors but no change in β_1- or α_2-receptors. However, no change occurs in the numbers of β_2-receptor-binding sites, which suggests the possible facilitation of G proteins[59]. More recently, a similar pattern of increased sensitivity has been reported for β_3-adrenoreceptors[24]. Weight loss is accompanied by a decrease in circulating insulin levels and a fall in plasma noradrenaline. The beneficial effects of these changes are a decrease in basal lipolysis (with decreased HSL function) and an increase in sensitivity to catecholamine stimulation of lipolysis. Thus, weight reduction appears to restore a more efficient regulation of lipolysis with less FFAs being released at rest and lower catecholamine levels required for lipolysis activation.

REFERENCES

1. Hartz AJ, Rupley DC Jr, Kalkhoff RD, Rimm AA. Relationship of obesity to diabetes: influence of obesity level and body fat distribution. *Prev Med* 1983; **12**:351–7.
2. Haffner SM, Stern MP, Hazuda HP et al. Do upper body and centralised adiposity measure different aspects of regional body fat distribution? Relationship to non-insulin-dependent diabetes mellitus in Mexican Americans and non-Hispanic whites. *Diabetes* 1987; **36**:43–51.
3. Haffner SM, Stern MP, Mitchell BD, Hazuda HP, Patterson JK. Incidence of type II diabetes in Mexican Americans predicted by fasting insulin and glucose levels, obesity and body fat distribution. *Diabetes* 1990; **39**:283–8.
4. Knowler WC, Pettit DJ, Saad MF et al. Obesity in the Pima Indians: its magnitude and relationship with diabetes. *Am J Clin Nutr* 1991; **53**:1543S–51S.

5. Colditz GA, Willett WC, Stamfer MJ et al. Weight as a risk factor for clinical diabetes in women. *Am J Epidemiol* 1990; **132**:501–13.
6. Chan JM, Stamfer MJ, Ribb EB, Willet WC, Colditz GA. Obesity, fat distribution and weight gain as risk factors for clinical diabetes in men. *Diabetes Care* 1994; **17** 961–9.
7. Edelstein SL, Knowler WC, Bain RP et al. Predictors of progression from impaired glucose tolerance to NIDDM: an analysis of six prospective studies. *Diabetes* 1997; **46**:701–10.
8. McKeigue PM, Pierpoint T, Ferries, JE, Marmot MG. Relationship of glucose intolerance and hyperinsulinaemia to body fat pattern in south Asians and Europeans. *Diabetologia* 1992; **35**:785–91.
9. Collins VR, Dowse GK, Toelupe PM et al. Increasing prevalence of NIDDM in the Pacific island population of Western Samoa over a 13 year period. *Diabetes Care* 1994; **17**:288–96.
10. Lundgren H, Bengtsson C, Blohme G et al. Adiposity and adipose tissue distribution in relation to incidence of diabetes in women: results from a prospective population study in Gothenburg, Sweden. *Int J Obesity* 1989; **13**:413–23.
11. Hodges AM, Dowse GK, Gareeboo H et al. Incidence, increasing prevalence, and predictors of change in obesity and fat distribution over 5 years in the rapidly developing population of Mauritius. *Int J Obesity* 1996; **20**:137–46.
12. Hodges AM, Zimmet PZ. The epidemiology of obesity. *Baillière's Clin Endocrinol Metab* 199; **8**:577–99.
13. McKeigue PM, Shah B, Marmot MG. Relation of central obesity and insulin resistance with high diabetes prevalence and cardiovascular risk in South Asians. *Lancet* 1991; **337**:382–6.
14. Chaturvedi N, McKeigue PM, Marmot MG. Relationship of glucose intolerance to coronary risk in Afro-Caribbeans compared with Europeans. *Diabetologia* 1992; **35**:785–91.
15. Frayn KN, Williams CM, Arner P. Are increased plasma non-esterified fatty acid concentrations a risk marker for coronary heart disease and other chronic diseases? *Clin Sci* 1996; **90**:243–53.
16. Smith CJ, Vasta V, Degerman E, Belfrage P, Manganiello VC. Hormone-sensitive cyclic GMP-inhibited cyclic AMP phosphodiesterase in rat adipocytes. Regulation of insulin- and cAMP-dependent activation by phosphorylation. *J Biol Chem* 1991; **266**:13385–90.
17. Lafontan M, Berlan M. Fat cell adrenergic receptors and the control of white and brown fat cell function. *J Lipid Res* 1993; **34**:1057–91.
18. Castan I, Valet P, Quideau N et al. Antilipolytic effects of α_2-agonists, neuropeptide Y, adenosine, and PGE_1 in mammal adipocytes. *Am J Physiol* 1994; **266**:1141–7.
19. Ong JM, Kern PA. Effect of feeding and obesity on lipoprotein lipase activity, immunoreactive protein and messenger RNA levels in human adipose tissue. *J Clin Invest* 1989; **84**:305–11.
20. Eaton RP, Berman M, Steinberg D. Kinetic studies of plasma free fatty acid and triglyceride metabolism in man. *J Clin Invest* 1969; **48**:1560–79.
21. Martin ML, Jensen MD. Effects of body fat distribution on regional lipolysis in obesity. *J Clin Invest* 1991; **88**:609–13.
22. Reynisdottir S, Ellerfeldt K, Wahrenberg H, Lithell H, Arner P. Multiple lipolysis defects in insulin resistance [metabolic] syndrome. *J Clin Invest* 1994; **93**:2590–9.
23. Krotkiewski M, Bjorntorp P, Sjostrom L, Smith U. Impact of obesity on metabolism in men and women: importance of regional adipose tissue distribution. *J Clin Invest* 1983; **72**:1150–62.

24. Lonnqvist F, Thorne A, Nilsell K, Hoffstedt J, Arner P. A pathogenic role of visceral fat β_3-adrenoceptors in obesity. *J Clin Invest* 1995; **95**:1109–16.
25. Martin ML, Jensen MD. Effects of body fat distribution on regional lipolysis in obesity. *J Clin Invest* 1991; **88**:609–13.
26. Dowling HJ, Fried SK, Pi-Sunyer FX. Insulin resistance in adipocytes of obese women; effects of body fat distribution and race. *Metabolism* 1995; **44**:987–95.
27. Kolterman OG, Insel J, Sackow M, Olefsky M. Mechanisms of insulin resistance in human obesity. *J Clin Invest* 1980; **65**:1272–84.
28. Kissebah AH, Vydelingum N, Murray R. Relation of body fat distribution to metabolic complications of obesity. *J Clin Invest* 1982; **54**:254–60.
29. Peiris AN, Mueller RA, Smith GA. Splanchnic insulin metabolism in obesity: influence of body fat distribution. *J Clin Invest* 1986; **78**:1648–57.
30. Evans DJ, Murray R, Kissebah AH. Relationship between skeletal muscle insulin resistance, insulin-mediated glucose disposal and insulin binding effects of obesity and body fat topography. *J Clin Invest* 1984; **74**:1515–25.
31. Rebuffe-Scrive M, Krotkiewski M, Elfverson J, Bjorntorp P. Muscle and adipose tissue morphology and metabolism in Cushing's syndrome. *J Clin Endocrinol Metab* 1988; **67**:1122–8.
32. Rebuffe-Scrive M, Andersson B, Olbe L, Bjorntorp P. Metabolism of adipose tissue in intraabdominal depots of non-obese men and women. *Metabolism* 1989; **38**:453–61.
33. Considine RV, Sinha MK, Heiman ML et al. Serum immunoreactive-leptin concentrations in normal-weight and obese humans. *N Engl J Med* 1996; **334**:292–5.
34. Cohen B, Novick D, Rubenstein M. Modulation of insulin activities by leptin. *Science* 1996; **274**:1185–8.
35. Maratos-Flier E, Goldstein BJ, Kahn CR. Insulin receptor and post-receptor mechanisms. In: Pickup JC, Williams G, eds. *Textbook of Diabetes*, 2nd edn. Oxford: Blackwell Science, 1997; 10.1–10.22.
36. O'Rahilly SP, Nugent Z, Rudenski AS et al. Beta-cell dysfunction rather than insulin insensitivity is the primary defect in familial type-2 diabetes. *Lancet* 1986; **ii**:360–4.
37. Bennett WM, Smith DM, Bloom SR. Islet amyloid polypeptide: does it play a pathophysiological role in the development of diabetes? *Diabetes Med* 1994; **11**:825–9.
38. Hattersley AT. Maturity-onset diabetes of the young. In: Pickup JC, Williams G, eds. *Textbook of Diabetes*, 2nd edn. Oxford: Blackwell Science, 1997; 22.1–22.10.
39. Hales CN, Barker DJP. Type 2 (non-insulin dependent) diabetes mellitus: the thrifty phenotype hypothesis. *Diabetologia* 1992; **35**:595–601.
40. Cigolin M, Smith U. Human adipose tissue in culture. VIII. Studies on the insulin-antagonistic effect of glucocorticoids. *Metabolism* 1979; **28**:520–10.
41. Bronnegard M, Arner P, Hellstrom L et al. Glucocorticoid receptor messenger ribonucleic acid in different regions of human adipose tissue. *Endocrinology* 1990; **127**:1689–96.
42. Rebuffe-Scrive M, Lundholm K, Bjorntorp P. Glucocorticoid hormone binding to human adipose tissue. *Eur J Clin Invest* 1985; **15**:267–71.
43. Bjorntorp P, Ottosson M, Rebuffe-Scrive M, Xu X. Regional obesity and steroid hormone interactions in human adipose tissue. *UCLA Symp Cell Biol* 1990; **132**:147–58.
44. Mayo-Smith W, Hayes CW, Biller BMK. Body fat distribution measured with CT: correlations in healthy subjects, anorexia nervosa and patients with Cushing's syndrome. *Radiology* 1989; **170**:515–18.

45. Laws A, Reaven GM. Evidence for an independent relationship between insulin resistance and fasting plasma HDL-cholesterol, triglyceride and insulin concentrations. *J Intern Med* 1992; **231**:25–30.
46. Kissebah AH, Peiris AN. Biology of regional body fat distribution: relationship to non-insulin-dependent diabetes mellitus. *Diabetes Metab Rev* 1989; **5**:83–109.
47. Pouliot MC, Despres JP, Nadeau A et al. Visceral obesity in men. Associations with glucose tolerance, plasma insulin and lipoprotein levels. *Diabetes* 1992; **41**:826–34.
48. Despres JP. Dyslipidaemia and obesity. *Baillière's Clin Endocrinol Metab* 1994; **8**:629–60.
49. Byrne CD, Brindle NPJ, Wang TWM, Hales CN. Interaction of non-esterified fatty acid and insulin control of triacylglycerol secretion by Hep G2 cells. *Biochem J* 1991; **280**:99–104.
50. Sniderman A, Cainflone K. Metabolic disruptions in the adipocyte–hepatocyte fatty acid axis as the cause of HyperapoB. *Int J Obesity* 1995; **19**(suppl 1): S27–33.
51. Durrington PN, Newton RS, Weinstein DB, Steinberg D. Effects of insulin and glucose on very low density lipoprotein triglyceride secretion by cultured rat hepatocytes. *J Clin Invest* 1982; **70**:63–73.
52. Sniderman A, Shapiro S, Marpole D, Skinner B, Teng B, Kwiterovich POJ. Association of coronary atherosclerosis with hypobetalipoproteinemia [increased protein but normal cholesterol levels in human plasma low density (beta) lipoproteins]. *Proc Natl Acad Sci USA* 1980; **77**:604–8.
53. Brindley DN, Rolland Y. Possible connections between stress, diabetes, obesity, hypertension, and altered metabolism that may result in atherosclerosis. *Clin Sci* 1989; **77**:453–61.
54. Campbell PJ, Carlson MG, Nurijhan N. Fat metabolism in human obesity. *Am J Physiol* 1994; **266**:E600–5.
55. Coppack SW, Evans RD, Fisher RM et al. Adipose tissue metabolism in obesity: lipase action in vivo before and after a mixed meal. *Metabolism* 1992; **41**:264–72.
56. Unger RH. Lipotoxicity in the pathogenesis of obesity-dependent NIDDM. Genetic and clinical implications. *Diabetes* 1995; **44**:863–70.
57. Svedberg J, Bjorntorp P, Smith U, Lonnroth P. Free fatty acids inhibition of insulin binding, degradation and action in isolated ra hepatocytes. *Diabetes* 1990; **39**:570–4.
58. Reaven GM. The fourth musketeer – from Alexander Dumas to Claude Bernard. *Diabetologia* 1995; **38**:3–13.
59. Reynisdottir S, Langin D, Carlstrom K, Holm C, Rossner S, Arner P. Effects of weight reduction on the regulation of lipolysis in adipocytes of women with upper-body obesity. *Clin Sci* 1995; **89**:421–9.

Part D

Prevention

12

Primary Prevention of Non-communicable Diseases

J. TUOMILEHTO

Diabetes and Genetic Epidemiology Unit, Department of Epidemiology and Health Promotion, National Public Health Institute, Mannerheimintie 166, FIN 00300 Helsinki, Finland

Cardiovascular disease, diabetes and other non-communicable diseases (NCDs) form the major health burden in the industrialized countries, and are a rapidly growing problem elsewhere. At the same time they represent the area where the greatest health gains can be achieved. In most of the developed world, three out of four deaths are the result of cardiovascular disease (CVD), cancer, accidents and other violent causes. As far as morbidity is concerned, disorders such as diabetes, hypertension, chronic respiratory disease, osteoporosis and some musculoskeletal disorders are also major problems.

Extensive medical research over the past few decades has probed the causes and mechanisms of these non-communicable diseases. There have been large epidemiological studies within and between populations, basic biochemical and animal studies, intervention trials, and large-scale community-based, preventive studies. Findings from this research have indisputably revealed that NCDs, or events leading to them, have their roots in unhealthy lifestyles or adverse physical and social environments. The major lifestyle factors implicated are unhealthy nutrition, smoking, physical inactivity, excess use of alcohol and psychosocial stress. Genetic susceptibility also plays an important role in the development of NCDs, particularly by interacting with the environmental exposures.

Although there is still much to learn, a wealth of knowledge for effective preventive action has already accumulated. Actually, the amount of information is so extensive that the main question in prevention of some NCDs is no longer 'what should be done?', but 'how should it be done?'.

Type 2 Diabetes: Prediction and Prevention. Edited by Graham A. Hitman

The key issue is indeed how best to apply our existing knowledge to effective prevention in real life.

FEATURES OF NON-COMMUNICABLE DISEASES

MULTIFACTORIAL AETIOLOGY

The environmental factors associated with the onset of disease do not seem to be very different for specific NCDs; they include cigarette smoking, high saturated fat intake, a low ratio of polyunsaturated to saturated fats in the diet, low fibre intake, high salt intake, low vitamin C and E intake, lack of physical activity, etc. Furthermore, these factors are also important for the successful resolution and prevention of severe complications related to NCDs. Therefore, not only does the prevention of these diseases have a common basis, but the treatment of these NCDs also has much in common, especially with regard to non-pharmacological therapeutic approaches, which are always aimed at reducing the levels of causal factors of diseases. Pharmacological treatment, in contrast, typically aims at controlling only the symptoms of the particular disease or blocking its natural history with actions that may sometimes even precipitate another disease, e.g. some forms of antihypertensive drug therapy may have a diabetogenic effect[1].

The concept of the multifactorial aetiology of NCDs is necessary to understand so that efficient prevention actions against them can be implemented. The central aspects of this issue are:

- Several simultaneous risk factors are required for disease to develop, even though in some extreme situations one factor may be enough.
- When present together, some risk factors operate additively, whereas others may increase the risk multiplicatively.
- Different risk factor combinations can result in development of the same disease within the population.
- The relative importance of some risk factors may vary between populations.
- Most of the risk factors and their combinations are quantitative traits with no evident threshold at which the risk starts to increase; the lower the risk factor profile the lower the probability of disease developing.
- Although the relative risk of NCDs increases with increasing risk factor levels, most incident cases of NCDs occur at intermediate levels of each risk factor.
- Efficient prevention of NCDs requires simultaneous control of several risk factors, in individuals and in populations.

In general, there is no single cause for any NCD. Nevertheless, for most NCDs a single risk factor can be identified that has the largest impact on development of the disease, e.g. smoking for lung cancer, high blood pressure for stroke; obesity for type 2 diabetes, low fibre intake for colon cancer, etc. Sometimes such a strong risk factor can on its own be the critical factor for development of the disease, although not a sufficient one. For instance, smoking is by far the most critical risk factor for lung cancer, but its effect is modified by dietary intake of oxidants and antioxidants. Extremely high blood pressure, say over 220/130 mmHg, can result in a stroke, or extremely high serum cholesterol concentration, say over 10 mmol/L, can result in acute myocardial infarction, but these situations are very rare, almost anecdotal, in the community.

Because not all subjects who are at high risk of developing an NCD have the same underlying risk factors, a prevention programme based on a single risk factor will never be efficient. Nevertheless, to modify any of the risk factors for NCDs, it is necessary to design and implement specific measures for this effect, although it should be done as part of a more comprehensive programme.

One of the most important issues in prediction and prevention of NCDs is that most of the risk factors are related quantitatively to disease development. The relative risk increases with increase in the level of risk factor in a linear or exponential manner. However, as the number of individuals who have a moderately elevated level of any risk factor is by far the largest, the absolute number of NCD events in this category is also the largest. Moreover, if one compares the probability of an incident event of any NCD in a person who has an extremely high value for just a single risk factor, it is the same as in a person who has only slightly raised levels in multiple risk factors. As, in the latter case, none of the risk factors is markedly elevated, it has been usual in clinical medicine to tell the person simply that his or her risk is not raised.

AN INTEGRATED APPROACH TO PREVENTION

Research into the aetiology of diseases has relied largely on an approach in which each disease has been considered separately. This approach has proved useful in defining the aetiology, treatment and potential for prevention of infectious diseases, genetic disorders and some relatively rare NCDs, but it has not solved the problem of the major NCDs that account for more than two-thirds of the world's mortality and severe morbidity. Typically, the major NCDs (such as cancer, CVD and diabetes) have a multifactorial aetiology, involving several environmental factors that interact with each other and with certain host factors, e.g. genetic susceptibility. It has been shown in many studies[2–7], that several NCDs have common aetiological factors, and this fact forms the scientific basis for the 'integrated approach' for prevention and control of NCDs[8]. Although these diseases were considered earlier as an indication of affluence, it is clear that today NCDs form a major public health problem in developing countries.

The case for an integrated approach to controlling NCD is based on the hypothesis of linked common causes of these diseases[9]. Irrespective of other considerations, community health programmes to prevent NCDs could be more cost-effective and efficient if several disease-specific programmes were integrated to make better use of available resources, in terms of both personnel and money. Furthermore, programmes aiming at the control of only one disease may persuade individuals to adopt healthier lifestyles in other ways, which could facilitate a broader NCD prevention; integration could be achieved simply by managerial unification of a set of preventive activities.

Diabetes may sometimes be directly associated with inconvenient and even serious health problems themselves, although diabetes is not usually the main cause of death[10]. Diabetes is, however, a major factor contributing – usually directly – to increased mortality and morbidity, especially in CVDs. In diabetic patients other known risk factors (smoking, hypertension, dyslipidaemia) play as important a part as, or even a more important part than, in non-diabetic subjects. Therefore, it is not wise (and probably not even justifiable) to start a community programme for diabetes without integrating it with interventions aimed at the more general prevention of CVDs.

INTERVENTION STRATEGIES FOR NCD PREVENTION

The primary goal of preventive programmes is the reduction of human suffering. In the development and implementation of a community control programme, a full *community analysis* is essential. Community analysis should provide as comprehensive an understanding as possible of the situation at the start of the programme; it should provide a basis for selecting priorities and appropriate methods of intervention. It should also indicate how continuous follow-up can be carried out through the programme and thereby help to determine the course of the activities. As the most important intervention methods in NCD control programmes are health education of the public, patient education and organization of primary health care, community analyis should be designed in such a way that these issues are covered satisfactorily. The review of existing data from earlier studies, statistics and other sources is invaluable.

Epidemiological knowledge about NCDs and their subsequent complications in the target population provides the essential basis for the programme: prevalence, incidence, mortality; the distribution within and between different population groups; the factors influencing the natural course of NCDs; and their prevalence[1]. It is also important to *understand the social and cultural features of the population* and the country. Information about health behaviour related to NCDs and their risk factors, about factors in the community influencing these behaviour patterns, and about community leadership and social interaction are essential for programme development and implementation.

Much of the success of any community programme depends on the *support of the population*. For this reason, information about how people and their official representatives see the problems, and how they feel about the possibilities of solving them, should be part of the community analysis. As the programme would also depend heavily on their cooperation, *the knowledge, attitudes and therapeutic practices of the health personnel* should also be surveyed. The main objectives of a programme are usually set by the perceived health needs of the community[12].

LEVELS OF PREVENTION

There are various levels or stages of prevention. Primary and secondary prevention are part of the established terminology in preventive medicine[13]. Primary prevention has been defined as all measures designed to reduce the incidence of a certain disease in the population, by reducing the risk of its onset. In practice, this means that attributable risk related to certain risk factors is modified by influencing the levels of such factors in order to reduce or remove the exposure. The selection of risk factors for intervention is always based on a good knowledge about the natural history of the disease and evidence-based information about the efficient intervention methods. Secondary prevention in a chronic disease includes all measures designed to reduce the morbidity and mortality in people who have the disease. Both types of prevention are needed to achieve effective control of chronic NCDs. The quality of the existing health care system will dictate which of the possible preventive methods will be selected and used.

Primary prevention can be implemented through a population strategy, i.e. changing the lifestyle and environmental determinants that are known to be the major risk factors for the disease, and through a high-risk strategy, i.e. identifying individuals or groups that are at high risk for the future development of the disease and targeting intervention measures only at those individuals[14]. In effective community-based programmes for primary prevention of NCDs, the population strategy and high-risk strategy complement each other and both must be employed concurrently.

The aim of the population strategy is to shift the entire distribution of the risk factor to the lower levels by actions that cover the entire population, or most of it. For instance, a reduction of sodium content or saturated fat content in commonly used foods may be an effective measure to influence the levels of blood pressure and serum cholesterol in the population. In the high-risk strategy, the aim is to lower the high levels of the selected risk factors with an individually designed intervention to 'normal' levels. It has been estimated that the high-risk strategy can reach only a proportion of subjects who are likely to develop an NDC in the community. Moreover, many interventions, such as antihypertensive drug therapy, antidiabetic drug therapy and weight reduction programmes, have not been shown to be fully successful in normalizing the risk factor levels; at best they provide only a partial solution[15]. Ideally, primary prevention should take precedence, because interventions after reaching the clinical stages of the disease will have only a limited impact on the mass epidemic of NDCs in many countries. Unfortunately, we cannot claim that such a priority setting has actually been obtained with regard to several NCDs, e.g. in diabetes care (Figure 12.1).

Although the high-risk strategy depends largely on the action of health workers, prevention of NCDs in the whole population requires action also from many other sectors of the community. Nevertheless, health personnel have an important role in increasing the public awareness through their leadership, their influence on national policy-making and their patient contacts. It is the health personnel who provide the necessary link between knowledge of the natural history of the NCD and selection of the intervention methods needed in primary prevention. In spite of gaps in our current knowledge, we probably understand the natural history of many NCDs sufficiently to justify various preventive actions. We must also remember that the history of public health is replete with examples of successful preventive actions that were not based on complete understanding of the aetiology and pathophysiology of the disease concerned. Actually, carefully planned and implemented prevention programmes have proved to be important in forming a link between basic laboratory and clinical research, and public health, often significantly adding to the knowledge of the disease aetiology.

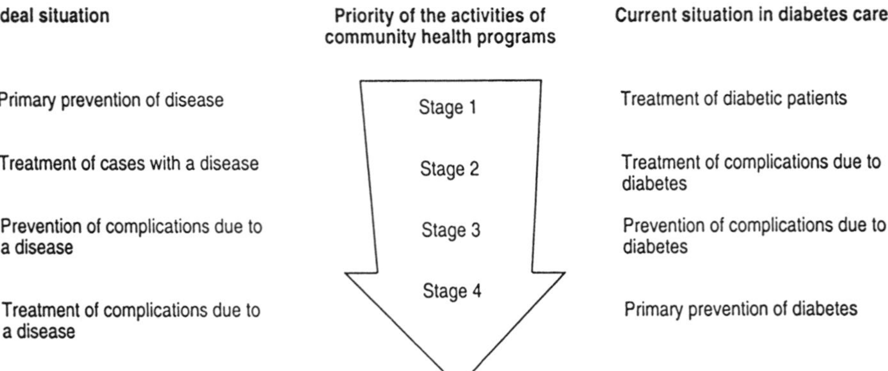

Figure 12.1. Order of priority of different intervention strategies in community health programmes, with special reference to diabetes care.

In the development of methods for modern community health programmes, CVD prevention has already become a self-evident concept. Diabetes-related activities can also serve as a model for more general NCD prevention and control, particularly in countries with a high prevalence of diabetes. This obviously becomes even more important since the occurrence of CVD in the middle-aged populations has decreased steeply[16], although the prevalence of diabetes is increasing in all populations worldwide[17]. Diabetes care has several important components that can be effectively incorporated into primary health care services. The components that form the basis of the population strategy in diabetes prevention and control include the following:

- health education of the public
- guided patient self-care
- continuous education of patients
- training of health personnel and lay workers
- community participation by people, various non-medical sectors and voluntary organizations
- organization and maintenance of primary diabetes health care supported by specialist consultations
- attempts to improve the environment
- social support
- development of diabetes registers or other relevant information systems.

PRACTICAL DEMONSTRATION PROGRAMMES FOR PREVENTION AND CONTROL OF NCDs

Community demonstration programmes for diabetes control are a key step in putting the current knowledge about proven effective prevention and control strategies into practice in the community. The prerequisite for a demonstration programme is an adequate level of health services in the community. Such a programme can be fully justified only when it is implemented within the existing health care system and social structure of the community. In countries where the health care system is heterogeneous, it has become obvious that lack of coordination among various resources and providers of care has contributed to inadequate prevention and primary care; this has also led to an ineffective use of resources.

It is important that community demonstration programmes adopt a problem-oriented planning process, in which problems and resources are first identified. This means that some level of community analysis will be carried out. Unfortunately, the database needed for a comprehensive community diagnosis of diabetes is completely, or almost completely, lacking in most communities[18,19]. It is, therefore, often the historical situation that determines the objectives and resources available, e.g. in the early 1970s mortality from CHD was the highest in the world in Finland[16,20]; the prevalence of type 2 diabetes is extremely high in the USA among some native tribes[24–26] and in Australia among the aboriginals; the population of the island republic of Nauru has developed a major diabetes epidemic during the past 50 years[24].

It must be borne in mind that community demonstration programmes are not planned, in the experimental sense, to test a formal hypothesis about the causal effects of risk modification. Rather, they test the feasibility and effects of complex but practical interventions, based on available knowledge. They should also be planned in such a way that they could be applied elsewhere, if successful. The great advantage of community demonstration programmes is that their findings are valid in real-life circumstances. It is clear that, when such programmes are carefully designed, their effectiveness and impact can be assessed.

The gap between existing medical knowledge and the situation in society stems from a host of formidable obstacles to healthy change – cultural, political, economic, psychological. The aim of community programmes is to build a bridge for people and communities to overcome these obstacles, or at least to minimize them. A powerful argument in favour of community-based preventive programmes is that the source of the mass epidemics of NCDs is unhealthy lifestyles, which often first emerge during periods of economic transition. Large portions of society are under at least some risk, so major reductions in disease rates call for widespread changes in the related lifestyles. Moreover, as these are embedded in the community in complex ways, major lifestyle changes are possible only if their determinants in the community are somehow modified.

Community demonstration programmes should simultaneously apply medical and epidemiological knowledge to identify health problems. This knowledge should also be used to set priorities in selecting objectives for such health programmes. Another principle of community demonstration programmes is that they use knowledge from social and behavioural sciences to design the actual programme content. This implies an interdisciplinary approach in the planning, implementation and evaluation of the programme. Many of these principles can be seen in existing diabetes control activities[25,27]. However, these principles have not been applied in a systematic way in community programmes for diabetes, but mainly for clinical management of individual diabetic patients[28–30].

THEORETICAL FRAMEWORK OF COMMUNITY DEMONSTRATION PROGRAMMES

Health-related lifestyles are largely determined by social forces and other environmental factors. Efforts towards major progress influencing disease rates in the community have to contend with environmental forces and structures. The natural and most effective way of changing a population's risk factor levels is to operate through the community; the entire community rather than its individual members should form the target.

Although the task of influencing people's behaviours and lifestyles lies in the domain of the social and behavioural sciences, a persistent and major problem has been the lack of a unifying theory to serve as a guide in health promotion. Action-oriented people often feel frustrated by the inability of behavioural scientists to tell them what to do in practice. In spite of this, there are sound principles in behavioural and social sciences to guide the planning, implemention and evaluation of community-based health programmes.

Behaviour Change Approach

This social–psychological approach deals with the determinants of an individual's behavioural changes, and is based on Bandura's work on the process of learning[31]. New behaviours tend to originate, at least on trial bases, from change exposure to powerful models; external and self-enforcement, plus cognitive control are the consequent determinants of continued new behaviours. This approach includes elements of the classic field theory of Lewin[32] and the behavioural intention model of Fishbein[33].

In another report, a framework compatible with this approach has been described in greater detail, using examples from the various activities in North Karelia[34]. This model emphasizes that programme planning and evaluation should include the following key steps to help individuals to modify their behaviour:

- Improved preventive services to help people identify their risk factors and to provide appropriate attention and services.
- Information to educate people about the relationship between their behaviour and health.
- Persuasion to motivate people and promote their intentions to adopt healthy action(s).
- Training to enhance skills of self-management, environmental control and necessary action.
- Social support to help people maintain the initial action.
- Environmental change to create the opportunities for healthy actions and improve unfavourable conditions.
- Community organization to mobilize the community for broad-ranging changes (through enhanced social support and environment modification) to support the adoption of the new lifestyles in the community.

The task of introducing new behaviours into the community is basically achieved by communicating: through popular media channels and via interpersonal approaches. A project disseminates its messages to the population through the mass media, in addition to maintaining direct communication with various community leaders. Well-documented theoretical backgrounds for this approach are provided by Bandura's social learning theory[31], the classic communication–persuasion model of McGuire[35], its modification by Flay et al.[36] and the belief–attitude–intention model of Ajzen and Fishbein[37].

INNOVATION–DIFFUSION APPROACH

New lifestyles are innovations that diffuse through the natural networks in a community by communication, and gradually lead to social change. The innovation–diffusion theory argues that, although the mass media are more effective in spreading knowledge about innovations and are useful for 'agenda-setting' purposes, interpersonal channels are more effective in actually changing attitudes and behaviours. The innovation process occurs in four stages (note the similarity to the previous approach): (1) knowledge; (2) persuasion; (3) decision and (4) confirmation.

The innovation–diffusion theory classifies people on the basis of their innovativeness: as innovators, early adopters, early majority, late majority, or laggards. The social structure has several norms (system effects) that exert a strong influence on rates of diffusion. Early adoption and a faster diffusion rate are more likely to occur with modern rather than with traditional community norms. Early adopters usually have the greatest social influence in the community and are thus in key positions to influence wider adoption of the innovation.

An agent of change can be a professional attempting to influence this innovation–decision process. The three main types of innovation decision are: (1) optional decisions (made individually); (2) collective decisions (by consensus) and (3) authority decisions (by a superordinate power). These central principles of innovation–diffusion theory were largely developed by Rogers[38], and complement the classic idea of a two-step flow of new ideas and attitudes through opinion leaders[39]. The simplified model holds that new ideas, often originating in the mass media, are mediated and modified by certain opinion leaders, and that most people are then mainly influenced by interpersonal contacts with these opinion leaders. Some opinion leaders can be identified by their particular expertise or position, whereas others cannot be distinguished by such formal criteria. Opinion leaders may either favour or resist a particular innovation–diffusion process.

The principles of innovation–diffusion are of great relevance to many community health programmes. A preventive project, as an agent of change, attempts to spread certain health innovations through the social network to members of the community by communication. The speed of diffusion is a vital aspect. Diffusion can be facilitated by the skilful application of the theoretical principles of the communication process. The degree of community resistance (system effect) is also obviously important.

COMPONENTS OF COMMUNITY DEMONSTRATION PROGRAMMES

Several components of the design of community demonstration programmes in NCDs have to be considered to strengthen the causal inference that the programme itself is responsible for changes observed during the programme's evaluation period. Blackburn[40] stated that, at the very least, the following issues require careful attention based on first principles.

Control

Experimental community health intervention has to be compared in reference populations that are similar in size and structure, but which should have separate trade and communication borders.

Repetition

Programme activities must be introduced in stages in the intervention communities. Staged introduction has not only practical managerial implications, but also amounts to a repetition of the experiment and generally strengthens the inference with each repetition, if the changes noted are in one direction.

Sensitive Trend Assessments

Cross-sectional, retrospective and prospective measurements of mortality, morbidity, levels of known risk factors, and social and behavioural indicators are used to characterize community risk and disease trends. Cohort analyses of those originally surveyed provide sensitive indicators of individual change. A number of other measurements, e.g. those of anthropological observations, medical care, community events, perceived health, personnel experiences, etc., are important to complete the trend data.

Dose–effect Measurement

The design of community demonstration programmes allows for a wide range of exposures to different intervention strategies, from those maximally exposed in the intensive intervention communities to those minimally exposed in the reference communities. A graded response strengthens the inference.

Maximal Intervention

A consistent series of activities using multiple strategies should continue at an intensive level for 5–10 years, providing a systematically planned intervention for prevention and control of diabetes by methods that are postulated to be synergistically effective.

Linkage

Links are established (1) between components of the intervention programme and its mass campaigns; (2) between short-term behaviour changes and their risk factor sequelae; and (3) between trends in population risk factors and disease trends.

Pooling

Pooling of results in several intervention communities within and between different health intervention programmes, compared with those of several reference communities, reduces variability and increases the power to detect trends. If this were not done, it might be difficult to separate the effects of the programme from changes occurring spontaneously in the community.

Design Limitations

There are many limitations in research related to demonstration programmes. It is usually not feasible to apply randomized assignment of multiple study units, i.e. entire communities, for several reasons. The characteristics to be dealt with in complete matching are possibly far more numerous than the analytical units involved. The nature of community health programmes precludes the experimental control of too many variables. It is not always certain whether the items chosen to be monitored in the programme are the best to reflect changes. Reliability of many interesting issues, such as the effects of socioeconomic factors associated with diet, exercise, smoking and drinking habits, etc., is often unknown.

THE PRACTICAL FRAMEWORK OF A COMMUNITY-BASED NCD DEMONSTRATION PROGRAMME

The practical framework of an NCD control programme is made up of three stages: (1) planning; (2) implementation of the intervention programme; and (3) evaluation. Although these usually occur sequentially in time, in many cases they operate simultaneously as the programme proceeds. The content is determined by the intelligent application and adaptation of existing medical, epidemiological, behavioural and social knowledge to local community settings and situations. The main issues that form the principles of community demonstration programmes are:

- These programmes serve as a link translating current knowledge of proven effective intervention measures into health care practice.
- There must be clear definition of objectives and methodologies to address the problems.
- They should not be planned only to test aetiological hypotheses.
- They should apply medical/epidemiological knowledge to identify problems, and should also use social/behavioural knowledge to design the actual intervention measures.
- Prerequisites are: adequate level of health care; commitment of the local health authorities to support the programme; community analysis at baseline; and identification of problems to be solved during the programme.
- Programmes should first be tested in pilot areas.
- Results (e.g. feasibility, effectiveness, costs, etc.) must be formally evaluated.

Planning

The major elements in programme planning are: (1) identification of the problem; (2) definition of objectives; (3) establishment of the programme organization; and (4) preparatory steps.

Identification of the problem in each community is carried out by means of the 'community analysis' (community diagnosis), which should provide a comprehensive understanding of the situation at the start of the programme. Data on risk factors and modifying factors contributing to the existence of the problem should be assessed by various means, sometimes by rapid surveys. Expert opinions are often very useful for review in the planning work[41].

The intermediate objectives are those requiring the expenditure of resources. They are designed on the basis of the available medical and epidemiological knowledge about methods of influencing the health problems identified. The practical objectives and actual intervention measures should then be based on careful community analysis and on understanding of the main determinants of the intermediate objectives. Usually the historic development of each community health programme dictates the programme organization, which has to be integrated into the existing health care and community structure. During the preparatory steps, various organizational and coordination aspects of the programme can be evaluated and adjusted accordingly.

Implementation

The goal is to implement the programme activities systematically according to its objectives and principles. Within the overall framework of the programme, its actual implementation can be sufficiently flexible to adjust in response to the local opportunities. Integrating the programme into the social organization of the community is necessary to ensure community participation and availability of various community resources, especially those outside the health sector[42]. The practical activities of the programme have to be carried out mainly by the community. However, expert advice and consultations by others are needed to support the community's efforts.

The programme activities have to be simple and practical to facilitate enactment in the entire community. Simple basic services for the largest possible proportion of the population are preferred to highly sophisticated services for a few people. Integration of several intervention measures will mean better use of the existing resources and avoid duplication of activities. To identify and mobilize all community resources, it is necessary to work closely with both official agencies and voluntary organizations.

The following groups of programme activities need to be considered and developed:

- Media-related and general educational activities.
- Training of local health personnel and other active groups.
- Organization of health services – primary health care, specialized supportive services, etc.
- Community activities for the modification of the environment.
- Information services for monitoring the development of the programme, and for providing feedback.

Many of these above-mentioned groups of activities have been used in diabetes care, but not very extensively in the framework of a community-based programme[26,30,41,43–45]. Experience from existing diabetes care projects can provide useful information for the community analysis, which is an essential step in the planning of integrated NCD prevention programmes.

It needs to be emphasized that, even when the framework of an intervention is well defined and structured on objectives, theoretical frameworks, local community diagnosis and practical considerations, the actual implementation must be flexible enough to respond to the changing community situations and to take advantage of any fresh opportunities that arise.

Evaluation

Any preventive or therapeutic action and its outcome must be continually evaluated to justify the programme's continuation[42,46,47]. Therefore, an evaluation component is needed for any efficient NDC prevention and control programme in order to carry out the following strategic actions:

- Add to the knowledge of disease aetiology.
- Evaluate the feasibility and effects of primary, secondary and tertiary prevention activities.

- Evaluate the effectiveness of secondary prevention activities.
- Devise and test new intervention strategies for disease prevention.

Evaluation can be divided into two components: (1) internal or formative evaluation; and (2) external or summative evaluation. The evaluation of community programmes for diabetes control must be distinguished from the more research-oriented clinical trials or those narrower interests that focus on one aspect of the intervention, such as diabetes patient education.

Internal evaluation is carried out during the programme to provide rapid feedback to the programme workers, management and public. Data are mainly used to develop the programme further. They are also used to assess the adequacy of the programme and provide information for the review of progress during the intervention.

The main aim of external evaluation is to assess the overall feasibiity, efficiency, effects, impact and other results of the programme over a given time. External evaluation is used to assess whether the main objectives have been attained and to what extent. It can also be used to identify the major factors contributing to the results, whether positive or negative. An expert group in some way external to the daily community activities is usually responsible for external evaluation. For national health policy, the assessment of cost-effectiveness of the programme is of great interest and significance, but it is usually very difficult to carry out[48,49].

SUMMARY OF FINDINGS FROM THE NORTH KARELIA PROJECT

The obvious role of CVD risk factors – serum cholesterol, blood pressure and smoking – was established in the 1960s and 1970s by biochemical and epidemiological studies, and by clinical trials. Twenty years ago Finland had the highest coronary mortality in the world[50] and, within Finland, the highest mortality was observed in the eastern province of North Karelia.

These observations led to the planning and launch of the North Karelia Project in 1972 – the first comprehensive community-based programme for the prevention of CVD through general lifestyle and risk factor changes, which included careful scientific evaluation[12]. Thereafter, in the 1970s and 1980s many community-based prevention programmes were started in several countries. In the 1980s, based on a general consensus about the role of risk factors, many countries started to develop national strategies to reduce mortality from CHD.

The original aim of the North Karelia Project was to test the feasibility and effects of a community-based programme for the prevention of CVD in North Karelia. Gradually, different kinds of activities aimed at preventing CHD were started over the whole country, and from 1977 the North Karelia

Project was actively involved in these activities. During the past few years North Karelia has been a national demonstration area for innovations in chronic disease prevention and health promotion.

The objectives of the project evolved from the public health needs of the community; the intervention strategies were designed using relevant theoretical considerations. Moreover, the project leaders and staff genuinely immersed themselves in the community and among the people, where they developed and adjusted programme activities according to available local options and circumstances.

After selection of the main objectives, the intermediate objectives were defined. These were derived from the medical/epidemiological/knowledge in the literature relating to the well-established risk factors for the diseases in question, and from the local prevalence rates of those factors. Clear definitions of the main and intermediate objectives helped also to decide on the respective indicators and data sources for monitoring and evaluation.

After settlement of the intermediate objectives, the immediate action plan or practical programme contents were decided upon. As the overall task largely concerned influencing the health behaviours and related lifestyles, behavioural and social theories were required. A sound understanding of the community ('community diagnosis') was also essential, so that all practical potentials and opportunities to this end could be pursued.

The main health goal of controlling CVD, or chronic disease in general, implies the application of all appropriate action to reducing the burden of disease, including primary prevention, treatment, rehabilitation and other secondary prevention, and related research. However, major success in controlling a chronic disease can be based only on primary prevention, because intervention during the clinical stages of the disease has a limited impact. The greatest potential for controlling most NCDs lies in primary prevention; in other words, a 'mass epidemic' should be tackled by 'mass prevention'.

In primary prevention the choice of the main risk factors for intervention was derived from the information about the prevalence of these factors in the target population. In the case of the North Karelia Project, this aspect was relatively easy. Back in the early 1970s several studies, along with their international conclusions, had identified three main CVD risk factors: elevated serum cholesterol, elevated blood pressure and smoking[51].

Five cross-sectional population surveys (in 1972, 1977, 1982, 1987 and 1992) assessed the levels of coronary risk factors in North Karelia and Kuopio at 5-year intervals. For each survey, an independent random sample was drawn from the national population register[12,50,51].

Initially (1972–1977), the effects of the North Karelia Project were compared with those in the neighbouring province of Kuopio. Among men, during the first 5 years, blood pressure and cholesterol fell more in North Karelia than in the reference area, and in the second 5-year period smoking also fell more markedly. After that the trend in risk factors was about the same in both areas. In 1982, blood pressure and cholesterol levels were still higher in the eastern part of the country than in south-western Finland. These differences have diminished over the last 10 years, and the risk factor profile in Finland appears to be becoming more homogeneous. From 1972 to 1992, serum total cholesterol decreased by 13.0% in men and 17.6% in women. Diastolic blood pressure fell by 9.2% and 13.3% in men and women, respectively. The prevalence of smoking declined among men from 53% to 37%, but rose among women from 11% to 20% (Table 12.1).

The findings show a marked decline in the mortality rate of the middle-aged population. The decline in IHD mortality started in North Karelia very soon after the intervention began. In the 1970s there was a significantly steeper decrease in North Karelia than in the whole of Finland or Kuopio[20,53], which corresponds with the clearly greater reduction in the risk factors there during the decade. Thereafter the trend levelled off somewhat in North Karelia, and was soon caught up by the steeper decline in the whole of Finland. Table 12.2 shows the average annual number of deaths from all causes and from CVD in North Karelia and the whole of Finland in 1969–71 and in 1990–92. It can be seen that, 20 years after the programme began, there were 2817 fewer deaths annually in all Finland and 202 fewer in North Karelia among men aged 35–74 years. For women, the respective figures were 2787 and 164. In North Karelia 82% of this decline and 89% in the whole of Finland was the result of reductions in cardiovascular deaths. Over the project period in this age group, the number of deaths was about 3800 less in North Karelia compared with the numbers if mortality had stayed at the pre-programme level. Life expectancy at birth rose in men from 66.4 in 1971 to 71.7 years in 1992 and in women from 74.6 years to 79.4 years.

During the last few years the decline has again been very steep in North Karelia. In 1992 the IHD mortality rate in North Karelia was 59% lower, and

Table 12.1. Changes in CHD risk factors levels in eastern Finland from 1972 to 1992

	1972	1977	1982	1987	1992
Men					
Serum cholesterol (mmol/l)	6.8	6.6	6.3	6.2	5.9
Diastolic blood pressure (mmHg)	92.8	91.0	87.8	88.4	84.2
Smoking (%)	53	47	42	39	37
Women					
Serum cholesterol (mmol/l)	6.7	6.4	6.1	5.9	5.5
Diastolic blood pressure (mmHg)	91.8	87.6	84.6	83.5	79.6
Smoking (%)	11	12	16	16	20

Table 12.2. Age-adjusted mean annual mortality rates (per 100 000) in 1969–71 in the whole of Finland and in North Karelia, and the 25-year changes among the 35- to 64-year-old population

Mortality	Males		Females	
	All Finland	North Karelia	All Finland	North Karelia
All causes				
1969–71	1272	1509	475	501
Change (%)	−45.0	−44.8	−41.1	−37.9
Cardiovascular diseases				
1969–71	647	855	205	262
Change (%)	−59.7	−60.5	−68.3	−64.5
Ischaemic heart disease				
1969–71	465	672	82	118
Change (%)	−62.4	−64.7	−65.9	−68.6
Cerebrovascular disease				
1969–71	93	90	69	65
Change (%)	−57.0	−47.8	−66.7	−50.8
Cancer				
1969–71	248	271	141	121
Change (%)	−39.9	−43.5	−15.6	−2.5
Lung cancer				
1969–71	105	147		
Change (%)	−57.1	−71.4		
Violent causes				
1969–71	201	227	41	31
Change (%)	−13.9	−10.6	+7.3	−41.9

in 1994 it was 65% lower, than the pre-programme rate in 1969–71. The decrease in mortality was larger in younger than in older age groups (Figure 12.2).

The average probability of an IHD death for each year of the risk factor survey was calculated by entering the mean risk factors values observed in the survey into the logistic regression function. The relative importance of each risk factor was also estimated separately by changing only the value of that risk factor in the logistic regression function, keeping the others unchanged according to the 1972 level. The percentage decline in predicted mortality compared to the 1972 level was then calculated for each survey year[54].

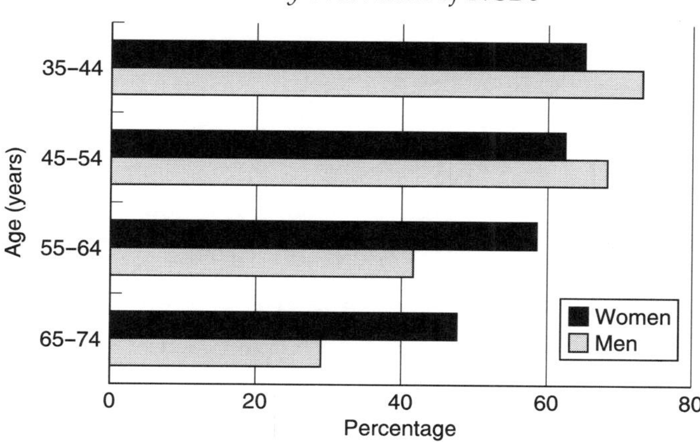

Figure 12.2. Percentage decline in CHD mortality in North Karelia from 1969–1971 to 1990–1992 in different age groups.

The observed decline in IHD mortality according to the mortality statistics is shown in Figure 12.3; in addition, Figure 12.3 shows the predicted decline in mortality based on the logistic function and the observed risk factor changes in men from 1972 to 1992. In men, observed mortality decreased by 55% (95% confidence limits of 95% CI 95%CI = 51–58) over the 20 years. The predicted decline, using the logistic regression model and the observed risk factor changes during the same period, was 44% (95%CI = 37–50). Until the mid-1980s the trend in observed mortality followed the predicted decline, but subsequently it accelerated faster than had been predicted by the risk factor changes. To estimate the relative importance of each risk factor separately, we computed three additional models. In men, the observed 13% decrease in serum cholesterol predicted a 26% decline in IHD mortality, the 9.2% decrease in diastolic blood pressure predicted a 15% decline, and the decrease in smoking from 53% to 37% predicted a 10% decline in IHD mortality. In women, the observed IHD mortality fell by 68% over the 20 years (Figure 12.4). The predicted decrease based on the risk factor changes was 49% (95%CI = 37–59). The 18% decrease in cholesterol predicted a 35% decline in IHD mortality, the 13% decrease in diastolic blood pressure predicted a 31% decline, and the increase in smoking from 11% to 20% predicted an 11% increase in IHD mortality.

The well-standardized population surveys every 5 years from 1972 to 1992, and the high qualtiy of mortality statistics in Finland, provided us with a unique opportunity to estimate the role of risk factor changes in the actual decline in IHD mortality. The results showed that we could predict about 75% of the decrease in IHD mortality by changes in the known risk factors among the men and women of the population. Almost half of the

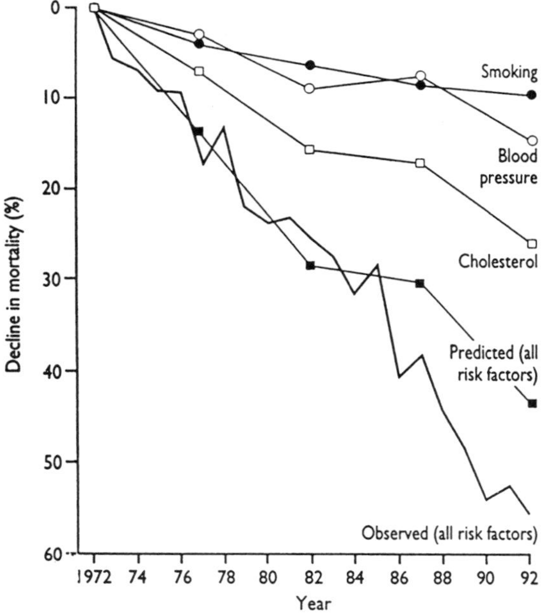

Figure 12.3. Observed decline in mortality from CHD and the decline predicted from the risk factor changes in eastern Finnish men aged 35–64 years.

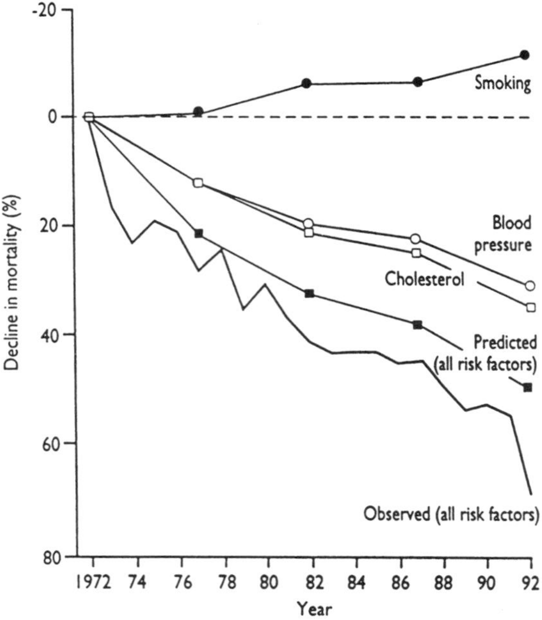

Figure 12.4. Observed decline in mortality from CHD and the decline predicted from the risk factor changes in eastern Finnish women aged 35–64 years.

decline in IHD mortality was explained by the falling serum cholesterol level. Our results confirmed, in the estimate derived from clinical trials[55], that a 1% decrease in serum cholesterol leads to a 2% decline in IHD risk. The marked decrease in serum cholesterol is obviously a consequence of the substantial concurrent dietary changes in Finland[56]. Use of saturated fats (mainly milk fat) has decreased by one-third from the early 1970s, whereas vegetable oil consumption has risen dramatically: in 1972, 90% of people in eastern Finland used butter on bread but, in 1992, only 10%. Vegetable oil was very rarely used for cooking 20 years ago, but now 30% of people use it regularly. Most people have switched from fatty milk to low-fat or skimmed milk, and the annual per capita consumption of vegetables has risen from about 20 kg to 50 kg.

On the basis of our results, the risk factor changes seem to explain almost all of the developments in mortality in the 1970s. In the 1980s, the decline in mortality was faster than predicted by the observed changes in risk factors in the population. Improved treatment of acute myocardial infarction may be one explanation; thrombolytic treatment, coronary bypass surgery and prophylactic use of acetylsalicylic acid became widespread during the late 1980s.

ADVANTAGES OF USING DIABETES AS A MODEL FOR INTEGRATION WITH OTHER NCDs

PUBLIC AWARENESS OF THE PROBLEM

It is well known that the public are aware of diabetes as a chronic, life-long disorder. A large body of data about the management of diabetes and the beneficial effects of treatment on diabetic patients has been accumulated. Therefore, relatively little community education is needed to make people aware of diabetes as a health problem. What people and decision-makers usually do not know is the magnitude of the diabetes problem in their own communities.

EXISTING MEDIA-RELATED AND GENERAL EDUCATIONAL ACTIVITIES

The strongest support for an integrated approach in prevention and control of major NCDs comes from the fact that these diseases have common causal factors, and that many recommendations for treatment include similar instructions for different diseases. This is a great advantage for health education. Numerous mass media activities on diabetes, especially those related to symptoms, diet, treatment and prevention of complications, are regularly seen in many countries. Thus, we have a number of media experts who could also provide assistance for more comprehensive educational activities related to other NCDs[58]. Health education concerning diabetes has a longer tradition than that relating to cancer or cardiovascular diseases in many countries. However, little attention has been paid so far to the primary prevention of diabetes[11], which was first advocated as early as the 1920s[59].

DIABETES PATIENT EDUCATION

Diabetes education has become an essential part of any modern diabetes control programme. The philosophy of self-care and health education for an improved long-term quality of life is probably nowhere better illustrated than when using self-management of diabetes as a model[25,29,30,43,44].

TRAINING OF HEALTH PERSONNEL AND OTHER ACTIVE GROUPS

Diabetes has been a major area for the continuous training of personnel in many medical and paramedical groups. This training has usually had clearly defined goals and is aimed at providing practical skills for the participants[25,26,60]. This is why it is an excellent model for integration with other NCDs[45]. Furthermore, not only specialist doctors, but also various other groups, including lay people in the community, have taken part in training about diabetes. Such training has traditionally stressed the importance of a multidisciplinary approach, which is one of the key strategies in the integrated prevention and control of NCDs[7,9,61].

ORGANIZATION OF HEALTH SERVICES

As diabetes is a disease usually of long duration, it is natural that health services for diabetes are fairly well organized in most developed countries. They are, in fact, sometimes too specialized and lack the strong support of primary health care that is the essential requirement for any community health programme. The comprehensive use of voluntary organizations and other non-medical community resources is well known in diabetes care. As treatment for diabetes is usually long term, the services developed also provide a good model for other NCDs. These activities include not only models for clinical services, but also educational programmes for families and community lay people[12,41].

MODIFICATION OF ENVIRONMENT

Traditionally, diabetes has been a disease with a visible impact on our environment. Food production, manufacturing and marketing have accepted the needs of diabetic citizens. The role of community organizations and active individuals in this development must be appreciated by all those who are dealing with diabetes care. The success of this development has confirmed that the modification of the environment is feasible. Moreover, not only are these achievements important for a small group of diabetic patients in the community, but the trend to produce healthier alternatives for the daily diet of the whole population has greatly benefited from the lead given by those interested in diabetes care. Recently, it has been realized that dietary guidelines for diabetes are, in fact, almost the same as those for prevention of cardiovascular diseases or cancer. On the topic of population-based strategies of disease control, Rose[62] has said, 'Once a social norm of behaviour has become accepted and once the supply industries have adapted themselves to the new pattern, then the maintenance of that situation no longer requires effort from individuals. The health education phase aimed at changing individuals is, we hope, a temporary necessity . . .'. This may be somewhat idealistic, but it underlines the importance and potential of environmental modification for health.

INFORMATION SYSTEMS FOR MANAGEMENT AND FEEDBACK

Until recently, information systems for diabetes care have not been very impressive when compared with those developed for cancer or cardiovascular diseases. The lack of systematic databases and international standardization in diabetes may reflect the earlier opinion of many experts that the diabetes problem could be solved by clinical and laboratory research alone, without public health involvement. Unfortunately, we now know that diabetes is rapidly increasing in most populations in the world[16,63]. As there has not been a systematic collection of data on possible causes of this increasing trend, we can only guess the reasons behind it.

CURRENT AIMS OF DIABETES CONTROL PROGRAMMES

Although diabetes control activities are being provided to some degree in most countries, objectives and strategies differ considerably, as do the outcomes of these control efforts. Countries will naturally differ in their approach to organizing, administering and financing health care. However, there are certain universal considerations in the provision of patient care and education. The following six assumptions are suggested as the foundation for diabetes programme development at the local, national and global level[27] :

1. Diabetes is a heterogeneous disease which requires detection, prevention and control measures, in individuals and communities, that are tailored to local cultural and practical considerations.

2. A substantial part of diabetes care is patient self-care. Thus, patients must be educated before having the responsibility for daily management of their condition delegated to them.
3. Optimal diabetes care by the patient and provider can prevent or delay the development of complications.
4. Properly designed and integrated diabetes care programmes may result in sizable reductions in morbidity, disability and mortality.
5. Diabetes health care costs may be reduced using a variety of cost-containment strategies.
6. Diabetes control programmes do not work in isolation. Their function is enhanced by intersectoral training/planning and integration of services at all levels in the health care system. Close linkage is encouraged with other chronic disease prevention and treatment programmes.

MAJOR CONSTRAINTS

Additional challenges posed by diabetes necessitate some vertical planning and programme development as well as formal linkage with the country's primary health care system. Specifically, diabetic individuals require considerable knowledge for daily self-care and disease management (e.g. adapting prescribed dietary, therapeutic and lifestyle actions), whereas their health care provider is required to apply complex cognitive and medical management skills, which may also require involvement of a number of professionals for extended periods of time.

The main constraints do not lie in the theoretical aspects of this issue of integrated prevention and control of diabetes, but concern more practical decisions and capabilities of working for a common goal. First of all, we are now faced with a historic decision that we could postpone with ease, using such commonly accepted excuses as 'We do not know enough', 'There is no final proof', 'Are you sure this action does not carry any risks?', etc.

Another constraint is that the resources will never be adequate to do all that needs to be done. However, many successful public health programmes may eventually even bring about cost reduction and lessen the burden to the community. The old adage is that prevention is better than cure (or at least less expensive than treatment). The programme for the integrated prevention and control of major NCDs could, in theory, save even more money than a programme designed for one disease only. In practice, however, such 'savings' may be difficult to identify because of the complex way in which the health care systems are developing, and because demands are usually much greater than the resources available.

Finally, among the major difficulties often encountered is the inadequate government support owing to: (1) low perception of priority of NCDs[57]; (2) no public health tradition for chronic disease control; (3) reluctance or resistance to cooperate in diabetes community programmes; and (4) general administrative barriers and bureaucracy. To overcome these problems, it is necessary to demonstrate that diabetes is a major public health problem in many countries and to motivate governments to set up national action programmes as recommended by the WHO[27].

REFERENCES

1. Amery A, Berthaux P, Bulpitt C et al. Glucose intolerance during diuretic therapy. Results from the European Working Party on Hypertension in the Elderly Trial. *Lancet* 1978; **1**:681–3.
2. Hinkle LE Jr, Wolff HG. Ecologic investigations of the relationship between illness, life experience and the social environment. *Ann Intern Med* 1958; **49**:1373–88.
3. Epstein FH, Francis T Jr, Hayner NS et al. Prevalence of chronic diseases and distribution of selected physiologic variables in a total community, Tecumsch, Michigan. *Am J Epidemiol* 1965; **81**:307–22.
4. Abrahamson JH, Gotin J, Peritz E, Hopp C, Epstein LM. Clustering of chronic disorders – a community study of coprevalence in Jerusalem. *J Chron Dis* 1982; **35**:221–30.
5. Manton KG, Patrick CH, Stallard E. Mortality model based on delays in progression of chronic diseases: alternative to cause elimination model. *Public Health Rep* 1980; **95**:580–5.
6. Fries FJ. Aging, natural death, and the compression of morbidity. *N Engl J Med* 1980; **303**:130–5.
7. Grabauskas V, Tuomilehto J. Integration of diabetes control with that of other non-communicable diseases. In: Tuomilehto J, Zimmet P, King H, Pressley M, eds. *Diabetes Mellitus. Primary health care prevention and control.* Singapore: International Press, 1982: 51–60.
8. Glasunov IS, Grabauskas V, Holland WW, Epstein FH. An integrated programme for the prevention and control of non-communicable diseases. A Kaunas report. *J Chron Dis* 1983; **36**:419–26.
9. Epstein FH, Holland W. Prevention of chronic diseases in the community-one-disease versus multiple-disease strategies. *Int J Epidemiol* 1983; **12**:135–7.
10. Fuller JH, Elford J, Goldblatt P, Adelstein AM. Diabetes mortality: new light on an underestimated public health problem. *Diabetologia* 1984; **24**:336–41.
11. Tuomilehto J, Tuomilehto-Wolf E, Zimmet P, Alberti KGMM, Knowler WC. Primary prevention of diabetes mellitus. In: Alberti KGMM, Zimmet P, DeFronzo RA, Keen H, eds. *International Textbook of Diabetes Mellitus*, 2nd edn. London: John Wiley & Sons, 1997: 1799–827.
12. Puska P, Nissinen A, Salonen JT et al. The community based strategy to prevent coronary heart disease: conclusions from the ten years of the North Karelia project. *Annu Rev Public Health* 1985; **6**:147–93.
13. Hogarth J. *Glossary of Health Care. Public health in Europe 5*. Copenhagen: WHO Regional Office for Europe, 1975: 302.
14. World Health Organization. *Prevention of Coronary Heart Disease. Report of WHO.* Techn Rep Ser 678. Geneva: WHO, 1982.

15. Marques-Vidal P, Tuomilehto J. Hypertension awareness, treatment and control in the community: is the 'rule of halves' still valid. *J Hum Hypertens* 1997; **11**: 213–20.
16. Uemura K, Pisa Z. Recent trends in cardiovascular disease mortality in 27 industrialized countries. *World Health Stat Q* 1985; **38**:142–62.
17. Amos AF, McCarty DJ, Zimmet P. The rising global burden of diabetes and its complications: estimates and projections to the year 2010. *Diabetes Med* 1997; **14**:S7–85.
18. King H, Rewers M, on behalf of the WHO Ad Hoc Diabetes Reporting Group. Diabetes in adults is now a Third World Problem. *WHO Bull* 1991; **69**:643–8.
19. Karvonen M, Tuomilehto J, Libman I, LaPorte R, for the WHO DIAMOND Project Study Group. A review of the recent epidemiological data on the worldwide incidence of type 1 (Insulin-dependent) diabetes mellitus. *Diabetologia* 1993; **36**:883–92.
20. Tuomilehto J, Geboers J, Salonen, JT, Nissinen A, Kuulasmaa K, Puska P. Decline in cardiovascular mortality in North Karelia and in other parts of Finland. *BMJ* 1986; **29**:1068–71.
21. Knowler WC, Bennett PH, Hamman RE, Miller M. Diabetes incidence and prevalence in Pima Indians, a 19-fold greater incidence than in Rochester, Minnesota. *Am J Epidemiol* 1978; **108**:497–505.
22. Gardner LI, Stern MP, Haffner SM et al. Prevalence of diabetes in Mexican Americans: relationship to percent of gene pool derived from native American sources. *Diabetes* 1984; **33**:86–92.
23. Brosseau J, Eelkema RC, Crawford AC, Abe TA. Diabetes among the three affiliated tribes: correlation with degree of Indian inheritance. *Am J Public Health* 1979; **69**:1277–8.
24. Zimmet P, Taft P, Guinea A, Guthrie W, Thoma K. The high prevalence of diabetes mellitus on a Central Pacific island. *Diabetologia* 1977; **13**:I11–15.
25. Leichter S, Allweiss P. National consensus standards for diabetic patient education programs: a first step in solving an important puzzle. *Arch Intern Med* 1984; **144**:1137–8.
26. Beaven DW, Dodge JS, Kilpatrick JA, Spears GFS. Education and diabetes: attitudes, opinions and needs of New Zealand doctors. *NZ Med J* 1975; **81**: 95–100.
27. Relber G, King H, eds. *Guidelines for the Development of a National Programme for Diabetes Mellitus*. Geneva: World Health Organization, 1991.
28. Stern MP, Pugh JA, Gaskill SP, Hazuda HP. Knowledge, attitudes, and behavior related to obesity and dieting in Mexican-Americans and Anglos: the San Antonio heart study. *Am J Epidemiol* 1982; **115**:917–28.
29. Rosenthal MM. Resistance to change: the case of the Swedish Diabetes Primary Care. In: Luft R, Bajaj JS, Rosenqvist U, eds. *WHG Workshop on Diabetes Care as a Model for Primary Health Care.* Kongl Carolinska Medico Chirurgiska Institutet, Stockholm, 1994: 229–45.
30. Vinicor F, Cohen SJ, Mazzuca SA et al. Diabeds: a randomized trial of the effect of physician and/or patient education on diabetes patient outcomes. *J Chron Dis* 1987; **40**:345–56.
31. Bandura A. *Social Learning Theory*. Englewood Cliffs, NJ: Prentice Hall, 1977.
32. Lewin K. Field theory in social science. In: Cartwright D, ed. *Selected Theoretical Papers*. New York: Harper & Row, 1951.
33. Fishbein M, Ajzen J. *Belief, Attitude, Intention, and Behaviour: An introduction to theory and research*. Reading, MA, Addison-Wesley, 1975.

34. McAlister A, Puska P, Salonen JT, Tuomilehto J, Koskela K. Theory and action for health promotion: Illustrations from the North Karelia Project. *Am J Public Health* 1982; **72**:43–50.
35. McGuire WJ. The nature of attitudes and attitude change. In: Lindsay G, Aronson E, eds., *Handbook of Social Psychology*, Vol. III. Reading, MA, Addison-Wesley, 1969.
36. Flay BR, Ditecco D, Schlegel RP. Mass media in health promotion. *Health Educ Q* 1980; **7**:127–43.
37. Ajzen I, Fishbein M. *Understanding Attitudes and Predicting Social Behavior*. Englewood Cliffs, NJ: Prentice Hall, 1980.
38. Rogers E. *Diffusion of Innovations*. New York: Free Press, 1983.
39. Katz E, Lazerfeld P. *Personal Influence: The part played by people in the flow of mass communications*. New York: Free Press, 1955.
40. Blackburn H. Research and demonstration projects in community cardiovascular disease prevention. *J Public Health Pol* 1983; **4**:398–421.
41. Smith CK, Taylor TR, Gordon MJ, WAMI Family Medicine Collaborative Research Group. Community based studies of diabetes control: program development and preliminary analysis. *J Fam Pract* 1982; **14**:459–67.
42. Tuomilehto J, Neittaanmäki L, Salonen JT, Puska P, Nissinen A. Community involvement in developing comprehensive cardiovascular control programs. A case study in North Karelia, Finland. *Yearbook Pop Res Finland* 1983; **21**:75–98.
43. WHO Expert Committee on Diabetes Mellitus. *WHO Technical Report Series 646*. Geneva: World Health Organization, 1980.
44. Wibell L, Walinder O. Success and failure in patient education in diabetes. *Skandia International Symposia: Recent trends in diabetes research*. Stockholm: Alrriqvist & Wiksell, 1981.
45. Beaven DW, Scott RS. The organization of diabetes care. In: Krall LP, Alberti KGMM, eds. *World Book of Diabetes in Practice*, vol. 2. Amsterdam: Elsevier, 1986: 284–7.
46. Cook T, Campbell D. *Quasi-experimentation. Design and analysis issues for field settings*. Chicago: Rand McNally, 1979.
47. World Health Organization. *Development of Indicators for Monitoring Progress towards Health for all by the Year 2000*. Geneva: WHO, 1981.
48. Jönsson B. Diabetes: the cost of illness and the cost of control. *Acta Med Scand Suppl* 1983; **67**:19–27.
49. Entmacher PS, Sinnock P, Bostic E, Harris MI. Economic impact of diabetes. In: *National Diabetes Data Group: Diabetes in America*. NIH Publication no. 85-1468. Bethesda, MD: NIH, 1985: XXX11-1–13.
50. Keys A. *Seven Countries: A multivariate analysis of death and coronary heart disease*. Cambridge, MA: Harvard University Press, 1980.
51. Puska P, Tuomilehto J, Salonen J et al. The North Karelia project: community control of cardiovascular diseases. Evaluation of a comprehensive community programme for control of cardiovascular diseases in North Karelia, Finland 1972–1977. WHO/EURO Monograph. Copenhagen 1981.
52. Vartiainen E, Puska P, Jousilahti P, Korhonen HJ, Tuomilehto J, Nissinen A. In: Puska P, Tuomilehto J, Nissinen A, Vartiainen E, eds. *The North Karelia Project: 20-year results and experiences*. Helsinki: University Printing House, 1995.
53. Salonen J, Puska P, Kottke T, Tuomilehto J, Nissinen A. Decline in mortality from coronary heart disease in Finland from 1969 to 1979. *BMJ* 1983; **286**:1857–60.
54. Vartiainen E, Puska P, Pekkanen J, Tuomilehto J, Jousilahti P. Changes in risk factors explain changes in mortality from ischaemic heart disease in Finland. *BMJ* 1994; **309**:23–7.

55. Lipid Research Clinics Program. The Lipid Research Clinics Coronary Primary Prevention Trial Results. 1. Reduction in incidence of coronary heart disease. *JAMA* 1984; **251**:351–64.
56. Pietinen P. Changing dietary habits in the population; the Finnish experience. In: Ziant G, ed. *Lipids and Health*. Amsterdam: Elsevier Science Publishers. B.V. (Biomedical Division), 1990: 342–56.
57. WHO. *From Alma-Ata to the Year 2000 – Reflections at the Midpoint*. Geneva: World Health Organization, 1988.
58. Davidson PO, Davidson SM. *Behavioral Medicine: Changing health lifestyles*. New York: Brunner Mazel, 1980.
59. Elliott PJ. The prevention of diabetes mellitus. *JAMA* 1921; **76**:79–84.
60. Weinberger M, Cohen SJ, Mazzuca SA. The role of physicians' knowledge and attitudes in effective diabetes management. *Soc Sci Med* 1984; **19**:965–70.
61. Mazzuca SA. Does patient education in chronic disease have therapeutic value? *J Chron Dis* 1982; **35**:521–9.
62. Rose G. Sick individuals and sick populations. *Int J Epidemiol* 1985; **14**:32–8.
63. WHO DIAMOND Project Group. WHO multinational project for childhood diabetes. *Diabetes Care* 1990; **13**:1062–8.

13

Screening and Prevention of Type 2 Diabetes

D. SIMMONS

Department of Rural Health, University of Melbourne, c/o Gouldburn Valley Base Hospital, Graham Street, Shepparton, Victoria 3630, Australia

'THE COMMUNITY'

The 'community' is an interesting concept. In its broadest perspective, it provides an impression of a large group of people acting together rather than as individuals. There is a sense of ongoing communication between the individuals involved and a commitment to an overall body. In reality, the 'community' is made up of a range of subgroups founded upon family, ethnic, religious, political, socioeconomic and cultural ties, each having its own subcomponents and priorities but with some shared values. Each issue that arises is prioritized to a different extent depending on the values held by the group or individuals concerned. In the case of diabetes, those with a diabetic family member or friend, or who are from ethnic groups that feel threatened by diabetes, may be more likely to take up diabetes interventions. Conversely, participation in interventions is less likely among those who consider themselves to be at low risk (e.g. the young) or those whose personal health is a low priority until ill-health occurs (e.g. those with a low socioeconomic status, care for a sick relative or who place religious demands above their own health)[1]. The take-up of primary and secondary preventive activities in the community therefore needs to be viewed with an understanding of personal and group priorities, if an effective programme is to be undertaken.

Within the community, there is a range of individuals who are able to influence the implementation of health initiatives. Their support can pro-

Type 2 Diabetes: Prediction and Prevention. Edited by Graham A. Hitman

mote 'success', while lack of support can undermine health interventions. For example, existing medical and health workers can provide conflicting advice if they are not aware of the programme content, or actively denigrate programmes if they disagree with the content or if there is a perceived threat to their livelihood or status[2]. Leaders of community organizations, at a variety of levels, can paint programmes as being useful or exploitative of the health needs of the community, if they have not been included during planning. Leaders are not necessarily those who have been visibly elected or selected and may not be 'elders'. They may be relatives of leaders (e.g. spouses) or have no recognizable qualification.

Thus, for the successful development and implementation of community-based programmes for the detection and prevention of type 2 or non-insulin-dependent diabetes mellitus, there is a need to define the 'community' concerned clearly, and thereby identify and enlist the assistance of local leaders and health workers[3]. Combining a review of screening and prevention is logical because the processes for each are intimately intertwined in the community. Lack of visible participation by leaders can undermine the status of programmes in the eyes of many community members. Screening of a leader can be an observed event which can attract other individuals into personal screening. As individuals are initially more concerned with their immediate risk of having type 2 diabetes, rather than adopting lifestyle changes, the initial screening session and return of results can be used as an educational session to promote the need for further education and participation in lifestyle programmes. Such screening sessions can also provide baseline information for evaluation and ongoing direction of programmes.

SCREENING FOR TYPE 2 DIABETES IN THE COMMUNITY

If screening is viewed purely from the impact of the direct benefits of screening asymptomatic individuals for undiagnosed type 2 diabetes, then it is a matter of controversy[4]. There are those who suggest that asymptomatic individuals should not be screened until an appropriate randomized controlled trial has been undertaken, although the outcome measures would need to be diverse and the duration extensive. On the other hand, it is clear that many of those with type 2 diabetes present with diabetic tissue damage or risk factors for complications[5,6]. Indeed, extrapolating backwards, it has been suggested that type 2 diabetes presents 9–12 years after development of the disease[7]. The growing evidence of the success of clinical intervention in type 2 diabetes, including glycaemic control[8], supports the contention that early diagnosis is worthwhile. Further benefits from screening would arise if impaired glucose tolerance (IGT) were to become a target for medical management or other successful interventions.

In view of the potential for improved health outcomes, there is general agreement that screening under certain circumstances would be worthwhile[9]. The methodology to be used to target groups remains a major subject for debate [9,10].

HOW NOT TO TEST IN THE COMMUNITY

In the community, there is a range of groups involved with people with diabetes. Although many follow a scientific doctrine, others apply a philanthropic, spiritual or commercial path without reference to the available data. So, although there appears to be a consensus among 'experts' that population screening, not linked to primary prevention programmes, is inappropriate[4], many community groups and pharmacies continue to provide a fingerprick glucose-testing service and claim to have diagnosed large numbers with diabetes. The low utility of such an approach is shown by a follow-up study from a lay screening programme in North Dakota[11]. Of 2016 people screened, 146 (7.2%) were referred for further evaluation, of whom 5.4% had newly diagnosed diabetes, i.e. the screening method used detected 4 per 1000 new cases. On the other hand, in a random sample not referred for further evaluation, 2% (i.e. 20 of 1000) had newly diagnosed diabetes. The study documented the following hazards associated with community-based diabetes screening:

- undocumented volunteer proficiency
- inherent inaccuracy of method
- handling of potentially infectious blood-contaminated supplies
- medical and legal ramifications.

Further risks are to provide reassurance to those with continued undiagnosed diabetes or with modifiable risk factors for type 2 diabetes. This may dissuade such individuals from attending lifestyle programmes or further diagnostic tests. There is also no certainty that reassurance will actually occur among the 'worried well'[12].

HOW TO TEST IN THE COMMUNITY

The underlying justification for screening in the community needs to be the direct or collateral benefits from the methodology chosen. There are four major outcomes:

- Early detection of diabetes linked with ongoing clinical and self-management.
- Identification of those at very high risk (e.g. IGT), linked with lifestyle programmes or ongoing medical care.

- Increased awareness of personal diabetes risk and linkage with lifestyle programmes.
- Increased awareness of diabetes without reassurance for those at risk of developing diabetes and without a future deterrent for ongoing screening.

Clearly, population-based screening is unable to address any of these outcomes, except as part of either ongoing care or a primary prevention programme linked to local clinicians.

In summary, screening for asymptomatic individuals therefore has the potential to increase the uptake of primary prevention programmes and to expedite the diagnosis of diabetes. Such screening should be undertaken by either of the following:

- Local clinicians who can provide ongoing care for those with diabetes and linked with local lifestyle programmes (e.g. the 'green prescription'[13])
- Integrated primary prevention programmes that can undertake the lifestyle programmes and link in with local primary and secondary diabetes services.

WHAT SCREENING TEST SHOULD BE USED?

Once the criteria for diagnosis have been agreed, the options for screening for type 2 diabetes can be reviewed. If the glycated haemoglobin (HbA_{1c}) becomes the diagnostic test for diabetes, this would probably alter the methods used. The aim of the screening test is either to be the first of two diagnostic tests or to determine who should proceed to a second test (e.g. the oral glucose tolerance test or OGTT). The assessment of screening tests must incorporate their cost and convenience (e.g. HbA_{1c} is more expensive than a glucose measurement), the underlying prevalence of type 2 diabetes in the population concerned, and the repeatability and validity of the method concerned[14].

The validity of the test is assessed using a 2×2 contingency table as shown in Table 13.1.

Generally, as the sensitivity increases, the specificity decreases and vice versa. This trade-off can be assessed using a receiver operator curve (ROC), where the true positive rate (sensitivity) can be plotted against a range of false-positive rates (1 − specificity)[9,14]. The area under the ROC for each screening method can then be compared.

The validity of each of the tests has been comprehensively reviewed[9]. Although there has been support for the fasting glucose as the screening method of choice[10], the inconvenience of the test minimizes its utility for many of those at the highest risk of diabetes. In the community, the best test is the least inconvenient and, for this reason, many general practitioners use a fingerprick test using a glucose meter. Unfortunately, the reliability, pre-

Table 13.1. Oral glucose tolerance test result

	Diabetes	No diabetes
Screening test		
Positive	True positives correctly identified (a)	False negatives (b)
Negative	False negatives (c)	True negatives correctly identified (d)
Test characteristics		
Sensitivity $= \frac{a}{a+c}$		Specificity $= \frac{d}{b+d}$
Positive predictive value $= \frac{a}{a+b}$		Negative predictive value $= \frac{d}{c+d}$

cision and accuracy of such machines outside the rigours of scientific studies are considered to be poor[9,15] and the method is therefore inappropriate. The HbA_{1c} appears to have a higher sensitivity than the fasting glucose and is also convenient (e.g. with an HbA_{1c} of 5.8–6.03%, there is a 60–92% sensitivity at a specificity of 89–91%). The sensitivity of a random glucose, if suitably adjusted for the postprandial period and the age, is currently the most convenient and relatively inexpensive test[16], e.g. in those aged 40–64 years, a random capillary glucose of 7.0 mmol/l had a sensitivity of 69.0% and specificity of 93.7% in UK Caucasians and test characteristics of 71.8% and 93.5% respectively in UK south Asians[17].

These one-off test characteristics need to be placed in to perspective within the continuum that applies in the community. Primary care services are in a position to repeat the screening test either opportunistically or in a planned way after a period of time for assessment of deterioration in glucose control. Rather than undertaking a more inconvenient test, it may be more suitable to repeat the convenient test after, for example, 12 months (any damage that may have occurred in this time period is unlikely to be significant[10]). The consensus statement for screening set by the New Zealand Society for the Study of Diabetes[18] recommends immediate referral for a second test if the random glucose measurement is 7.0 mmol/l or more. However, for those with a random glucose of 5.5–6.9 mmol/l, there is a recommendation to repeat the test after 12 months.

WHO SHOULD BE SCREENED?

In high-risk ethnic groups (which includes most non-Caucasian ethnic groups once they have adopted a Western lifestyle), there is general agreement that all adults should be screened at regular intervals. The recommended frequency of such screening varies (e.g. every 3 years). Among low-risk ethnic groups, it has been recommended that screening is carried out only in high-risk individuals (those who are obese, older, or have a family history, a sedentary lifestyle or have had a baby over 4 kg (9 lb)[9,10]). In a community setting, repeat screening should be used as an opportunity to address risk factors for developing diabetes in the same manner as the initial screen.

PREVENTION OF TYPE 2 DIABETES IN THE COMMUNITY

Therapeutic options for the prevention of type 2 diabetes can use either pharmacological agents or lifestyle approaches (or a mixture). Although many pharmacological agents are under investigation, there is currently no support from studies in humans for any particular agent. However, there are a growing number of non-randomized studies that describe changes in prevalence or describe predictors of diabetes in association with lifestyle interventions[19]. Whether these are temporal or secular trends or result from the interventions themselves can be assumed only from a mixture of qualitative data (formative and process evaluation) and from knowledge of the underlying trend.

There has been one major randomized controlled trial of a lifestyle programme in Da Xing in China [20]. That study involved the screening of 100 000 of the population using urine testing. The subsequent identification of over 500 Chinese with IGT (presumably in the high range for IGT) provided subjects for a 2×2 factorial study with exercise and nutrition as the two interventions. All bar the control group had a reduction in diabetes incidence of more than 30% over the 6-year period.

As the therapeutic options (diet, exercise and pharmacological agents) are discussed elsewhere, the purpose of this chapter is to discuss the approaches required in the community, i.e. how to apply the therapeutic options.

ECOLOGICAL APPROACHES FOR THE PREVENTION OF DIABETES

Ecological intervention for the prevention of type 2 diabetes is the alteration of the general environment to make diabetogenic activities less and anti-diabetogenic activities more accessible. There are many examples and the numbers are increasing[21]. The growth of cycle lanes, walking tracks, improved lighting for recreational areas, televised fitness programmes, fitness centres and workplace programmes are designed to increase access to more acceptable exercise activities. Crêche facilities would allow young parents greater access to the exercise activity of their choice. Reduced (or absent) fees would remove the cost barrier for some (although cost can be used as an excuse rather than being a genuine barrier to exercise).

One of the more interesting ecological approaches is to reduce access to elevators and escalators by siting them at the rear of new buildings and placing the stairs in a more readily accessible and visible position. The concept of compelling private industry to implement work place safety procedures with a low health benefit yield (far lower than many health interventions that are inaccessible because of their cost) is already in place[22].

Influencing the food supply is another ecological approach increasingly being implemented as part of preventing other non-communicable diseases (NCDs). World War II and its associated rationing provided an excellent example of the speed with which such an intervention could work[23]. In the modern age, such rationing would be unacceptable, and more subtle forms of food supply manipulation have been used. The growth in 'low-fat' foods has been a helpful consumer-led phenomenon. In the North Karelia Project, a popular local sausage was adapted by replacing some meat and fat with mushrooms[24]. Increased awareness of foods likely to be low in fat is provided not only as a direct marketing point through the sale of 'low-fat' foods, but also by labelling and public benchmarking programmes. The latter involves signposting of the lowest fat products in a range using a specific symbol (e.g. the 'Pick the Tick' programme in New Zealand)[25]. The importance of benchmarking foods and promoting the cooperation of food producers, regulatory bodies and health groups provides a major opportunity in improving access to, and uptake of, less diabetogenic foods in the long term. One example of this was the Norwegian Nutrition and Food Policy programme ratified in 1976[26]. Although the dietary changes achieved were modest, the model provides a sound basis for further development.

Controlling the food supply in local areas has also been attempted. In the small, isolated Australian Aboriginal community of Minjilang, the adjustment of foods available in a local monopoly store reduced obesity, blood pressure and serum cholesterol, and favourably altered other blood micronutrients[27]. However, this was a community-initiated programme, implying that an awareness of the need to alter food consumption was already in place.

HIGH-RISK APPROACH, POPULATION APPROACH OR BOTH?

The aim of a primary prevention programme is to prevent the maximum number of individuals developing diabetes. In practical terms, this also needs to be at the lowest cost. The impact of a prevention programme is dependent upon the efficacy of the intervention, the numbers of those at risk who take up the programme and adherence to the programme. If the programme is to be targeted only at those who are at high risk, then there needs to be a means of identifying these individuals, and this depends upon the sensitivity of the detection programme and its penetration into the community.

The high-risk approach has a number of advantages. It motivates the subject and physician and utilizes the patient–doctor relationship. The intervention is appropriate for that individual and the risk–benefit ratio can be tailored to that individual's needs. The disadvantages are the difficulties and cost of screening and the potential hazards of labelling asymptomatic individuals as 'sick'. The other major disadvantage of the approach is that the development of the high-risk status has not been addressed. With the increasing incidence of type 2 diabetes, it is clear that the incidence of risk factors (especially obesity) is increasing and that the high-risk approach cannot prevent the epidemic of risk factors. As none of the available interventions can be absolute (because of uptake and adherence and associated problems), the epidemic will continue and the costs of prevention will escalate.

The population approach addresses the root causes of the increase in incidence of both type 2 diabetes and its risk factors. The cost of interventions with pharmacological agents on a personal basis would generally be prohibitive and hence the population approach is more applicable to lifestyle programmes (or one-off/infrequent treatments such as immunization). A major advantage is that a large number of individuals are involved at an earlier stage in the development of risk factors. A disadvantage is that, although the physician can play a role in the overall strategy, the interventions are generally not tailored to the individual and there is a greater chance of a problematic risk–benefit ratio. If the perception of health-promoting behaviour approaches the population-preferred behaviour (as is becoming the case with smoking), then there is a greater motivation for change.

Three hypothetical situations are shown in Figure 13.1 that compare the cumulative numbers with new diabetes and IGT over a 10-year period in a population of 10 000. The model assumes no death, no new subjects, and a fixed progression from normal to IGT and IGT to diabetes of 3% per annum. The baseline data are for south Asians with a 10% baseline prevalence of IGT[28]. The situations assume a one-third reduction in progression rates per annum in both normal subjects (population approach) and those with IGT (population and high-risk approach). A high-risk approach will reduce the numbers developing diabetes by 31%, but the numbers with IGT will increase by 6%. The population approach would reduce the numbers developing diabetes by 42% and those developing IGT by 16%. The modelling approach applied by Eastman et al.[29], incorporating mortality rates, estimated that a delay in onset of type 2 diabetes by 6 years was associated with an approximately 45% reduction in the incidence of proliferative diabetic retinopathy by the age of 65 years.

From this model, the population approach would appear to be more sustainable over time. However, there is a range of caveats. The estimated annual cost of the average person with either diabetes or IGT (with intervention and screening), or without either (with intervention) would deter-

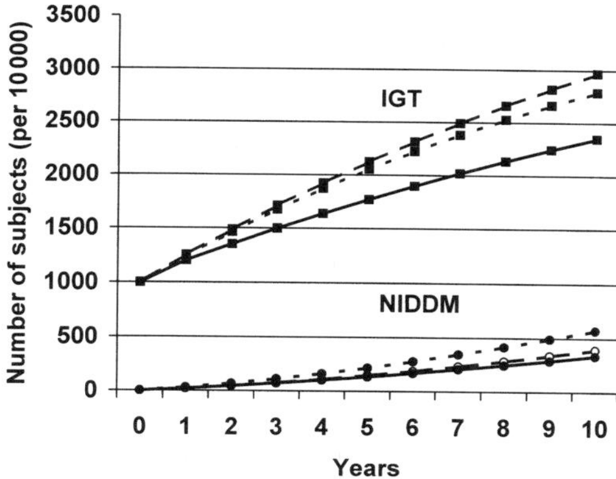

Figure 13.1. Hypothetical increase in numbers of subjects with IGT and type 2 diabetes over a 10-year period in south Asians with a baseline prevalence of IGT of 10%. Three crude models are presented: No intervention (- - -), high-risk intervention reducing the rate of progression from IGT to type 2 diabetes by one-third (— — —) and population-based intervention reducing the rate of progression from normal to IGT to one-third and from IGT to type 2 diabetes by one-third (——).

mine which approach would be most viable in the short term. One of the major costs in the high-risk approach, screening, has a sensitivity, assumed to be 100% in Figure 13.1, but it is far less than this in practice. This would result in fewer high-risk subjects receiving the intervention. On the other hand, population-based interventions require an infrastructure and development costs, whereas those for high-risk interventions (through pre-existing medical services) can be taken up rapidly (albeit with variable adoption by physicians and adherence by patients). The models in Figure 13.1 assume that the adherence to and efficacy of the interventions are the same in the population and high-risk approaches, and this is unlikely to be the case. The potential for a lower benefit from a population intervention could reduce adherence (not only in proportions adopting the intervention, but also in the degree of adoption). Rose calls this the 'prevention paradox'[30]. However, if lifestyle change is the intervention, then there are a range of collateral benefits for the individual in terms of symptoms and general well-being[31]. Collateral benefits from a lifestyle programme in the population would also offset costs from other obesity-related diseases such as coronary heart disease, hypertension, cholelithiasis, and breast and colon cancer[32]. Modelling programmes such as those of Eastman et al. could be used to assess theoretical outcomes from a range of high-risk and population scenarios.

Behind both the high-risk and the population approach is the need to maximize uptake and adherence to the intervention. Developing strategies to address this requires an understanding of how and why people change their behaviour.

HOW DO PEOPLE SEEK CHANGE?

The traditional medical model functions with patients seeing their doctor for a real or perceived health problem. The doctor 'treats' (this may be reassurance or other clinical intervention) and the patient decides whether or not to adhere to the treatment. This medical model, based upon the relationship and trust between patient and doctor, can be well utilized for reducing risk of diabetes (Table 13.2). The model combines decisions by both patient and doctor. The former decides that they are at risk and that they will attend for an assessment and for advice, and the degree to which they will adhere to therapy. The latter decides what the therapy should be and monitors the progress in risk factor reduction. In many cases, the decision that a patient is at risk will be declared within a consultation, and hence the only decision by the patient may be the extent of adherence to therapy.

The empowerment approach puts the person concerned as the only decision-maker. This requires an adequate knowledge base, an acceptance of personal risk, a high self-efficacy (belief in personal ability to achieve) and an understanding of the scientific validity of the interventions. If a doctor is visited (and in many cases the practitioner may be an allied health professional or a provider of alternative remedies), then this is strictly on the basis of acquiring knowledge, an assessment and/or Western therapy.

There remains a heterogeneous group comprising people who remain unaware of their risk and are unwilling to attend for assessment or unwilling or unable to adhere to treatment. Other more complex concepts also enter into the arena, e.g. the degree of personal risk may help to determine the priority given to addressing the risk, and the degree of misinformation can mislead individuals and undermine genuine attempts to reduce modifiable risk factors.

The 'transtheoretical model' provides a framework for addressing participation in risk-reduction strategies within these groups[33]. The readiness to change concept proposes that the decision by an individual to adopt a particular behaviour is based on a balance of its perceived benefits and disadvantages. This decision-making is often subconscious. The stages of change concept proposes that there is a standard path by which decision-making progresses, which in turn is dependent upon the readiness to change status. There are five stages of change:

1. Precontemplation: not considering changing behaviour.
2. Contemplation: thinking about changing.
3. Preparation: making plans to change.
4. Action: initiating behaviour change.
5. Maintenance: continuing with changed behaviour.

Table 13.2. Personal approaches for the prevention of diabetes in those perceiving they are at high risk

Medical model										
Patient perceives is at high risk of diabetes	→	Patient attends doctor, assesses risk	→	'Prescribes' intervention (advice, drug referral, surgery)	→	Patient adheres to an extent	→	Risk factor reduction	→	Reduced risk of diabetes
Empowered model										
Person perceives is at risk of diabetes	→	Person identifies possible strategies	→	Attends practitioner whom he feels is appropriate	→	Seeks treatment which he thinks is appropriate	→	Overall better adherence	→	Risk factor reduction if effective intervention

These concepts provide a framework from which to address issues of risk perception and then adherence to appropriate therapeutic options. Difficulties (or strengths) may lie in immovable health beliefs, which are based on interpretations of past experiences and spiritual values. Attempting to address issues that are seen to hold a major disadvantage for the individual can undermine the advisory and advocacy role of a 'practitioner' and can lead to alienation. This may explain the higher predominance of smokers among diabetic patients who do not attend diabetes services[34].

EMPOWERMENT

The success of the Minjilang study demonstrates the underlying complexity and synergies behind the population approach. The community initiated the change in food supply. Had this been imposed, it is unlikely that change would have occurred. To make this decision, the community needed to be aware of their risk and that altering the food supply could be one successful way of reducing their risk. They were willing, as a community, to make a positive balance between the benefits of the healthier food and the disadvantage of less access to food that provided some degree of pleasure. If this process had been easy, then similar changes in other small communities would have occurred. In general, they have not. The implication behind Minjilang is that an empowered community, which has adequate information and collectively believes that change is worthwhile, can achieve change at little cost. How can Minjilang be reproduced? What else happened to support and stimulate the process?

Support for the community empowerment approach comes from a study in Rarotonga[35]. As part of a research study, a village, consisting mainly of migrants from other islands in the Cook Islands, was chosen to participate in an obesity control pilot. The pilot area received nutrition education, practical support and training, in order to improve nutritional choices and to adopt exercise. A control area on the other side of the (small) island comprised mainly Rarotongans who were disappointed that they were not in the pilot area. They received intermittent media reports about progress in the intervention village. After 1 year, the pilot area had gained, on average, 1 kg and the control area had lost 1 kg! On further investigation, it transpired that the control village had established their own programme.

The empowerment model can therefore be a powerful force for change. If an individual patient is empowered (e.g. one with IGT), then this is likely to be associated with improved self-care behaviours and greater adherence to interventions. This approach is now the preferred method for diabetes education[36]. However, empowerment is itself an interesting concept. An empowered individual with high self-efficacy, but with inadequate knowledge, can adopt ineffective strategies and view expert advice as a threat to his or her cultural and personal integrity. This may apply in community groups as well as in individuals. It is clear that a great deal more research is required in order to determine methods for maximizing effective empowerment.

A fundamental requirement for effective empowerment is knowledge and the media is one source of information. The early studies of the use of media, such as the three-city study in California[37], demonstrated an increase in knowledge and had a major influence on some health behaviours. This included some self-reported eating habits (e.g. fat consumption), although these were not confirmed by anthropometric measures. An evaluated poster campaign on the symptoms of diabetes in the UK increased knowledge but did not measurably increase the uptake of screening for diabetes[38]. In Mauritius, a national campaign to control diabetes had no measurable impact on the incidence of obesity, IGT or diabetes within 5 years[39]. Thus, media campaigns appear to increase knowledge but do not generally change behaviour sufficiently to lead to a reduction in obesity.

Although knowledge is a prerequisite for effective empowerment, increased knowledge may itself not lead to any change in behaviour. At a community level, participation in the process of change (either directly or by an acceptable proxy) appears to be necessary to achieve the changes required. Such changes are likely to occur only in the action and maintenance stages of change. Community development as a public health process enhances participation in 'change', and early results suggest that it may be a useful public health practice for contributing to the prevention of type 2 diabetes[19].

COMMUNITY DEVELOPMENT MODELS

Community development has been defined as 'the process of organising and/or supporting community groups in identifying their health issues, planning and acting upon their strategies for social action/change, and gaining increased self reliance and decision making power as a result of their activities'[40]. Clearly, empowerment of the community and of the individuals within that community are at the heart of the community development process.

The growth of community development programmes for the control of diabetes in New Zealand, North America and Australia reflects the growing appreciation by high-risk communities that a diabetes epidemic exists and needs to be addressed[19]. Although none of the programmes has yet been completed to the stage of being able to demonstrate a reduction in the incidence of diabetes or IGT, the South Auckland Diabetes Project pilot programme has demonstrated positive changes in intermediate outcomes[41]. In a pilot programme in two urban Pacific Islands churches, a reduction in waist circumference and stable weight occurred in the intervention church (of about 80 congregants) and a gain in waist circumference and weight occurred in the control church (of about 125 congregants). The control church even had its own exercise group for a while.

The components of the community development programmes have overlapped markedly in those that have been described to date. Before any action is planned, it is essential that community leaders are identified and invited into the planning group. It would be preferable if health workers had also been invited in to assist them. If such an invitation arrives, it should be taken up, even if there had initially been no consideration of such a programme by health workers. Priorities in the community often change and knowledge of a refusal to assist can persist and influence events for a remarkably long time.

Involvement of a joint health worker and community team ensures that, where possible, cultural aspects of the interventions can be considered and addressed early. The cultural and local expertise of the community representatives needs to be respected in the same way that they respect the scientific and health skills of health workers. The synergy between primary, secondary and tertiary prevention strategies needs to be appreciated and utilized. Those with a diabetic relative are at high risk themselves (for primary and secondary prevention strategies), and can support their diabetic relative to attend and adhere to tertiary prevention strategies.

One of the great opportunities within a community development project comes from training community members to train others (train the trainers) and to lead lifestyle change. The Minnesota Heart Health 'Shop Smart for your Heart' Grocery programme had the grocers participating in the planning and implementation of their programme[42]. By training local, culturally appropriate people in leading groups and by training others the participation rates by high-risk communities can increase; this is another process used in diabetes education[43]. It is essential to have trained local people committed to their own community as part of the implementation and planning teams in order to make programmes meaningful for those being targeted. Once participation rates are high, many communities will run their own interventions; this has happened in the South Auckland Diabetes Project pilot church described earlier. This immediately reduces costs and can increase participation rates further.

Further growth of programmes can be achieved through diffusion of the information to, and programme implementation by, other groups[44]. The study in Rarotonga was one example of this, and a similar diffusion happened in North Karelia[45].

PRACTICAL ASPECTS OF COMMUNITY-BASED PROGRAMMES

Programmes are usually a mix of educational sessions, nutritional modules (e.g. cooking demonstrations, supermarket tours), a range of exercise programmes and training in other life skills, including how to use local health services. Although specific lifestyle strategies are described elsewhere, there are two further practical aspects of programmes that need to be considered. First, the venue for group sessions needs to be easily accessible, culturally acceptable and inexpensive. Because of the internal divisions that may exist within a community, venues either need to be 'neutral' or in a variety of sites. Second, integration with other prevention and health programmes can enhance diabetes-related interventions by reducing boredom and increasing relevance to a larger number of people.

EVALUATION

Ongoing evaluation of programmes is essential to optimize the chance of success. Cost analyses are of particular importance in the current health climate. Any new programmes will generally be judged on their short-term marginal cost. Although the potential for long-term savings will be a consideration, immediate personal health demands will usually take priority where health is a major political issue. In view of this, it may be difficult to obtain adequate resources for a population approach. The failure of most population-based approaches to control obesity[19] also serves to promote the short-term, high-risk approach. Therefore, if a population approach is to be used (and this is probably the most sustainable approach), this needs to have the maximal impact at the lowest cost, which requires careful monitoring and continual fine tuning.

There are a range of tools available for evaluating the progress and outcomes from a primary prevention programme[46]:

- formative evaluation
- quality assurance
- assessment of delivered dose
- assessment of received dose
- component programme impact
- intermediate outcomes
- community impact
- cost analysis.

Evaluation costs can be high in small programmes. However, as these roll out to larger proportions of the populations and measures become more restricted, these costs will be relatively smaller as has happened in the cardiovascular disease prevention programmes[47]. In general, outcome measures (either intermediate such as weight or disease measures such as type 2 diabetes) will help to demonstrate the value of the programme. Formative and other evaluation help to tailor the intervention to the needs and expectations of the community, and maximize the ability to achieve useful outcomes.

REFERENCES

1. Ockene IS. The rationale for intervention. In: Ockene IS, Ockene JK, eds. *Prevention of Coronary Heart Disease*. Boston: Little, Brown & Co., 1992: 103–22.
2. Hagey, R. The native diabetes program: Rhetorical process and praxis. *Med Anthropol* 1989; **12**:7–33.
3. Kreuter MW. PATCH: its origin, basic concepts and links to contemporary public health policy. *J Health Educ* 1992: **23**:135–9.
4. WHO Study Group. *Prevention of Diabetes Mellitus. WHO Technical Series* no. 844. Geneva: WHO, 1994: 35–40.
5. Hillson RM, Hockaday TDR, Newton DJ, Pim B. Delayed diagnosis of non-insulin dependent diabetes is associated with greater metabolic and clinical abnormality. *Diabetic Med* 1985; **2**:383–6.
6. Harris MI. Undiagnosed NIDDM: clinical and public health issues. *Diabetes Care* 1993; **16**:642–52.
7. Harris MI, Klein RE, Welbourn TA, Knuiman MW. Onset of NIDDM occurs at least 4–7 years before clinical diagnosis. *Diabetes Care* 1992; **15**:815–19.
8. Ohkubo Y, Kishikawa H, Araki E et al. Intensive insulin therapy prevents progression of diabetic microvascular complications in Japanese patients with non-insulin dependent diabetes mellitus: a randomised prospective 6 year study. *Diabetes Res Clin Pract* 1995; **28**:103–17.
9. Engelgau MM, Aubert RE, Thompson TJ, Herman WH. Screening for NIDDM in non-pregnant adults. *Diabetes Care* 1995; **18**:1606–18.
10. Expert Committee on the Diagnosis and Classification of Diabetes Mellitus. Report of the expert committee on the diagnosis and classification of diabetes mellitus. *Diabetes Care* 1997; **20**:1183–97.
11. Newman WP, Nelson R, Scheer K. Community screening for diabetes. *Diabetes Care* 1994; **17**:363–5.
12. McDonald IG, Daly J, Jelinek VM, Panetta F, Gutman JM. Opening Pandora's box: the unpredictability of reassurance by a normal test result. *BMJ* 1996; **313**: 329–32.
13. Swinburn BA, Walter LG, Arroll B, Tilyard MW, Russell DG. The Green Prescription Study: a randomised controlled trial of written exercise advice in general practice. *Am J Public Health* (in press).
14. Barker DJP, Rose G. Screening. In: *Epidemiology in Medical Practice*, 2nd edn. New York: Churchill Livingstone, 1982: 116–24.
15. Patterson KR. Population screening for diabetes mellitus. *Diabetic Med* 1993; **10**:77–81.
16. Engelgau MM, Thompson TJ, Smith PJ et al. Screening for diabetes mellitus in adults. *Diabetes Care* 1995; **18**:463–6.
17. Simmons D, Williams DRR. Random blood glucose as a screening test for diabetes in a biethnic population. *Diabetic Med* 1994; **11**:830–5.

18. NZSSD Consensus statement on screening for diabetes in asymptomatic individuals. *NZ Med J* 1995; **108**:464–5.
19. Simmons D, Voyle J, Swinburn B, O'Dea K. Community-based approaches for the primary prevention of non-insulin dependent diabetes mellitus. *Diabetic Med* 1997; **14**:519–26.
20. Pan X, Guangwei L, Yinghua H. et al. Effect of dietary and/or exercise interventions on incidence of diabetes in 530 subjects with IGT: The Da-Wing IGT and Diabetes Study. In: *15th International Diabetes Federation Congress Abstracts*. Kobe, Japan, 1994: 489.
21. Egger G, Swinburn BA. An ecological approach to the obesity pandemic. *BMJ* 1997; **315**:477–80.
22. Tengs TO, Adams ME, Pliskin JS et al. Five hundred life-saving interventions and their cost-effectiveness. *Risk Anal* 1995; **15**:369–90.
23. Himsworth PH. Diet and the incidence of diabetes. *Clin Sci* 1935; **2**:117–48.
24. McAlister A, Puska P, Salonen JT, Tuomilehto J, Koskela K. Theory and action for health promotion: Illustrations from the North Karelia Project. *Am J Public Health* 1982; **72**:43–50.
25. Scott V, Worsley AF. Ticks, claims, tables and food groups: a comparison for nutrition labelling. *Health Prom Int* 1994; **9**:27–36.
26. Klepp KI, Forster JL. The Norwegian Nutrition and Food Policy: An integrated policy approach to a public health problem. *J Public Health Policy* 1985; **6**:447–63.
27. Lee AJ, Bailey APV, Yarmirr D, O'Dea K, Mathews JD. Survival tucker: improved diet and health indicators in an Aboriginal community. *Aust J Public Health* 1994; **18**:277–85.
28. Simmons D, Powell MJ. Metabolic and clinical characteristics of South Asians and Europeans in Coventry. *Diabetic Med* 1993: **10**:751–8.
29. Eastman RC, Silverman R, Harris M, Javitt JC, Chiang YP, Gorden P. Lessening the burden of diabetes. *Diabetes Care* 1993; **16**:1095–102.
30. Rose G. Strategy of prevention: lessons from cardiovascular disease. *BMJ* 1981 **282**:1847–51.
31. Simmons D, Fleming C, Cameron M. Evaluation of a diabetes and exercise programme in a multiethnic work force. *NZ Med J* 1996; **109**:268–70.
32. Segal L, Carter R, Zimmet P. The cost of obesity: The Australian perspective *PharmacoEconomics* 1994; **5**(suppl 1):45–52.
33. Prochaska JO. Strong and weak principles for progressing from precontemplation to action on the basis of twelve problem behaviours. *Health Psychol* 1994; **13**:47–51.
34. Graver AL, Davidson P, Brown AW, McRae JR, Wooldridge K. Dropout and relapse during diabetes care. *Diabetes Care* 1992; **15**:1477–83.
35. In: Swinburn B, Matenga Smith T, Daniel R, Craig P, Mantagi H. *Tutakimoa Lifewise Project*. University of Auckland, Auckland, 1995.
36. Arnold MS, Butler PM, Anderson RM, Funnell MM, Feste C. Guidelines for facilitating a patient empowerment programme. *Diabetes Educator* 1995; **21**:308–12.
37. Farquar JW, Maccoby N, Wood PD et al. Community education for cardiovascular health. *Lancet* 1997; **i**:1192–5.
38. Singh BM, Prescott JJW, Guy R, Walford S, Murphy M, Wise PH. Effect of advertising on awareness of symptoms of diabetes among the general public: the British Diabetic Association Study. *BMJ* 1994; **308**:632–6.
39. Dowse GK, Gareeboo H, Alberti KG et al. Changes in population cholesterol concentrations and other cardiovascular risk factor levels after five years of the

non-communicable disease intervention programme in Mauritius. *BMJ* 1995; **311**:1255–9.

40. Labonte R. Community development and partnerships. *Can J Public Health* 1993; **84**:237–40.
41. Simmons D, Fou F, Leakehe L, Voyle J, Dee J, Gatland B, Fleming C. A pilot church based diabetes control programme among Pacific Islands people: The South Auckland Diabetes Project. *Ann d'Endocrinol* (in press).
42. Mullis RM, Hunt MK, Foster M, Hachfield L, Lansing D, Snyder P, Pirie P. The shop smart for your heart grocery program. *J Nutr Educ* 1987; **19**:225–8.
43. DePue JD, Wells BL, Lasater TM, Carleton RA. Training volunteers to conduct heart health programs in churches. *Am J Prev Med* 1987; **3**:51–7.
44. In: Winett RA. *Information and Behaviour, Systems of Influence*. New Jersey: Lawrence Erlbaum Associates, 1986: 59–82.
45. Puska P, Nissinen A, Tuomilehto J et al. The community based strategy to prevent coronary heart disease: Conclusions from the ten years of the North Karelia Project. *Annu Rev Public Health* 1985; **6**:147–93.
46. Pirie P, Stone E, Assaf A, Flora J, Masehewsky-Schneider V. Programme evaluation strategies for community based health promotion programmes: perspectives from the cardiovascular disease community research and demonstration studies. *Health Educ Res* 1994; **9**:23–36.
47. Shea S, Basch CE, Lantigua R, Wechsler H. The Washington Heights–Inwood Healthy Heart program: A third generation community based cardiovascular disease prevention programme in a disadvantaged urban setting. *Prev Med* 1992; **21**:203–17.

14

Dietary Risk Factors

B.J. BOUCHER

Medical Unit, St Bartholomew's and the Royal London School of Medicine and Dentistry, Royal London Hospital, London E1 1BB, UK

It is increasingly recognized that there are environmental triggers for the development of type 2 diabetes in the individual, although the individual's susceptibility to the diabetogenic effects of such factors is likely to be determined largely by their genetic make-up[1,2]. The evidence for environmental triggering is as compelling as that for type 1 diabetes, where 60% of the risk of disease has been calculated as being environmentally determined[3]. The five WHO criteria for environmental triggering of disease[4], designed for the study of smoking and lung cancer, are fulfilled for type 2 as well as type 1 diabetes. Most of the recent literature in this area simply refers to 'diet' in the causation of this condition, with the implication that intake in excess of basic requirement is the main culprit[5]. A brief review of the available data in relation to the five criteria for environmental causation suggests that a more sophisticated approach may be required if optimal recommendations on healthy diet are to be produced[2].

1. *It should be possible to produce type 2 diabetes in animals by exposure to environmental agents*. Excess intake can certainly do this but so can variation in composition in the diet, excess vitamin A, vitamin D depletion, and exposure to low-dose diabetogenic nitrosamines such as streptozotocin, those found in smoked cured mutton and those produced from the betel nut (*Areca catechu*)[6–12].
2. *There should be considerable geographical differences in the incidence of type 2 diabetes*. In the UK itself, 3% of Caucasians and 10–15% of various Asian groups have this form of diabetes as do 40–66% of Nauruans and older Pima Indians[13–15].

Type 2 Diabetes: Prediction and Prevention. Edited by Graham A. Hitman

3. *Some populations should have rapid temporal changes in incidence in less than a generation that cannot be accounted for by genetic change*. This has been true in Western Samoa and Nauru[16,17] where a rapidly increasing prevalence has been described. We have found a drop in east London in the last 8 years[18].
4. *The risk to immigrants should rapidly rise to that of the host country*. This has been a feature for southern Asians migrating to Western countries and from rural to urban lifestyles[19,20]. The converse should also happen for immigrants with a high prevalence of disease and we have early evidence for this as shown in (3).
5. *There should be strong epidemiological evidence that certain environmental agents cause type 2 diabetes in humans*. The rat poison Vacor produces type 1 diabetes in survivors of high doses whereas 80% of survivors of lower doses develop type 2 diabetes with only a low incidence of type 1 diabetes[21]. Obesity, increasing affluence, lack of exercise, reduced fibre intake and excessive fat intake were the first well-substantiated risk factors for type 2 diabetes to be appreciated in humans[22-24].

Wholesale dietary restriction is not an option welcomed by affluent populations although, at the other end of the spectrum, malnutrition is a major problem worldwide. Some Europeans, in social classes 1 and 2, have taken current health promotional advice on low-fat, vegetarian and high-fibre meals to such extremes as to induce iron, protein and vitamin malnutrition in their children[25]. Very specific information about individual aspects of diet is therefore needed for the formulation of advice to both populations and individuals. The rest of this chapter reviews current knowledge with regard to both macro- and micronutrients and dietary 'toxins', and their influence on risk for type 2 diabetes.

PROTEINS AND AMINO ACIDS

Variation in the proportions of proteins, carbohydrates and fats in the diet has been investigated in relation to the risk of development of type 2 diabetes. Protein–energy malnutrition in young animals, and in humans, in whom it causes kwashiorkor, is often followed by diabetes mellitus. In rats, this is associated with reduced β-cell mass and reduced insulin secretory capacity which does not recover with adequate feeding later in life[26]. Indeed, re-feeding in this situation leads to abnormally large deposition of fat[27], similar in distribution to that of human syndrome X. The more recent appreciation that maternal protein malnutrition is followed by increased risk of diabetes later in life, and that small-for-dates babies have increased risks of ischaemic heart disease, hypertension and increased insulin resistance, as well as type 2 diabetes, should not therefore come as a surprise (see Chapter 9).

Catch-up in longitudinal growth can be achieved with restoration of an adequate diet in humans, up to the early or mid-20s, provided that puberty has been delayed. The catch-up growth seen with re-feeding early in childhood is, however, associated with premature puberty and subsequent stunting[28]. For this reason it has been suggested that cross-generational re-feeding will be required before optimal growth can be achieved by deprived population groups[29]. This proposition also implies that transgenerational re-feeding should reduce the prevalence of type 2 diabetes that is now being seen in Nauruans[17] and in Asians living in east London[18]. Explanations for stunting and development of type 2 diabetes in the offspring of protein-malnourished mothers include genetic imprinting or fetal programming of organs, such as the liver, with permanent metabolic derangement (see Chapter 9)[30]. A high-protein diet is, however, a recent development in primate life and one to which humans are not well adapted because the resultant low-carbohydrate intake induces insulin resistance[31]. Although an 'adequate' protein intake is likely to be desirable, an excessive intake is equally undesirable, both for protection of normal carbohydrate metabolism and for reduction in risk of cancer and hypertension[32]; in this respect, moderation in consumption of red meat is currently being considered by the Committee on the Medical Aspects of food policy of the Department of Health. Certain dietary amino acids may, however, be particularly 'essential' for protection of the developing pancreas and in maintenance of β-cell efficiency. In cats, taurine is essential for healthy islet function[33] whereas leucine is a well-known insulin secretogogue in animals and humans. Detailed information on the importance of other amino acids to the β-cell is not yet available for humans. It is not yet possible, therefore, to produce a specification for the profile of the 'ideal' protein contribution to the human diet in early or even in later life.

CARBOHYDRATES

It is generally advised that 60% of the diet should be made up of carbohydrates in affluent Western countries, to match the diets of early humans; there should be adequate fibre or other non-adsorbed starches, at more than 25 grams daily. This advice appears to be based as much on the need to keep fat intake down (see below) as on the specific 'virtues' of carbohydrates[35] apart from the high fibre or complex starch that some such foods contain. Increasing carbohydrate intake does, however, relate to a reduction in insulin–resistance experimentally and also relates to reduction in risk of type 2 diabetes in humans[35–38]. Different sources of carbohydrate in the diet can differ widely in the degree to which blood glucose rises after consumption. For example, isocaloric portions of legumes such as lentils (dahl) raise blood glucose levels less than cereal products, vegetables or fruit[38,39]. These differences relate to the slower rates of digestion of legumes (and of complex starches generally) than of cereals, by amylases, rather than to non-absorption or non-availability of their calorific content. Insulin responses to leguminous foods are less than to other complex carbohydrate foods in healthy people. Insulin response to 'white', or fibre-reduced, bread is less in healthy people than that to intact cereals fed after being similarly cooked. These effects are independent of the effects of variation in fibre content, although clearly such factors interact during digestion[37–40].

The practical value of a reversion to traditional high-carbohydrate and high-fibre low-fat diets, for improvement in insulin secretion and glucose utilization, has been demonstrated in Pima Indians[41]. It is difficult to separate the effects of a variation in proportion of any single major nutrient on insulin resistance, secretion and glucose tolerance because one cannot be altered without another being changed as well. It has been suggested that dietary sucrose has a deleterious effect on glucose tolerance. When sucrose is taken together with natural fruit potassium, delivery of glucose to the bowel from the stomach is progressively slowed over the range of 0.84–4.18 MJ/l; this is the range of sugar concentrations in fruit. Hyperglycaemia only occurs in normal mammals when sucrose is fed at concentrations above 4.18 MJ/l. The use of sucrose concentrates in affluent societies is a recent development to which humans have not yet adapted[42].

ALCOHOL

Alcohol consumption can induce hypoglycaemia in the fasting state as a result of inhibition of gluconeogenesis in the liver, although alcoholic pancreatitis can cause destruction of the islets with resultant diabetes, usually progressing more or less rapidly to insulin requirement. One recent study reports an increased incidence of type 2 diabetes with alcohol consumption of more than 30 g/day in men and women. Interestingly, there was also an inverse relationship of glucose tolerance to alcohol use at less than 30 g/day in men and women, i.e. a protective effect[43]. It is therefore possible that the beneficial effects reported for moderate alcohol/wine intake on mortality and incidence of heart disease may relate in part to reduction in the prevalence of type 2 diabetes. Further studies in this area will be helpful.

DIETARY FATS

Increasing dietary intake of animal fat, either of dairy origin or in meat products, is associated with an increased prevalence of type 2 diabetes across a wide range of populations[44]. Several mechanisms contribute to this effect, including increases in insulin resistance. One mechanism for this is impairment of insulin-stimulated recruitment of GLUT4 from the cytoplasm to the cell membrane in skeletal muscle, reducing glucose transport into muscle with high-fat diets[45]. This effect is independent of contraction (i.e. exercise)-induced recruitment. These findings help to explain the beneficial effect of exercise on insulin resistance, even in obese subjects who have not reduced their weight, and the beneficial effects seen soon after cutting down on excessive fat intake, even before weight loss, in obese people who do or do not have type 2 diabetes[46]. The adverse effects described related mainly to high intakes of saturated fats. The exception appears to be fish; in European studies increasing consumption of fish protects against heart disease and type 2 diabetes[46,47].

The effects of fish oil have therefore been investigated widely: taken in a high-lard (bovine fat) diet, it prevents obesity, hyperlipidaemia and abnormal increases in insulin resistance in rats[48], and protects the liver from the enhancement of pyruvate dehydrogenase activity otherwise induced by diets high in saturated fats[47,48]. Fish oil also reduces insulin resistance[49,50]. The mechanism for these beneficial effects may lie with the ω3-fatty acids found in fish oils[51], although vitamin D, plentiful in most oily fish, may be a contributing factor (see section on Vitamins below). Circulating concentrations of free fatty acids (FFAs) are increased in obesity. FFAs impair peripheral glucose utilization and promote increased hepatic gluconeogenesis. These phenomena were described early on as the glucose–fatty acid cycle[52]. Many mechanisms contribute to this effect, ranging from direct effects on the citrate cycle in the liver, reduction in insulin secretion, increases in insulin resistance (caused by inhibition of pyruvate kinase in muscle), to the recently described effect of tumour necrosis factor in increasing insulin resistance[53,54]. Epidemiological findings in humans strongly suggest that increasing fish consumption is protective against type 2 diabetes and heart disease[46,55] (see also Vitamins below). For polyunsaturated fats, usually thought to be beneficial agents in terms of risks of heart disease[56], in one recent Dutch study[43], increasing consumption has been reported to be associated with worsening glucose tolerance in men. Thus, the ideal profile for dietary fat intake is emerging but is still incomplete. What is certain is that no amount of information on healthy eating appears to make it any easier to interest people, or indeed governments, in ensuring that such diets are chosen by individuals or conformed to by the food industry.

DIETARY TOXINS

Many dietary toxins have been suspected of causing chronic pancreatic β-cell damage and type 2 diabetes. Cassava is one such food. It contains cyanide and consumption is associated with an increased risk of type 2 diabetes, although fortunately adequate cooking by boiling destroys the cyanide[57].

Streptozotocin administration induces type 1 diabetes in animals and, when used to treat malignant insulinomas in humans, has the same effect. Low-dose administration of streptozotocin in very young rodents can induce a non-insulin-requiring type of diabetes[10]. A large number of other nitroso compounds are diabetogenic[58–60]. Carcinogenic nitrosamines target specific tissues according to their individual chemical structure. Alloxan reaches the β cell because it contains a chair-shaped glucose-like moiety[61], and the same is true for streptozotocin. When type 1 diabetes was found to have an increased incidence in Icelandic teenage boys born in October, Helgasen[62] conceived the idea that the consumption, preconception, of the local delicacy of smoked cured mutton, eaten mainly over the weeks of Christmas and New Year, might be responsible. When this hypothesis was tested in mice, it was found to induce diabetes not in the fed animals but in their offspring, especially males and especially those born to fed fathers rather than to fed mothers, i.e. the effect was independent of any maternal glucose intolerance. This effect in mice was then shown to be the result of the nitrosamines specific to this foodstuff[63].

Increasing consumption of nitrites, nitrates and nitrosamines from protein in the diet was subsequently demonstrated to be associated with increasing incidence of type 1 diabetes in children in Europe[64]. Although the carcinogenicity of nitrosamines has been widely studied and levels in processed food, babies' teats, beer, bacon and many other foods are controlled by legislation in most countries, there appear to have been no epidemiological studies to investigate whether there might be similar associations for type 2 diabetes. As type 2 diabetes has a much greater prevalence than type 1, and as it carries huge risks to health and costs in health care, it is to be hoped that such studies will be forthcoming. The fact that nitroso-induced diabetogenicity may be apparent only in offspring of fed adults and that it may be passed to subsequent generations is a serious problem that could confound such studies; both streptozotocin and betel nut-specific arecal nitrosamines can induce inheritable diabetes[12,63] and other such agents may yet be discovered. The high prevalence of type 2 diabetes in Asians living in the UK, together with the high prevalence of oropharyngeal and foregut cancers caused by chewing betel nut, with or without chewing tobacco, suggested a study of betel nut feeding in CD1 mice, a non-diabetic strain used in the work on smoked cured mutton. Five days of betel nut feeding, completed 2 weeks preconception, induced glucose intolerance in significant numbers of adults and their control-fed offspring. Significant numbers of the subsequent F2–F4 generations of mice not fed betel nuts also developed glucose intolerance[12]. This effect has been reproduced by the specific arecal nitrosamine 3-(methylnitrosamino)propionaldehyde (MNPN), the most carcinogenic of its products[65]. An epidemiological study of betel nut usage and glycaemia in Bangladeshis living in east London has shown increasing betel usage to be associated with increases in weight and waist size, which are good markers for hyperglycaemia. Although total life-long consumption of betel nut correlated with glycaemia, this relationship was dependent on age and not on betel usage[66]. Any degree of inheritance of betel nut-related diabetes, in a population using this traditional foodstuff for thousands of years, would invalidate such cross-sectional studies, illustrating the difficulties of work in this area. Similar difficulties apply where type 2 diabetes is common because material hyperglycaemia can itself induce diabetes. Most nitroso compounds derived from proteins have been introduced into the diet only recently (by new techniques for food preservation and storage). It will therefore be easier to investigate newer toxins of this type for possible diabetogenicity than those in traditional foods. Cigarette smoking has been shown to be associated with increasing risk of type 2 diabetes, notably in a prospective study of 40 000 American female nurses[67]. Although chewing tobacco is banned in most Western countries, many Asians who chew betel nut quids add imported tobacco to them. Such tobacco is much stronger than products such as cigarettes or the Skol bandits that have been banned[68]. There is as yet no evidence about whether chewing tobacco confers similar risks, but work in progress may answer this question.

VITAMINS

Certain vitamins have direct or indirect roles in insulin metabolism. Vitamin D has been shown experimentally to be necessary for normal insulin secretion. Deficiency, or experimental depletion, leads to failure in insulin release and, if prolonged, to failure of insulin secretion and diabetes. Such diabetes becomes irreversible if depletion is continued[69–73]. Similar changes occur in humans; thus in renal failure the replacement of activated (1,25-dihydroxy)-vitamin D can correct glucose intolerance and lipid abnormalities, and reduce both the hypertension and the increased insulin resistance found in uraemia[74,75]. These changes may result directly from lack of vitamin D or from secondary hyperparathyroidism. Type 2 diabetes has been reversed by surgical correction of hyperparathyroidism in humans and improved by prolonged replacement treatment in osteomalacia. In a few cases, type 2 diabetes was corrected by calcium replacement[76–81]. Both mechanisms are probably important. Insulin secretory response to glucose relates directly to vitamin D status in a deficient Asian population without overt diabetes whereas glucose tolerance is inversely associated with vitamin D status[82]. Insulin secretion increased significantly with short-term treatment of deficiency with no improvement in impaired glucose tolerance.

As the risk of type 2 diabetes falls with increasing fish intake[83] a subgroup of Dutchmen from the study mentioned earlier were examined for vitamin D status. Both glucose tolerance and insulin resistance related inversely to vitamin D status although only 39% of this elderly Caucasian population suffered vitamin D deficiency, compared with 95% of the Asians who had minor degrees of glucose intolerance and 45% of those with no defect in glucose tolerance[82,84]. In populations with a high prevalence of vitamin D deficiency, early and continued repletion should contribute to prevention of type 2 diabetes and such a clinical trial is in progress (N Mannan and BJ Boucher, unpublished data, 1997). Vitamin D supplementation of non-deficient subjects has no specific effects directly relevant to type 2 diabetes, though it does lower blood pressure[85]. It is, however, clear that avoidance of vitamin D deficiency protects islet β-cell function. In populations with a high risk of type 2 diabetes, and a high prevalence of vitamin D deficiency, oral supplementation aimed at achieving the minimum daily recommended intake (or adequate exposure to sunlight) is clearly desirable although excessive intake should not be encouraged because of the risk of vitamin D toxicity and adverse effects on serum lipids[86]. Populations at risk include Asians living in northern countries, Asians or Blacks whose lifestyle keeps them out of the sun (e.g. Saudi men, prosperous women living in cities, Asians in the UK[87,88]). Older Caucasians suffered marked degrees of vitamin D deficiency, present in 36% of men and 47% of women living in 19 towns in 12 countries, who formed the SENECA study[89]. Fasting glucose (reflecting glucose tolerance) and insulin concentrations (reflecting insulin resistance) were inversely related to vitamin D status in this population, none of whom were vitamin D deficient (A Teuscher, 1996, personal communication).

Vitamin D action is effected through a ligand-bound vitamin D receptor (VDR) after dimerization with the retinoid X receptor, activated by 9-*cis*-retinoic acid. Both these receptors are present in islet β-cells[90,91]. Large intakes of vitamin A are known to antagonize the actions of vitamin D, reducing toxicity in overdose, and producing rachitic changes when given to otherwise normal animals[92,93]. Experimentally, vitamin A depletion induces glucose intolerance and increasing amounts can inhibit insulin release and secretion, inhibit secretion but not release or stimulate of biphasic insulin releases depending on concentration[94–96]. It is not surprising, as β-cells contain receptors to both vitamins and these receptors need to dimerize to be effective, that glucose intolerance can follow intravenous vitamin A administration in humans[97]. Feeding of vitamin A induces glucose intolerance in CD1 mice, comparable in incidence and severity to that induced by feeding betel nut or MNPN[64]. Avoidance of deficiency or excessive intake of vitamin A is therefore desirable. General guidance should be available rather than being restricted to pregnant women as it is at present in the UK, especially in populations with a significant prevalence of vitamin D depletion.

DIETARY METALS

Zinc is an integral part of the insulin molecule and a high groundwater content is reported to be associated with reduction in risk of type 1 diabetes, although this has not been examined in relation to type 2 diabetes[98]. Increasing arsenic content in drinking water is associated with increased risk of diabetes in copper smelters, independent of copper itself[99,100]. Iron deficiency impairs absorption of fat and fat-soluble vitamins, including vitamins A and D. Iron deficiency can therefore add to the problems that result from deficiency of these vitamins[101]. Calcium is an essential ion for β-cell function, for both membrane and cytosolic processing. It is essential for one of the endopeptidases that splits insulin from proinsulin[102]. Calcium deficiency reduces insulin secretory responses and correction restores these functions as discussed above. Magnesium is also essential for healthy β-cell function[103,104]. Vanadium is unusual in that it has a useful therapeutic effect in experimental animals as a result of insulin-like effects on enzyme activity[105].

OTHER FACTORS

The role of foods that have hypoglycaemic effects is rarely included in work on diet in the aetiology of type 2 diabetes. Several foods fall into this category, but it is not known whether their use in the diet is protective against islet dysfunction, abnormal insulin resistance or other disorders that lead to glucose intolerance. The bitter gourd, karela, used widely by Asians as a treatment for diabetes, onions, garlic, the piper betel leaf used as a wrapping in betel nut quids worldwide and the betel nut alkaloid arecoline all have this effect experimentally and in humans[106,107]. Many spices potentiate insulin action[108]. Fat substitutes (such as olestra) in use in the USA, and being introduced in Europe, induce malabsorption, which is theoretically capable of leading to hyper- or hypoglycaemia. Guar gum, reducing food breakdown and sugar absorption[109], is widely used to thicken foods commercially in every kind of pre-prepared food from soup to ice-cream. The effects of the intake of these foods and fillers warrants more epidemiological attention to the aetiology of chronic disease such as type 2 diabetes than has been given.

CONCLUSIONS

The question of what constitutes a healthy diet, in terms of reduction of risk of type 2 diabetes, has to reflect current knowledge and to remain open to modification as our knowledge in this area improves. It is already clear that it is not simply a question of avoidance of excess calorie intake over requirement, or of excess intake of fats over complex carbohydrates; detailed knowledge of the roles and effects of macro- and micronutrients has to be considered. Earlier reports on this subject have recommended avoidance of obesity, excessive intake of energy or excessive (> 30%) fat intake of animal origin and an increased intake of fibre and complex starches and, in Asians, reduction of free sugar intake[46,110–115]. All these points remain valid. Recent reviewers have suggested that avoidance of a high intake of saturated fats and maintenance of a high intake (> 60% of calorific value) of carbohydrates with high-fibre content are especially protective[116]. A change from an animal-based to a plant-based diet is recommended for the avoidance of degenerative disorders, such as hypertension, heart disease, diabetes and cancer, in the Policy Watch document, 'American Diet Performance and Healthy People 2000'[117].

The combination of a return to traditional lifestyles, to include regular physical work and adequate amounts of a balanced diet free of excess, would appear to sum up the best advice that we can give at the present time[118–121], although it is not clear who will be listening to this advice in a world where starvation is still rife. Perhaps a balancing out between the 'haves', with their excessive food intake and more than their share of consumption of material things, and the 'have-nots,' with their continuing cycles of deprivation, in terms of food above all, would be the ideal way to achieve health for all by the year 2000.

REFERENCES

1. Leslie RDG, ed. *Causes of Diabetes: Genetic and environmental factors*. Chichester: John Wiley, 1993.
2. Boucher BJ. Strategies for reduction in the prevalence of NIDDM; the case for a population-based approach to the development of policies to deal with environmental factors in its development. *Diabetologia* 1995; **38**:1125–9.
3. Diabetes Epidemiology Research International. Preventing insulin dependent diabetes mellitus: the environmental challenge. *BMJ* 1987; **295**:479–81.
4. Doll R, Peto R. The causes of cancer: quantitative estimates of avoidable risks of cancer in the United States today. *J Nat Cancer Inst* 1981; **66**:1191–308.
5. Florez H. Steps toward the primary prevention of type 2 diabetes mellitus. Various epidemiological considerations. *Invest Clin* 1997; **38**:39–52.
6. Adler AI, Schraer CD, Boyko EJ, Murphy NJ. Lower prevalence of impaired glucose tolerance and diabetes associated with daily seal oil or salmon consumption among Alaskan natives. *Diabetes Care* 1994; **17**:1498–501.
7. Chertow BS, Baker GR. The effects of vitamin A on insulin release and glucose oxidation in isolated rat islets. *Endocrinology* 1978; **103**:1562–72.
8. Billaudel B, Faure A, Labriji-Mestaghanmi H, Sutter B Ch J. Direct in vitro effect of 1,25-dihydroxyvitamin D3 on islet insulin secretion in vitamin deficient rats: Influence on vitamin D3 pre-treatment. *Diabete Metab* 1989; **15**:85–7.
9. Voss C, Harman K, Hartmann H et al. Diabetogenic effects of N-Nitrosomethylurea. *Exp Clin Endocrinol* 1988; **92**:25–31.

10. Bonner-Weir S. Leahy JL. Induced rat models of non-insulin-dependent diabetes. In: Shafrir E, Renold AE, eds. *Frontiers in Diabetes Research: Lessons from animal diabetes*. London: John Libby, 1988; 295–300.
11. Helgason T, Ewen SWB, Jaffrey B et al. N-Nitrosamines in smoked meats and their relation to diabetes. *IARC Scientific Publications* 1984; **57**:11–920.
12. Boucher BJ, Ewen SWB, Stowers JM. Betel nut (Areca catechu) consumption and the induction of glucose intolerance in adult CD1 mice and in their F1 and F2 offspring. *Diabetologia* 1994; **37**:49–55.
13. Simmons D, Williams DR, Powell MJ. Prevalence of diabetes in different regional and religious South Asian communities in Coventry. *Diabetic Med* 1992; **95**:428–31.
14. Zimmet P, Dowse G, Finch C et al. The epidemiology and natural history of NIDDM: lessons from the South Pacific. *Diabetes Metab Rev* 1990; **6**:91–124.
15. Bennett PH, Knowler WC. Increasing prevalence of diabetes in the Pima (American) Indians over a ten-year period. In: Waldhouse WK, ed. *Proceedings of the 10th Congress of the International Diabetes Federation*. Amsterdam: Excerpta Medica, 1979; 507–11.
16. Collins VR, Dowse GK, Toelupe PM et al. Increasing prevalence of NIDDM in the Pacific island population of Western Samoa over a 23-year period. *Diabetes Care* 1994; **17**:288–96.
17. Dowse GK, Zimmet PZ, Finch CF, Collins CR. Decline in incidence of epidemic glucose intolerance in Nauruans: implications for the 'thrifty genotype' hypothesis. *Am J Epidemiol* 1991; **133**:1093–104.
18. Prasad P, Balarajan B, Boucher BJ. Falling prevalence of NIDDM in Asians living in two East London Boroughs. In Preparation. 1999.
19. Ramachandran A, Jali MV, Mohan V et al. High prevalence of diabetes in an urban population in South India. *BMJ* 1988; **297**:587–90.
20. Ramachandran A, Jali MV, Mohan V et al. Prevalence of glucose intolerance in Asian Indians: urban–rural differences and significance of upper body adiposity. *Diabetes Care* 1992; **15**:1348–55.
21. Karam JH, Lewitt PA, Young CW et al. Insulinopenic diabetes after rodenticide (Vacor) ingestion. *Diabetes* 1980; **29**:971–8.
22. Trowell H. Diabetes mellitus death-rates in England and Wales 1920–70 and food supplies. *Lancet* 1974; 998–1002.
23. Henry RR. Prospects for primary prevention of type 2 diabetes mellitus. *Diabetes Rev Int* 1994; **3**:2–5.
24. Trovati M, Carta Q, Cavalot F et al. Influence of physical training on blood glucose control, glucose intolerance, insulin secretion and insulin action in non-insulin-dependent diabetic patients. *Diabetes Care* 1984; **7**:416–20.
25. Sanders TA, Reddy S. Vegetarian diets and children. *Am J Clin Nutr* 1994; **59**:1176S–1181S.
26. Swenne I, Borg LA, Crace CJ, Schnell Landstrom A. Persistent reduction of pancreatic cell beta-cell mass after a limited period of protein–energy malnutrition in the young rat. *Diabetologia* 1992; **35**:939–45.
27. Harris PM, Widdowson EM. Deposition of fat in the body of the rat during rehabilitation from starvation. *Br J Nutri* 1978; **39**:201–11.
28. Tuvemo T, Proos LA. Girls adopted from developing countries: a group at risk of early pubertal development and short final height. Implications for health surveillance and treatment [editorial]. *Ann Med* 1993; **25**:217–19.
29. Golden MH. Is complete catch-up possible for stunted malnourished children? *Eur J Clin Nutr* 1994; **48**:S58–70.

30. Desai M, Bryne J, Zhang SJ, Petry A, Lucas A, Hales CN. Programming of hepatic insulin-sensitive enzymes in offspring of rat dams fed an isocaloric protein restricted diet. *Am J Physiol* 1997; **272**:G1083–90.
31. Brand-Miller JC, Clagiuri S. The carnivore connection: dietary carbohydrate in the evolution of NIDDM. *Diabetologia* 1994; **37**:1280–6.
32. Barnard ND, Nicholson A, Howard JL. The medical costs attributable to meat consumption. *Prev Med* 1995; **24**:646–55.
33. Hayes KC, Trautwein EA. Taurine deficiency syndrome in cats [Review]. *Vet Clin North Am [Small Anim Pract]* 1989; **19**:403–13.
34. Cherif H, Reusens B, Dahri S, Remacle C, Hoet JJ. Stimulatory effects of taurine on insulin secretion by fetal rat islets cultured in vitro. *J Endocrinol* 1996; **151**:501–6.
35. Zimmet PZ. Kelly West Lecture 1991; from West to the rest. *Diabetes Care* 1991; **15**:232–52.
36. Walker AR, Walker BF. Glycaemic index of South African foods determined in rural blacks – a population at low risk of diabetes. *Human Nutri Clin Nutr* 1984; **38**:215–22.
37. Jenkins DJ, Jenkins AL, Wolever TM, Collier GR, Rao AV, Thompson LU. Starchy foods and fiber: reduced rate of digestion and improved carbohydrate metabolism [Review]. *Scand J Gastroenterol* 1987; **120**:132–41.
38. Himsworth HP. Diabetes mellitus: its differentiation into insulin-sensitive and insulin-insensitive types. *Lancet* 1936; **i**:127–30.
39. Karlstrom B, Vessby B, Asp NG, Ytterfors A. Effects of four meals with different kinds of dietary fibre on glucose metabolism in healthy subjects and non-insulin-dependent diabetic patients. *Eur J Clin Nutri* 1988; **42**:519–26.
40. Shukla K, Narain JP, Gupta A, Bijlani RL, Mahapatra SC, Karmarkar MG. Glycaemic responses to maize, bajra and barley. *Ind J Physiol Pharmacol* 1991; **35**:249–54.
41. Boyce VL, Swinburn BA. The traditional Pima Indian diet. *Diabetes Care* 1993; **16**:369–71.
42. Baschetti R. Sucrose metabolism. *NZ Med J* 1997; **110**:43.
43. Mooy JM, Grootenhuis PA, de Vries H et al. Prevalence and determinants of glucose intolerance in a Dutch Caucasian population. *Diabetes Care* 1995; **18**: 1270–73.
44. Marshall JA, Hoag S, Shetterly S, Hamman RF. Dietary fat predicts conversion from impaired glucose tolerance to NIDDM. The San Luis Valley Diabetes Study. *Diabetes Care* 1994; **17**:50–6.
45. Zierath JR, Houseknecht KL, Gnudi L, Kahn BB. High-fat feeding impairs insulin-stimulated GLUT4 recruitment via an early insulin-signalling defect. *Diabetes* 1997; **46**:215–23.
46. Kromhout D, Bosschieter EB, De Lezenne Coulander C. The inverse relationship between fish consumption and 20-year mortality from coronary heart disease. *N Engl J Med* 1985; **312**:1205–9 (Abstract).
47. Sugden MC, Holness MJ, Orfali KA, Fryer LGD. Fish oil attenuates long-term enhancement of hepatic pyruvate dehydrogenase kinase activity by dietary saturated fat. *Proc Nutri Soc* 1995; **54**:38A.
48. Hainault I, Carolotti M, Hajduch E, Guichard C, Lavau M. Fish oil in a hard lard diet prevents obesity, hyperlipemia, and adipocyte insulin resistance in rats. *Ann NY Acad Sci* 1993; **683**:98–101.
49. Increasing fish oil intake – any net benefits? *Drug Therapeut Bull* 1996; **34**: 60–2.

50. Delarue J, Cuet C, Cohen R, Brechot JF, Antoine JM, Lamisse F. Effects of fish oil on metabolic responses to oral fructose and glucose loads in healthy humans. *Am J Physiol* 1996; **270**:E353–62.
51. Sanders TA. Marine oils: metabolic effects and role in human nutrition. *Proc Nutri Soc* 1993; **52**:457–72.
52. Randle PJ, Garland PB, Hales CN, Newsholme EA. The glucose fatty-acid cycle: its role in insulin sensitivity and the metabolic disturbances of diabetes mellitus. *Lancet* 1963; **i**:785–9.
53. Boden G. Role of fatty acids in the pathogenesis of insulin resistance and NIDDM. *Diabetes* 1997; **46**:3–10.
54. Randle PJ. Mechanisms modifying glucose oxidation in diabetes mellitus. *Diabetologia* 1994; **37**:S155–61.
55. Feskens EJM, Kromhout D. Hyperinsulinaemia, risk factors, and coronary heart disease. The Zutphen Elderly Study. *Arterioscler Thrombosis* 1995; **14**:1641–47.
56. Shaper AG. Reflections on the Seven Countries Study. *Lancet* 1996; **347**:208.
57. WHO Study Group on Diabetes. *Diabetes Mellitus: Report of a WHO study group on diabetes mellitus.* WHO Technical Report Series 727. Geneva: WHO, 1985.
58. Wilson GL, Leiter EH. Streptozotocin interactions with pancreatic beta cells and the induction of insulin-dependent diabetes [Review]. *Curr Topics Microbiol Immunol* 1990; **156**:27–54.
59. Portha B, Giroix MH, Cros JC, Picon L. Diabetogenic effect of N-nitrosomethylurea and *N*-nitrosomethylurethane in the adult rat. *Ann Nutri Aliment* 1980; **34**:1143–51.
60. Wilson GL, Mossman BT, Craighead JE. Use of pancreatic beta cells in culture to identify diabetogenic *N*-nitroso compounds. *In Vitro* 1983; **19**:25–30.
61. Singh C. The structure of the pyrmidines and purines. 8. The crystal structure of alloxan. *Acta Crystallograph* 1965; **19**:759–67.
62. Helgasen T, Jonasson MR. Evidence for a food additive as a cause of ketosis-prone diabetes. *Lancet* 1981; **ii**:716–18.
63. Stowers JM, Ewen SWB. Possible dietary factors in the induction of diabetes and its inheritance in man, with studies in mice [Review]. *Proc Nutri Soc* 1991; **50**:287–98.
64. Dahlquist G, Blom LG, Persson LA, Sandstrom AI, Wall SG. Dietary factors and the risk of developing insulin dependent diabetes in childhood. *BMJ* 1990; **300**:1302–6.
65. Motahar V, Boucher BJ. Induction of hyperglycaemia in CD1 mice by the betel-nut (*Areca catechu*) nitrosamine MNPN, inhibition by beta-carotene and enhancement by vitamins A and E. *Clin Sci* 1997; **14p**. M47Abst.
66. Boucher BJ, Mannan N, Evans SJW. Anthropomophic markers for risk of type 2 diabetes in relation to betel nut consumption in East London Asians. *Clin Sci* 1995; **45**:P14, m55.
67. Rimm EB, Manson JE, Stampfer MJ et al. Cigarette smoking and the risk of diabetes in women. *Am J Public Health* 1993; **83**:211–4.
68. Bedi R, Gilthorpe MS. Betel-quid and tobacco chewing among the Bangladeshi community in areas of multiple deprivation. In: Bedi, R, Jones, P, eds. Betel-quid and Tobacco Chewing among the Bangladeshi Community in the United Kingdom. London: Centre for Transcultural Health, 1995; 37–72.
69. Frankel BJ, Heldt AM, Grodsksy GM. Vitamin D deficiency inhibits pancreatic secretion of insulin. *Science* 1980; **209**:823–5.
70. Labriji-Mestaghanmi H, Billaudel B, Garnier PE, Sutter BCJ. Vitamin D and pancreatic islet function. 1. Time course for changes in insulin secretion and

content during vitamin D deprivation and repletion. *J endocrine Invest* 1988; **11**:577–87.

71. Bikle DD. Clinical counterpoint: Vitamin D: New actions, new analogs, new therapeutic potential. *Endocrine Rev* 1992; **13**:765–84.
72. Reichel H, Koeffler HP, Norman AW. The role of the vitamin D endocrine system in health and disease. *N Engl J Med* 1989; **32**:980–91.
73. Gedik O, Akalin S. Effects of vitamin D deficiency and repletion on insulin and glucagon secretion in man. *Diabetologia* 1986; **29**:142–5.
74. Inomata S, Kadowaki S, Yamatani T, Fukase M, Fujita T. Effect of 1 alpha (OH)-vitamin D3 on insulin secretion in diabetes mellitus. *Bone and Mineral* 1986; **1**:187–92.
75. Orwoll E, Riddle M, Prince M. Effects of vitamin D on insulin and glucagon secretion in non-insulin-dependent diabetes mellitus. *Am J Clin Nutr* 1994; **59**:1083–7.
76. Mak R. Renal disease, insulin resistance, and glucose intolerance. *Diabetes Rev* 1994; **2**:19–28.
77. Lind L, Lithell H, Wengle B, Wrege U, Ljunghall S. A pilot study of metabolic effects of intravenously given alpha-calcidol in patients with chronic renal failure. *Scand J Urol Nephrol* 1988; **22**:219–22.
78. Beaulieu C, Kestekian R, Havrankova J, Gascon-Barre M. Calcium is essential in normalising intolerance to glucose that accompanies vitamin D depletion in vivo. *Diabetes* 1993; **42**:35–43.
79. Quinn JD, Gumpert JR. Remission of non-insulin-dependent diabetes mellitus following resection of a parathyroid adenoma. *Diabetic Med* 1997; **14**:80–1.
80. Kumar S, Davies M, Zakaria Y et al. Improvement in glucose tolerance and beta-cell function in a patient with vitamin D deficiency during treatment with vitamin D. *Postgrad Med J* 1994; **70**:440–3.
81. Kocian J. Diabetic osteopathy. Favourable effect of treatment of osteomalacia with vitamin D and calcium on high blood glucose levels. [Czech]. *Vnitrni Lekarstvi* 1992; **38**:352–6.
82. Boucher BJ, Mannan N, Noonan K, Hales CN, Evans SJW. Glucose intolerance and impairment of insulin secretion in relation to vitamin D deficiency in East London Asians. *Diabetologia* 1995; **38**:1239–45.
83. Feskens EJM, Bowles CH, Kromhout D. Inverse association between fish intake and risk of glucose intolerance on normoglycaemic elderly men and women. *Diabetes Care* 1991; **14**:935–41.
84. Baynes K, Boucher BJ, Feskens EJM, Kromhout D. Vitamin D, glucose tolerance and insulinaemia in elderly men. *Diabetologia* 1997; **40**:344–7.
85. Ljunghall S, Lind L, Lithell H et al. Treatment with one-alpha-hydroxycholecalciferol in middle-aged men with impaired glucose tolerance – a prospective randomised double-blind society. *Acta Med Scand* 1987; **222**:361–7.
86. Davies H. Coronary heart disease: The significance of coronary pathology in infancy and the role of mitogens such as vitamin D. [Review]. *Med Hypotheses* 1989; **30**:179–85.
87. Iqbal SJ, Kaddam I, Wassif W, Nichol F, Walls J. Continuing clinically severe vitamin D deficiency in Asians in the UK (Leicester). *Postgrad Med J* 1994; **70**:708–14.
88. Boucher BJ. Poor vitamin D status, a risk factor for Syndrome X? *Br J Nutr* 1999; **79**:315–27.
89. van der Wielen RPJ, Lowik MRH, van den Berg H et al. Serum vitamin D concentrations among elderly people in Europe. *Lancet* 1995; **346**:207–10.

90. Chertow BS, Driscoll HK, Goking NQ, Primareno D, Cordle MB, Mathews KA. Retinoid-X receptors and the effects of 9-*cis*-retinoic acid on insulin secretion from RINm5F cells. *Metabolism* 1997; **46**:656–60.
91. Ozono K, Seino Y, Yano H, Yamaoka K. 1,25-Dihydroxyvitamin D3 enhances the effect of refeeding on steady state preproinsulin messenger ribonucleic acid levels in rats. *Endocrinology* 1990; **126**:2041–5.
92. Metz AL, Walser MM, Olson WG. The interaction of dietary vitamin A and vitamin D related to skeletal development in the turkey poult. *J Nutr* 1985; **115**:929–35.
93. Chertow BS, Baker GR. The effects of vitamin A on insulin release and glucose oxidation in isolated rat islets. *Endocrinology* 1982; **103**:1562–72.
94. Chertow BS, Baranetsky NG, Sivitz WI, Meda P, Webb MD, Shih JC. Cellular mechanisms of insulin release. Effects of retinoids on rat islet cell-to-cell adhesion, reaggregation, and insulin release. *Diabetes* 1983; 32:568–74.
95. Chertow BS, Blaner WS, Rajan N et al. Retinoic acid receptor, cytosolic retinol-binding and retinoic acid-binding protein mRNA transcripts and proteins in rat insulin-secreting cells. *Diabetes* 1993; **42**:1109–14.
96. Blaizot S, Bonmort J, Garcin H, Higueret P. Glycaemia and insulinaemia of vitamin A deficient rats after administration of glucose. *Ann Nutri Aliment* 1978; **32**:93–109.
97. Chertow BS, Sivitz WI, Baranetsky NG et al. Vitamin A palmitate decreases intravenous glucose tolerance in man. *Acta Vitaminol Enzymol* 1982; **4**:291–8.
98. Haglund B, Ryckenberg K, Selinus O, Dahlquist G. Evidence of a relationship between childhood-onset type 1 diabetes and low ground water concentration of zinc. *Diabetes Care* 1996; **19**:873–5.
99. Rahman M, Axelson O. Diabetes mellitus and arsenic exposure: a second look at case–control data from a Swedish copper smelter. *Occup Environ Med* 1995; **52**:773–4.
100. Salonen JT, Salonen R, Korpela H, Suntioinen S, Tuomilheto J. Serum copper and risk of acute myocardial infarction: a prospective population study in men in eastern Finland. *Am J Epidemiol* 1991; **134**:268–76.
101. Heldenberg D, Tenenbaum G, Weisman Y. Effect of iron on serum 25-hydroxyvitamin D and 24,25-dihydroxyvitamin D concentrations. *Am J Clin Nutri* 1997; **56**:533–6.
102. Rhodes CJ, Alarcon C. What B-cell defect could lead to hyperproinsulinaemia in NIDDM?; some clues from recent advances made in understanding the proinsulin-processing mechanism. *Diabetes* 1994; **43**:511–17.
103. Kimura J. Role of essential trace elements in the disturbance of carbohydrate metabolism [Review]. *Nippon Rinsho – Jpn J Clin Med* 1996; **54**:79–84.
104. Milner RDG, Hales CN. The role of calcium and magnesium in insulin secretion from rabbit pancreas studied in vitro. *Diabetologia* 1967; **3**:47–9.
105. Sekar N, Li J, Schecter Y. Vanadium salts as insulin substitutes: mechanisms of action, a scientific and therapeutic tool in diabetes research. [Review]. *Crit Rev Biochem Mol Biol* 1996; **31**:339–59.
106. Platel K, Srinavasan K. Plant foods in the management of diabetes mellitus: vegetables as potential hypoglycaemic agents [Review]. *Nahrung* 1997; **41**: 68–74.
107. Boucher BJ. Betel-quid, smokeless tobacco and general health. In Bedi R, Jones P, eds, *Betel-quid and Tobacco Chewing among the Bangladeshi Community in the United Kingdom*. London: Centre for Transcultural Health, 53–60.

108. Khan A, Bryden NA, Polansky MM, Anderson RA. Insulin potentiating factor and chromium content of selected food and spices. *Biol Trace Element Res* 1990; **24**:183–8.
109. Gatenby SJ, Ellis PR, Morgan LM, Judd PA. Effect of partially depolymerized guar gum on acute metabolic variables in patients with non-insulin-dependent diabetes. *Diabetic Med* 1996; **13**:358–64.
110. Mann JL. A prudent diet for the nation. *J Hum Nutr* 1979; **33**:57–63.
111. Sevak L, McKeigue PM, Marmot MG. Relationship of hyperinsulinaemia to dietary intake in South Asian and European men. *Am J Clin Nutr* 1994; **59**:1069–74.
112. Snowden DA, Phillips RL. Does a vegetarian diet reduce the occurrence of diabetes? *Am J Public Health* 1985; **75**:507–12.
113. Feskens EJM, Bowles CH, Kromhout D. Carbohydrate intake and body mass index in relation to the risk of glucose intolerance in an elderly population. *Am Clin Nutri* 1991; **54**:136–40.
114. Marshall JA, Wiess NS, Hamman RF. The role of dietary fiber in the etiology of non-insulin-dependent diabetes mellitus. the San Luis Valley Diabetes Study. *Ann Epidemiol* 1993; **3** 18–26.
115. Keen H. Insulin resistance and the prevention of diabetes mellitus. *N Engl J Med* 1994; **331**:1226–7.
116. Virtanen SM, Aro A. Dietary factors in the aetiology of diabetes. *Ann Med* 1994; **26**:469–78.
117. Pickett G. American dietary performance and healthy people 2000 [policy watch]. *Am J Med* 1996; **100**:11–111.
118. Torjesen PA, Birkeland KI, Anderssen SA, Hiermann I, Holme I, Urdal P. Lifestyle changes may reverse development of the insulin resistance syndrome: the Oslo diet and exercise study; a randomised trial. *Diabetes Care* 1997; **20**:26–31.
119. James WP. A public health approach to the problem of obesity. [Review]. *Int J Obesity Related Dis* 1995; **19**(suppl 3): S37–45.
120. Gopalan C. Current food and nutrition situation in south Asian and south-east Asian countries. *Biomed Environ Sci* 1996; **9**:102–6.
121. WHO Study Group on Diabetes. *Report, Prevention of Diabetes.* Technical Report Series 844. Geneva: WHO, 1994.

15

Prevention Strategies: Diet and Exercise

R.R. WING

Obesity/Nutrition Research Center, Western Psychiatric Institute and Clinic, University of Pittsburgh School of Medicine, 3811 O'Hara Street, Pittsburgh, PA 15213, USA

Type 2 diabetes is increasing worldwide, primarily as a result of changes in lifestyle. Several 'natural' experiments are available, in which ethnic groups, who are genetically susceptible to diabetes, have experienced rapid Westernization and, with it, dramatic increases in the rates of obesity and type 2 diabetes[1,2]. Thus, it is logical that, by reversing these lifestyle changes, it would be possible to prevent the development of this disease. O'Dea[3] demonstrated this empirically by showing that after just 7 weeks of reversion to a traditional lifestyle, diabetic Australian Aborigines experienced marked improvements in carbohydrate and lipid metabolism.

The purpose of this chapter is to discuss the recent studies that have used lifestyle interventions to prevent development of type 2 diabetes. Most of these studies have focused on individuals with impaired glucose tolerance because of their high conversion rates to diabetes[4] and have examined both physical activity and dietary changes, either singly or in combination. Before discussing these intervention studies, the evidence supporting these two intervention strategies is reviewed briefly.

DEFINING TARGET BEHAVIOURS FOR LIFESTYLE INTERVENTION

DIETARY GOALS

Obesity is a well-established risk factor for diabetes. The reader is referred to Chapter 11 of this volume for a discussion of the relationship between

Type 2 Diabetes: Prediction and Prevention. Edited by Graham A. Hitman

obesity and Type 2 diabetes. Recent studies suggest that even modest degrees of being overweight may increase the incidence of diabetes. In the Nurses' Health Study[5], for example, the relative risk of developing diabetes increased linearly with body mass index (BMI), but even a BMI of 23–25 increased the risk of diabetes threefold compared with a BMI of less than 21.

There is also evidence to indicate that weight reduction in those who are overweight will decrease the risk of developing diabetes. The strongest evidence is from the study by Long et al.[6] which used gastrointestinal surgery to produce large weight losses in a group of 109 individuals with impaired glucose tolerance (IGT) who were followed for 6 years. Surgical weight reduction reduced the progression from IGT to diabetes thirtyfold.

More modest weight losses also appear to be beneficial. Weight losses of approximately 10% of initial weight have been shown to lower glucose levels and reduce insulin resistance both in individuals with established diabetes[7,8] and in those at risk for this disease[9,10].

The exact magnitude of weight loss required to reduce the risk of diabetes is unclear; whether weight loss will be beneficial in all ethnic groups (e.g., in Japanese–Americans who have high abdominal obesity but are not typically overweight) remains to be established.

Most of the dietary interventions focus specifically on lowering fat intake in the diet. This emphasis is based on the literature that suggests that fat intake may be related to both the risk of diabetes[11] and the development/maintenance of obesity[12,13]. However, the evidence relating dietary fat intake to prevention of diabetes is far less consistent than that concerning obesity or exercise[14].

EXERCISE

Exercise is a key component of lifestyle intervention for the prevention of diabetes. Increased physical activity is expected to modify the risk of developing diabetes directly through improvements in insulin sensitivity[15,16], and indirectly through promoting long-term weight loss and maintenance[17].

Epidemiological studies suggest that the frequency and intensity of exercise required for prevention of diabetes may be relatively modest. In two large prospective studies on the incidence of diabetes[18,19], one conducted with women and one with men, respondents were asked to indicate how often they exercised vigorously enough to work up a sweat. In both studies, individuals who reported vigorous exercise just once a week had about a 25% reduction in their risk of developing diabetes (age-adjusted relative risk of 0.74 in women and 0.77 in men) relative to those with no vigorous exercise. More frequent exercise reduced the risk further (to 0.58–0.63) but the largest changes occurred by increasing from zero to one bout of vigorous exercise/week. Similarly, Helmrich et al.[20] found that modest increases in leisure-time physical activity reduced the risk of developing diabetes. In this study, the risk was reduced 6% for every 500 kcal increment in physical activity. The protective effect of vigorous exercise was greater than that of moderate exercise, but both were effective. Moreover, in each of these studies cited above, the benefits of exercise were comparable or even greater in those who were overweight or at increased risk for developing type 2 diabetes.

PREVIOUS STUDIES OF LIFESTYLE INTERVENTIONS TO PREVENT DIABETES

Evidence to support the effectiveness of a lifestyle intervention is found in several trials, which are reviewed below. Bourne and colleagues in New Zealand[21] studied 32 individuals who were required to have persistent IGT at baseline, i.e., at least two out of three oral glucose tolerance tests (OGTTs) indicating IGT, using WHO criteria. These individuals were then given a diet and exercise intervention. The dietary goals were to increase complex carbohydrates to 50–55% of energy intake and fiber to 20 g/1000 cal, to decrease fat to 30% of energy intake (and increase the ratio of polyunsaturated fat to saturated fat), and to minimize intake of sugars. As many of the participants were overweight, calorie restriction was also discussed, but no information was provided on the specific weight loss goals for the study. The diet messages were reinforced by group meetings at 3-month intervals and 'phone contacts between meetings. The exercise goal was to complete low-impact aerobic exercise (e.g., walking or swimming) for at least 30 min three times a week. A 1-hour weekly exercise class was available to help participants achieve this goal. These interventions were maintained for 2 years, with assessments of diet and exercise and repeat OGTTs at 3-month intervals.

Of the 32 subjects who started this program, 26 (81%) completed 12 months and 22 (69%) completed 24 months. Forty percent of the 22 subjects had a normal 2-hour glucose level at 2 years. As there is no control group of untreated subjects, it is difficult to interpret this finding. However, as subjects were tested three times for IGT before entering the study, it is unlikely that so many would have normalized their blood sugars without the intervention. BMI decreased over the first 3 months of the program (29.8 to 28.7 kg/m^2), but then gradually returned toward baseline. Dietary changes were greater in women than in men, and again were most impressive at 3 months. Physical activity level also improved: 14% of the subjects met the exercise goal at baseline, whereas 20–30% met this goal during the study.

Recently, a 3-year follow-up of this study was reported[22]. Nineteen of the 22 IGT subjects tested at 24 months were re-studied. Weight increased significantly from 79.1 kg at 24 months to 80.6 kg at 3 years, but still remained below the baseline level of 82.9 kg. Twenty-six percent of the subjects continued to meet the physical activity goal (30 min, 3 days/week). Fifty-three percent had 2-hour glucoses in the normal range (comparable to 47% of these same 19 subjects at 2 years). Thus the beneficial changes seem to have been maintained through this longer follow-up interval.

A second study, which utilized a non-randomized control group and included a far larger sample of subjects with IGT, is the Malmö Study[23]. This study included 181 subjects with IGT (161 completed the 5-year study) who were interested in participating in a diet–exercise intervention. IGT was defined by a fasting glucose of less than 6.7 mmol (120 mg/dl) and a 2-hour value between 7.0 and 11.0 mol/l (126–200 mg/dl). These subjects were compared with 79 other individuals with IGT (56% of whom completed the study) who, for various reasons, chose not to be in the treatment arm of the study. Thus, interpretation of this study is complicated by the lack of random assignment and possible baseline differences between two groups.

Subjects in the lifestyle intervention were given the option of participating in the treatment program on their own or as a group. Thirty-eight percent chose the group format and participated in a 6-month period of supervised physical training followed by 6 months of dietary instruction or vice versa. All subjects then continued to follow the diet and exercise protocol on their own or as part of a group. Participants were seen every 6 months by the physician. No further information is provided on the specific diet or exercise intervention used in this study.

At follow-up, which was completed after 6 years, IGT subjects in the intervention group maintained a weight loss of 3.3 kg, whereas the control subjects had increased their weight by 0.2 kg. Similarly, estimated oxygen uptake increased 8% in lifestyle subjects, but decreased 2% in controls. Although changes in weight and fitness were greatest at 6–12 months of follow-up, at the 6-year follow-up 71% of the lifestyle participants maintained some weight loss and 47% showed improvements in oxygen intake compared with baseline. Thus, this study was successful in producing at least modest behaviour changes through a 6-year follow-up period.

These changes in weight and exercise led to marked reductions in development of diabetes. Whereas 28.6% of IGT subjects in the control group developed diabetes, only 10.6% of the intervention subjects had diabetes. Moreover, 2-hour glucose decreased from 8.2 mmol/l at baseline to 7.1 mmol/l at follow-up in the treated subjects ($p < 0.001$). Both changes in estimated oxygen uptake and changes in body weight were found to be independently related to changes in 2-hour glucose levels, with the greatest changes observed in those who had the greatest improvements in weight and fitness.

Recently, we reported results from a study of lifestyle intervention in 154 individuals at high risk for diabetes because they were overweight and had one or both parents with diabetes[24,25]. Intervening in subjects with a family history of diabetes may be an effective strategy, because it allows for recruitment without extensive screening, it may help to identify highly motivated subjects, and it allows intervention even before the development of IGT.

These subjects were randomly assigned to a control group, diet only, exercise only, or a combination of diet plus exercise. The control group was given a self-help manual with information on healthy eating and exercise, but were not invited to any treatment meetings. The other three groups participated in 6 months of weekly meetings, followed by 6 months of bi-weekly meetings, and two 6-week refresher courses during the second year. The diet intervention was designed to reduce intake to 1200–1500 kcal/day (5.04–6.3 MJ/day), with 20% energy as fat. They began with an initial period of even greater calorie restriction and structural meal plans, but then moved to a more flexible eating plan. The exercise goal increased gradually to a goal of 1500 kcal/week (3-mile walk on 5 days/week). Supervised exercise sessions were held initially to help participants achieve these goals. Results at the end of 6 months were extremely positive, especially for the groups given diet and diet plus exercise. These subjects reported decreases in calorie intake of 600–700 kcal/day (2.52–2.94 MJ/day) and decreases in fat of 5–10%. Weight losses in these two groups averaged 9.1–10.3 kg at 24 weeks, which were associated with positive changes in glucose, lipids, and blood pressure. The exercise groups also experienced significant improvements in oxygen consumption ($V\text{O}_{2\,\text{max}}$), and weight loss of 2.1 kg. However, these changes were not sustained over time. The diet group maintained a non-significant weight loss of 2.1 kg at 24 months and the diet plus exercise group maintained a significant loss of 2.5 kg. Self-reported calorie and fat intake also remained significantly below baseline, although differences between conditions were far smaller. Estimated $V\text{O}_2$ max was no longer improved over baseline and subjects in the exercise group averaged a 1 kg weight gain. At 2 years, 7% of the control, 30% of the diet, 19% of the exercise, and 15.6% of the diet plus exercise group ($p < 0.08$) had developed diabetes.

Despite these discouraging between-group differences, there was evidence that long-term weight loss positively affected diabetes risk. A 4.5-kg weight loss at 2 years reduced the risk of diabetes by 25% in those with IGT at baseline, and by 31% in those with normal glucose tolerance. This study found no evidence that changes in exercise or fitness were related to risk of diabetes.

The largest study of the effects of diet and exercise in preventing progression from IGT to type 2 diabetes was reported recently from Da Qing, China[26]. In this study, 577 subjects, classified by WHO criteria as having IGT, were randomly assigned by clinics to either a control condition or interventions involving diet, exercise, or a combination of diet plus exercise. All subjects were then followed for 6 years. In the diet intervention group, subjects with a BMI of less than 25 were prescribed a diet of 35–30 kcal/kg body weight, with 55–65% carbohydrate, 10–15% protein, and 25–30% fat.

Subjects with a BMI of more than 25 were encouraged to reduce their intake to lose weight gradually at a rate of 0.5–1.0 kg/month. Participants received individual counselling from physicians regarding their intake, and participated in small group counselling sessions held weekly for 1 month, monthly for 3 months, and then once every 3 months for the remainder of the study.

The exercise group participated in counselling sessions on the same schedule as the diet group and were encouraged to increase their activity by 1 unit/day or by 2 units for those aged under 50 and healthy. One unit of activity was defined as 30 minutes of mild exercise (slow walking or housecleaning), 20 minutes of moderate exercise (faster walking, cycling), 10 minutes of strenuous activity (slow running, climbing stairs), or 5 minutes of very strenuous activity (jumping rope, basketball, swimming).

Outcome assessments were completed every 2 years. The endpoint (development of type 2 diabetes) was defined by two OGTTs. Of the 577 subjects entering the study, 530 completed the trial. In the control group, cumulative incidence of diabetes was 67.7%. In each of the intervention groups, the incidence of diabetes was significantly lower than in the control group (43.8% in diet only, 41.1% in exercise only, and 46.0% in diet plus exercise), but the incidence did not differ by treatment condition. The group given diet plus exercise instruction appeared to reduce their intake to the greatest degree (−242 cal/day or −1.02 kJ/day) and increased their exercise the most (from 3.1 to 3.9 units/day), but data were not presented on the relationship between changes in behaviour and the development of diabetes.

DIABETES PREVENTION PROGRAM

The literature reviewed above suggests that lifestyle interventions, which produce modest changes in diet, exercise, and body weight, are effective in reducing the risk of the conversion of IGT to type 2 diabetes. However, there are methodologic limitations to each of these studies and none compared lifestyle to pharmacologic approaches to diabetes prevention.

The Diabetes Prevention Program (DPP), funded primarily by the National Institute of Diabetes and Digestive and Kidney Diseases (NIDDK), is a randomized clinical trial to test whether it is possible to prevent or delay the development of type 2 diabetes in those at high risk by virtue of having IGT[27]. The DPP includes 27 clinical centers, that will recruit a total cohort of at least 3000 participants, with about 50% minorities, 20% aged 65 or over, and about 50% of each sex. To be eligible, participants must be age 25 or older and have IGT with fasting levels of 5.3-6.9 mmol/l (95–125 mg/dl) and 2-hour levels of 7.8–11.0 mmol/l (140–199 mg/dl). Participants were initially randomly assigned to one of four intervention groups: intensive lifestyle or standard lifestyle combined with metformin, troglitazone, or placebo. Later, the troglitazone arm of this study was discontinued. Recruitment is currently ongoing and will last approximately 3 years. Subjects will be followed for 3 years after the end of recruitment, resulting in a 3- to 6-year follow-up interval. The primary endpoint is development of diabetes according to 1997 criteria of the American Diabetic Association (ADA)[28] for fasting glucose or 2-hour plasma glucose during an OGTT. Secondary endpoints include cardiovascular disease and its risk factors, insulin sensitivity and secretion, and obesity.

The Intensive Lifestyle Intervention was developed based on the literature described above, suggesting that both weight loss and exercise may be important in preventing the conversion from IGT to type 2 diabetes. After careful consideration of what may be effective in preventing diabetes, and also feasible for participants to achieve and maintain over a 3–6-year trial, the following goals were identified:

1. To achieve a weight loss of at least 7% of initial body weight through healthy eating and activity and maintain this weight loss throughout the trial.
2. To expend at least 700 kcal/week (2.94 MJ/week) in physical activity through moderately intense activities such as biking and brisk walking, and maintain this level of activity throughout the trial.

To help participants achieve and maintain these lifestyle changes, all participants in the intensive lifestyle intervention condition are assigned a lifestyle coach who meets with the participant 16 times over the initial 24 weeks, and then arranges at least monthly contact thereafter (with in-person contacts at least every 2 months). All participants receive a 'core curriculum' that provides general information about diet and exercise, and behavioral strategies such as self-monitoring, goal-setting, stimulus control, and problem-solving. A fat gram goal designed to reduce fat to less than 25% of the energy intake is prescribed and a calorie goal is given as needed to achieve a weight loss of 7% of initial weight within the first 24 weeks of the program.

The exercise intervention focuses on activities of moderate intensity, such as brisk walking, but can be individually tailored to identify activities enjoyed by each participant. Participants are helped to gradually increase their activity until they achieve 150 min/week of brisk activity (which should represent an expenditure of approximately 700 kcal/week or 2.94 MJ/week). Supervised sessions are offered at each clinic to help participants achieve these goals.

Although the goals are the same for all subjects, there is a great deal of flexibility in the approaches that can be used to help participants achieve these goals. The intervention is conducted individually to allow lifestyle coaches to tailor the mode of presentation and pacing of new material to fit the needs of the participant. The diet and exercise interventions are flexible and allow lifestyle coaches to be sensitive to cultural differences among participants. For individuals who have difficulty in achieving the weight and exercise goals, a "tool box" approach is used to provide new strategies to help the participant. Tool box approaches to weight loss include use of more structured eating plans, liquid formula, or home visits. Tool box approaches to exercise include loaning the participant exercise tapes or home exercise equipment.

The individual contact with the participant is supplemented by group maintenance activities held quarterly each year. These courses, which are optional for participants, will allow for further discussion, practice, and modelling of healthy eating, exercise, and behaviour change strategies.

CONCLUSION

The increasing rates of diabetes worldwide have led to new interest in prevention of this disease. Initial studies of lifestyle intervention suggest positive results from relatively modest changes in eating and exercise behaviour. Such studies have focused on high-risk individuals, usually those who already have IGT. Whether similar interventions can be used effectively with larger groups and communities of individuals at risk for diabetes remains an important next step.

REFERENCES

1. Ravussin E, Valencia ME, Esparza J, Bennett PH, Schulz LO. Effects of a traditional lifestyle on obesity in Pima Indians. *Diabetes Care* 1994; **17**:1067–74.
2. Dowse GK, Zimmet P, Collins V et al. Obesity in Pacific populations. In: Bjorntorp P, Brodoff BN, eds. *Obesity*. Philadelphia: JB Lippincott Co., 1992; 619–39.
3. O'Dea K. Marked improvement in carbohydrate and lipid metabolism in diabetic Australian aborigines after temporary reversion to traditional lifestyle. *Diabetes* 1984; **33**:596–603.
4. Edelstein SL, Knowler WC, Bain RP et al. Predictors of progression from impaired glucose tolerance to NIDDM: An analysis of six prospective studies. *Diabetes* 1997; **46**:701–10.
5. Carey VJ, Walters EE, Colditz GA et al. Body fat distribution and risk of non-insulin-dependent diabetes mellitus in women: The Nurses' Health Study. *Am J Epidemiol* 1997; **145**:614–19.
6. Long SD, O'Brien K, MacDonald KG et al. Weight loss prevents the progression of impaired glucose tolerance to type II diabetes: A longitudinal interventional study. *Diabetes Care* 1993; **17**:372–5.
7. Wing R, Koeske R, Epstein LH, Nowalk MP, Gooding W, Becker D. Long-term effects of modest weight loss in type II diabetic patients. *Arch Intern Med* 1987; **147**:1749–53.

8. Kanders BS, Blackburn GL. Reducing primary risk factors by therapeutic weight loss. In Wadden TA, Van Itallie TB, eds. *Treatment of the Seriously Obese Patient*. New York: Guilford, 1992; 213–30.
9. Olefsky J, Reaven GM, Farquhar JW. Effects of weight reduction on obesity: Studies of lipid and carbohydrate metabolism in normal and hyperlipoproteinemic subjects. *J Clin Invest* 1974; **53**:64–77.
10. Farinaro E, Stamler J, Upton M et al. Plasma glucose levels: Long-term effect of diet in the Chicago Coronary Prevention Evaluation Program. *Ann Intern Med* 1977; **86**:147–154.
11. Marshall JA, Shetterly S, Hoag, S, Hamman RF. Dietary fat predicts conversion from impaired glucose tolerance to NIDDM: The San Luis Valley Diabetes Study. *Diabetes Care* 1994; **17**:50–6.
12. Tucker LA, Kano MJ. Dietary fat and body fat: A multivariate study of 205 adult females. *Am J Clin Nutr* 1992; **56**:616–22.
13. Rolls BJ, Shide DJ. The influence of dietary fat on food intake and body weight. *Nutr Rev* 1992; **50**:283–90.
14. Manson JE, Spelsberg A. Primary prevention of non-insulin-dependent diabetes mellitus. *Am J Prev Med* 1994; **10**:172–84.
15. Kriska AM, Blair SN, Pereira MA. The potential role of physical activity in the prevention of non-insulin-dependent diabetes mellitus: The epidemiological evidence. *Exerc Sport Sci Rev* 1994; **22**:121–43.
16. Wallberg-Henriksson H. Exercise and diabetes mellitus. In Holloszy JO, ed. *Exercise and Sports Sciences Reviews*. Baltimore: Williams & Wilkins: 1992; 339–68.
17. Pronk NP, Wing RR. Physical activity and long-term maintenance of weight loss. *Obesity Res* 1994; **2**:587–99.
18. Manson JE, Nathan DM, Krolewski AS, Stampfer MJ, Willett WC, Hennekens CH. A prospective study of exercise and incidence of diabetes among US male physicians. *JAMA* 1992; **268**:63–7.
19. Manson JE, Rimm EB, Stampfer MJ et al. Physical activity and incidence of non-insulin-dependent diabetes mellitus in women. *Lancet* 1991; **338**:774–8.
20. Helmrich SP, Ragland DR, Leung RW, Paffenbarger RS. Physical activity and reduced occurrence of non-insulin-dependent diabetes mellitus. *N Engl J Med* 1991; **325**:147–52.
21. Bourn DM, Mann JI, McSkimming BH, Waldron MA, Wishart JD. Impaired glucose tolerance and NIDDM: Does a lifestyle intervention program have an effect? *Diabetes Care* 1994; **17**:1311–19.
22. Bourne DM, Mann JI. The 3-yr follow-up of subjects with impaired glucose tolerance or non-insulin dependent diabetes mellitus in a diet and exercise intervention programme. *Diabetes Nutr Metab* 1996; **9**:240–6.
23. Eriksson KF, Lindgärde F. Prevention of type 2 (non-insulin-dependent) diabetes mellitus by diet and physical exercise. *Diabetologia* 1991: **34**:891–8.
24. Wing RR, Venditti EM, Jakicic JM et al. Lifestyle intervention in those at risk for NIDDM: Lack of a long-term benefit [Abstract]. *Diabetes* 1996; **45**(suppl): 173A.
25. Wing RR, Venditti EM, Jakicic JM et al. Onset of NIDDM in high risk subjects in a lifestyle intervention [Abstract]. *Diabetes* 1996; **45** (suppl): 217A.
26. Pan XR, LI GW, Hu YH et al. Effects of diet and exercise in preventing NIDDM in people with impaired glucose tolerance. *Diabetes Care* 1997; **20**:537–44.
27. Diabetes Prevention Program Research Group. The Diabetes Prevention Program Design and Methods for a clinical trial in the prevention of Type 2 diabetes mellitus. *Diabetes Care* (in press).
28. American Diabetes Association. Report of the Expert Committee on the Diagnosis and Classification of Diabetes Mellitus. *Diabetes Care* 1997; **20**: 1183–97.

16

Prevention Strategies: the Use of Drugs

R.J. HEINE

Department of Endocrinology, Vrije Universiteit, University Hospital, P.O. Box 7057, 1007 MB Amsterdam, The Netherlands

Abnormal glucose tolerance, including impaired glucose tolerance (IGT) and diabetes is a frequently occurring condition affecting 20–30% of the adult European and US population in the age range 40–70 years[1-3]. The major consequence of this condition is the severely elevated risk of vascular disease. These vascular complications include the classic microvascular complications (eye and kidney disease), neuropathy and cardiovascular disease. The severely (four to six times) elevated mortality risk conferred by type 2 diabetes is not only related to chronic hyperglycaemia, but also, and possibly mainly, to the coexistence of a cluster of cardiovascular risk factors, including hypertension, dyslipidaemia and high plasminogen activator inhibitor-1 (PAI-1) levels; this is the so-called insulin resistance syndrome or syndrome X[4-6].

At the time of diagnosis of type 2 diabetes, micro- and macrovascular complications can already be demonstrated in an estimated 20–30% of patients[7]. The delay between the occurrence of hyperglycaemia and the diagnosis of the disease has been estimated to be 7–10 years[8]. Moreover, treatment of type 2 diabetes is often unsuccessful in achieving the metabolic targets that are thought to be necessary to prevent the occurrence of the devastating complications. Achieving glycaemic targets by implementing structured care in most people with type 2 diabetes patients does not, to a significant extent, affect the cardiovascular risk factors and, more particularly, the serum lipid levels[9].

Type 2 Diabetes: Prediction and Prevention. Edited by Graham A. Hitman.

Thus, lowering of the burden of type 2 diabetes-related complications requires early detection, and intensive and targeted management of hyperglycaemia, dyslipidaemia and hypertension. Prevention of the disease seems therefore to be a reasonable objective, and possibly the most effective way to reduce the cardiovascular disease rate in people at risk.

PATHOPHYSIOLOGY OF ABNORMAL GLUCOSE TOLERANCE

The term 'type 2 diabetes' is, according to the new classification, reserved for individuals with insulin resistance and relative, rather than absolute, insulin deficiency[10]. Impaired glucose tolerance is a stage intermediate between normal glucose tolerance and diabetes. This condition is considered to be a transitory phase between normal glucose tolerance and frank hyperglycaemia. Both insulin resistance and insulin secretion defects have been demonstrated already at the stage of IGT[11,12]. The β-cell dysfunction includes loss of pulsatility and a lower first-phase insulin response to glucose, and enhanced secretion of metabolically less effective precursors of insulin, in particular proinsulin and 32,33 split-proinsulin[13]. It seems therefore that the almost generally accepted, but simplified, model, which assumes that insulin resistance is primarily involved in the development of IGT and that β-cell abnormalities causes further progression to diabetes, does not hold true[14]. Several prospective studies in subjects with IGT have demonstrated that parameters that reflect deteriorated β-cell function are predictive of progression to type 2 diabetes[15,16]. Also, recent studies in Mexican–Americans have demonstrated that elevated proinsulin levels, reflecting compromised β-cell function, and the proinsulin:insulin ratio predict the development of type 2 diabetes, after adjustment for glucose tolerance and body mass index at baseline[17]. The data suggest that the pre-diabetic state, including the obese high-risk subjects, can be characterized not only by insulin resistance but also by compromised β-cell function.

Type 2 diabetes has a strong genetic, probably multigenetic, component which interacts with several environmental determinants. Obvious examples of this are obesity, lack of physical activity, and high intake of different nutrients, particularly saturated fat[3,18]. Taken together, strategies to prevent the development of type 2 diabetes should be targeted at one or a combination of the above-mentioned factors, including restoration of β-cell function and/or diminishing insulin resistance.

POTENTIAL TARGETS FOR INTERVENTION (Figure 16.1)

The insulin secretory defect includes a relative overproduction of insulin precursors and a lower first-phase insulin response. One of the consequences

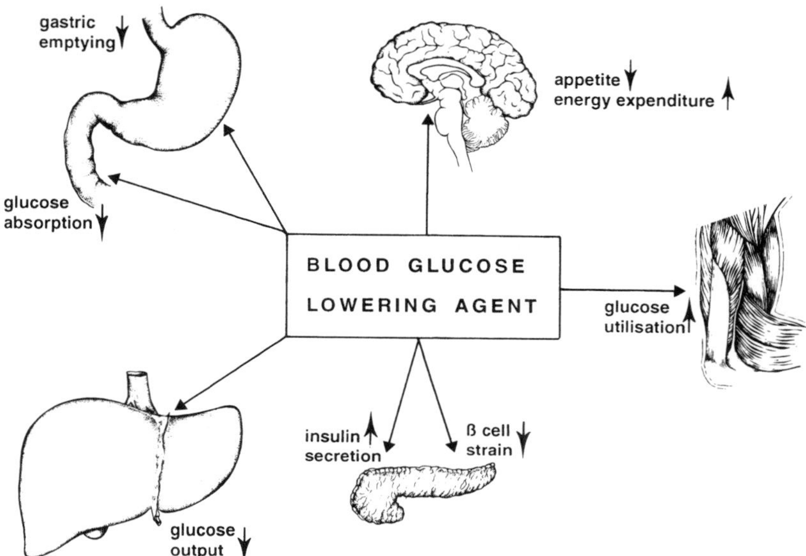

Figure 16.1. Schematic representation of the various actions of blood-glucose-lowering agents by which the plasma concentration of glucose can be lowered, directly (e.g. lowering of hepatic glucose production by metformin) or indirectly (e.g. the suppression of appetite by leptin).

of the deficit is a less than normal suppression of hepatic glucose production[11-13]. This β-cell dysfunction and/or its metabolic consequences can theoretically be corrected by several interventions, such as

- stimulation of insulin secretion
- lowering of glucose production by the liver
- retardation of intestinal glucose absorption
- improvement in insulin sensitivity.
- lowering of the glycaemic burden on the β cell.

STIMULATION OF INSULIN SECRETION

Sulphonylureas

Currently, the most widely used drugs to promote insulin secretion are the sulphonylureas[19]. These drugs have been in use since the 1950s. The prime mode of action is to sensitize β cells to glucose, thereby increasing insulin secretion. Sulphonylureas bind to specific receptors on the β cell which leads to closure of potassium channels. The resulting rise in intracellular concentration of calcium ions promotes exocytosis of insulin.

Sulphonylureas, in particular tolbutamide, have in the past been tested for the prevention of type 2 diabetes[20-23]. Some of these studies were able to demonstrate a reduction of the conversion rate from IGT to diabetes (Table 16.1). A Swedish study demonstrated during a 12-year follow-up a preventive effect of 500 mg tolbutamide given three times daily on the occurrence of diabetes, compared with dietary advice alone[20]. In the 23 of 49 subjects who were randomized to tolbutamide and continued to take these tablets, no diabetes emerged, whereas diabetes developed in 29 of 59 subjects with IGT who received no therapy. In the group treated with placebo plus diet and those who discontinued medication, an intermediate conversion rate was seen. The Malmöhus study suffered a large drop-out rate and lack of compliance to allocated treatment: 26 of 49 patients on tolbutamide and 22 of 48 subjects on placebo stopped taking the tablets. Remarkably, despite the small number of subjects participating in the study, a significant higher mortality rate was found among those who developed diabetes: 11 of 35 vs 26 of 171 who remained non-diabetic ($p < 0.05$).

Recently, the Malmöhus study has been reanalysed by Knowler et al.[24]. The main question was whether IGT conferred a higher mortality risk. The 2500 individuals studied in Malmöhus were followed for 12–15 years. The age- and sex-adjusted mortality rates were, as expected, almost twice as high in those with diabetes as in the controls (70 ± 3.6 vs 37.9 ± 1.9 deaths per 1000 person-years) and intermediate in the IGT group: 53.6 ± 4.2 deaths. In addition, the 20-year cumulative mortality rates were analysed, also for a period of 12 years after the end of the trial. The results suggest that, whether diabetes was prevented or just delayed, randomization to tolbutamide may have lowered mortality rates by 34%. As a result of the small sample size, no firm conclusions could be drawn. Nevertheless, these results argue against the findings of the University Group Diabetes Program (UGDP), which reports excess mortality in those treated with tolbutamide[25]. These findings also provide an argument for carrying out a large-scale trial with a sulphonylurea derivative in subjects with IGT.

These existing results have so far not been confirmed in other trials. In the Bedford Study, middle-aged individuals were randomized to 1 g tolbutamide or placebo with a follow-up of 10 years. During the follow-up, 10% of the subjects on placebo developed diabetes versus 11% on tolbutamide[21]. The lack of efficacy in the Bedford Study can possibly be explained by the use of a suboptimal dose of tolbutamide and no assessment of compliance with the allocated drug therapy. A small-scale study comparing glibenclamide with diet alone in 45 subjects with IGT, and a follow-up duration of 2 years, showed an improvement of glucose tolerance in the subjects who were classified as low insulin responders[26].

Since the UGDP study, there has been a lingering fear for an increased risk of cardiovascular disease with the use of sulphonylureas. Recent experimental evidence has also fuelled this anxiety, by demonstrating an impairment of the recovery of the contractile function and an increase of the infarct size in animal models pretreated with sulphonylureas[27,28]. These experimental

Table 16.1. Intervention trials for the prevention of type 2 diabetes

	Country	Participants	Interventions	Duration of follow-up (years)	Efficacy	Reference
Previous trials						
Bedford	UK	241	Tolbutamide 1000 mg or diet	10	No effect	Keen et al.[21]
Malmöhus	Sweden	267	Diet or tolbutamide 500 mg three times daily	10	No diabetes in tablet-taking subjects	Sartor et al.[20], Knowles et al.[24]
Whitehall	UK	200	Phenformin 50 mg or diet	5	No effect	Jarrett et al.[58]
Ongoing trials						
EDIT (Early Diabetes Intervention Trial)	UK	640	Acarbose or metformin	3		Johnson and Taylor[64]
FHS (Fasting Hyperglycaemia Study)	UK	227	Lifestyle or gliclazide	3		
DAISI (Dutch Acarbose Intervention Study in IGT)	The Netherlands	120	Acarbose	3		
Stop NIDDM (Study to prevent NIDDM)	Canada, Germany, Scandinavia	750	Acarbose	3		
DPP (Diabetes Prevention Trial)	USA	4000	Lifestyle or metformin or troglitazone	3–6		Fujimoto[59]

findings warrant proper evaluation of cardiovascular endpoints in glucose-intolerant subjects treated with sulphonylurea drugs. The adverse effects of sulphonylureas have been attributed to binding to cardiovascular $K^{+}{}_{atp}$ channels. There is, therefore, a growing interest in developing so-called pancreas-specific sulphonylureas[29]. Another factor associated with the use of sulphonylureas, which may confer an excess risk of cardiovascular disease, is the recent finding that they stimulate the secretion not only of insulin but also of proinsulin[30].

Sulphonylurea therapy has been associated with significantly higher levels of proinsulin and PAI-1 antigen levels[31,32] which may be the result of the propensity of proinsulin to augment PAI-1 expression in vascular tissue[31,32]. These findings have raised the awareness of a potential 'problem' with sulphonylureas which urgently needs to be addressed in future studies.

GLP-1

Much interest has been targeted on GLP-1, a gut hormone that has been shown to be a potent insulin secretagogue[33–37]. Insulin responses to glucose could almost be normalized in patients with so-called moderate type 2 diabetes, after intravascular administration of GLP-1[37]. Moreover, in several studies, a marked improvement of fasting and postprandial glucose levels could also be demonstrated in patients with type 2 diabetes[34–37]. The major problem with GLP-1 is the short duration of action and low bioavailability after subcutaneous injections[33].

An additional effect of GLP-1 is a marked retardation of gastric emptying[38]. This may contribute to an improved control of postprandial glycaemia. However, in other circumstances, e.g. autonomic neuropathy, this may be regarded as an adverse effect.

One of the major potential advantages of GLP-1 over sulphonylureas is the lower risk of hypoglycaemia, because the stimulating effect of the insulin response becomes self-limiting with lowering of the glycaemia. In subjects with IGT this is an important and serious consideration. The applicability of GLP-1 will depend heavily on the possibility of creating a pharmaceutical preparation with adequate bioavailability and duration of action[33]. Gutniak et al.[39] recently reported the pharmacokinetics of GLP-1 administered via a buccal tablet. This study demonstrated that it is feasible to achieve therapeutic levels of this hormone by this mode of administration. Further studies are required, using preparations with a prolonged duration of action, before this drug can be considered in diabetes prevention studies.

Non-sulphonylurea Insulin-releasing Drugs

Two novel oral hypoglycaemic agents are now being tested in clinical studies. One is a benzoic acid derivative (repaglinide) and the other is a phenylalanine derivative (A4166)[40]. The mode of action of these drugs is similar to that of the sulphonylureas; these compounds occupy a common receptor site with glibenclamide and close ATP-dependent K^+ channels[41]. The results presented suggest that these non-sulphonylurea insulin-releasing drugs have both a fast and a short duration of action, and the insulin response is partly dependent on the prevailing glycaemia[40]. These characteristics are of potential interest when considering their usage in early type 2 diabetes or in IGT. However, as was also discussed for sulphonylureas, we need more information about the influence of these drugs on the various cardiovascular risk factors, including possible extrapancreatic effects and, more particularly, the effects on vascular ATP-dependent K^+ channels[27].

Antioxidants

Chronic hyperglycaemia has been associated with increased oxidation of proteins and lipids[42]. Reactive oxygen species are generated from, among others, the glycation process; these in turn enhance the cross-linking of different proteins, a process that may also involve DNA damage[43]. As several epidemiological studies have suggested a relationship between antioxidant consumption and several chronic diseases, treatment with antioxidants seems to be a targeted approach to inhibit damage caused by increased oxidation[44–46]. Glutathione (GSH) plays an important role in the antioxidant defence of the cell, including the islets of Langerhans. This has led to several studies assessing the effect of antioxidants on glucose homeostasis in rats and on stimulated insulin secretion in humans[47,48]. Infusion of GSH in subjects with IGT resulted in a potentiation of the insulin secretion after a glucose load and during a hyperglycaemic clamp[48]. In normal glucose-tolerant subjects, no effect was found. These intriguing findings are supported by the recent observations of an antioxidant deficiency in subjects with IGT[49]. Glutathione and ascorbic acid were reduced by 15% in IGT. Moreover, there were elevated peroxidation products in plasma, red blood cells and red blood cell membranes. In diabetic rats, a glucose-lowering effect of another antioxidant, lipoic acid, has been demonstrated[47]. The mechanism leading to the glucose lowering has not, however, been elucidated. These very preliminary findings, although fascinating, need to be confirmed, and more work should be done on the mode of action of antioxidants with respect to glucose homeostasis.

HEPATIC GLUCOSE PRODUCTION

Biguanides

In most countries, metformin is the only available biguanide. The main mechanism of action by which this drug lowers the blood glucose level is the inhibition of glucose production by the liver[50,51]. Metformin enhances the suppressive effect of insulin on gluconeogenesis. An improvement of insulin sensitivity has been demonstrated in studies using the euglycaemic clamp technique, and this is probably secondary to the glucose lowering[51].

Metformin does not affect the insulin secretion process. The blood-glucose-lowering efficacy is similar to that seen with sulphonylureas, but at a lower level of insulinaemia[51,53]. The main advantages over sulphonylureas are the absence of hypoglycaemia risk and the lack of weight gain. These characteristics render this drug suitable for obese patients, although metformin has also been shown to be effective in lean ones[54].

Furthermore, in contrast to what is seen with sulphonylurea therapy, metformin lowers plasma concentrations of PAI-1 and proinsulin[55,56]. These changes may lower the risk of cardiovascular disease[28]. One study in which proinsulin was used as a study drug, and the UKPDS render support to this assumption[53,57].

The most feared side-effect of this drug is lactic acidosis which occurs rarely, with an estimated incidence of 0.03/1000 patient-years[51]. Even then, it almost always happens only when the contraindications are neglected.

Taken together, metformin seems to be a suitable candidate for a diabetes prevention trial. As such, in 1977 Jarrett et al.[58] had already reported, from the Whitehall study, on a 5-year therapeutic trial of carbohydrate restriction with or without another biguanide, phenformin (50 mg/day), in men with 'borderline' diabetes. In this study, cardiovascular disease and the conversion to diabetes were not affected by either treatment (see Table 16.1). This somewhat disappointing result has not discouraged the investigators in the now ongoing Diabetes Prevention Program (DPP) from including one study arm in which metformin is given[59]. Support for this choice comes from a recent French study demonstrating favourable effects of metformin in 324 middle-aged subjects with upper-body obesity[60]. One year of treatment with metformin, compared with placebo, resulted in weight loss, better maintenance of fasting blood glucose and cholesterol levels, and lower insulin and PAI-1 concentrations. The researchers concluded that long-term trials are warranted in well-defined high-risk populations.

RETARDATION OF INTESTINAL GLUCOSE ABSORPTION

α-Glucosidase Inhibitors

Type 2 diabetes is characterized by insulin resistance and the inability of the β cells to compensate for the enhanced insulin requirements. At the early stage of abnormal glucose tolerance, i.e. IGT, these defects are already present, albeit to a lower degree[11,12]. Theoretically, therefore, drugs that correct the postprandial abnormalities may alleviate the β-cell distress and thereby alleviate the adverse sequelae of postprandial hyperglycaemia (glucose toxicity) the β-cell function and insulin sensitivity[61].

α-Glucosidase inhibitors prevent the conversion of poly- and disaccharides to monosaccharides in the small intestine, and thus delay glucose absorption[62]. This effect on glucose absorption should therefore reduce the postprandial glucose excursions and lower the demand on the insulin secretory process. One compound, acarbose, is the most well-known representative of this class of drug; it is now widely used as a blood-glucose-lowering agent for the treatment of type 2 diabetes. The major side-effects are, understandably, of a gastrointestinal nature, affecting about 30% of those taking it[62]. A recent study suggested that α-glucosidase inhibitors may improve insulin sensitivity[63]. Treatment with 100 mg three times daily for 16 weeks resulted in a significant reduction of the steady-state plasma glucose level during an insulin suppression test in eight subjects, while this value was not affected by placebo treatment in ten subjects. However, a similar study in type 2 diabetic patients, using another α-glucosidase inhibitor, miglitol 50 mg three times daily, could not demonstrate any beneficial effect on insulin sensitivity[64]. There was also no apparent effect on HbA_{1c} (glycated haemoglobin), fructosamine or fasting blood glucose. The authors therefore concluded that lowering of the postprandial glucose in itself does not ameliorate insulin sensitivity[64]. The main differences between these studies are the patient population and probably, of greater importance, the duration of the intervention: 4 months vs 2 months.

The beneficial effects of acarbose on postprandial control of blood glucose levels and plasma insulin concentrations, and the impact on insulin sensitivity, make the α-glucosidase inhibitors potentially useful for the prevention of diabetes in people at high risk, e.g. people with IGT. This hypothesis is now tested in several studies in subjects with IGT or so-called fasting hyperglycaemia in different countries (see Table 16.1).

Amylin

In 1987, the amylin molecule, which makes up a major proportion of the amyloid deposits in the pancreas of patients with type 2 diabetes, was identified[66]. Amylin is a hormone comprising 37 amino acids which is co-secreted with insulin by the β cells[67]. This hormone has been shown to be a potent inhibitor of gastric emptying and, in rats, also of food intake. Initial studies in animals have shown a reduction in postprandial blood glucose levels that could be attributed to a retardation of gastric emptying[68,69].

To inhibit the inherent tendency of native human amylin to self-aggregate, analogues have been developed[70]. One of these is pramlintide, Pro-25,28,29-human amylin. Substitution of proline at positions of 25, 28 and 29 results in a molecule that does not self-aggregate. In recent years, several studies have been carried out in patients with type 1 and type 2 diabetes. Invariably, these studies have demonstrated a lowering of the postprandial blood glucose levels and a modest decrease of HbA_{1c} with three or four daily preprandial injections of pramlintide. A 4-week study in patients with insulin-treated type 2 diabetes resulted in a reduction in HbA_{1c} values of about 0.5% and a trend towards reduced body weight[71].

Moreover, it has been shown that amylin inhibits glucagon secretion, thus lowering glucagon-stimulated glucose production by the liver. This effect is abolished by lowering blood glucose levels. Preliminary experimental studies have shown no impairment of hypoglycaemia-induced glucagon responses.

The effects described above are of great interest and they all contribute to an improvement of glucose tolerance, but particularly the weight-lowering effect. The obvious disadvantage of this compound is the required mode and frequency of administration; most human studies so far have used three or more injections daily. Notwithstanding its highly interesting modes of action and efficacy, it is therefore premature to include this drug at this time for prevention of diabetes in a high-risk population. We must await more data from ongoing studies in type 2 diabetic patients, to assess in greater detail the longer-term effects on glycaemic control, body weight and patient tolerability of this new drug.

ENHANCERS OF INSULIN SENSITIVITY

Thiazolidinediones

Troglitazone is the first representative of a new class of drugs, the thiazolidinediones, to reach the market place. These drugs act mainly by improving insulin sensitivity of the peripheral tissues, in particular the fat and skeletal muscle cells[72,73]. The first thiazolidinedione, ciglitazone, was developed in the 1980s[74]. There have since been other compounds including pioglitazone and englitazone. Troglitazone is synthesized with an α-tocopherol substitution, rendering it bifunctional because, as a result of this substitution, it also has a strong antioxidant property[72].

The main molecular action of troglitazone involves the peroxisome proliferator-activated receptor γ (PPARγ), a member of the steroid/thyroid hormone receptor superfamily of transcription factors. After binding of thiazolidinediones to PPARγ the activated receptor activates or represses transcription of responsive genes. PPARγ is expressed in several tissues, particularly adipose tissue, but also skeletal muscle and the immune system[72]. In obese subjects with or without IGT, who were treated with troglitazone for 3 months, insulin sensitivity, as assessed by an euglycaemic clamp, improved markedly. This was also reflected by a 41% reduction in fasting and postprandial insulin levels and a normalization of glucose tolerance in 80% of the subjects who were IGT at baseline[73]. In addition, a modest improvement of blood pressure was noted.

The long-term efficacy of high doses of troglitazone (800 mg) has recently been compared with that of glibenclamide titrated to a dose of 20 mg. An interesting and potentially important difference was found in both the onset and time course of action between these drugs[75]. For glibenclamide, the glycaemic response was observed earlier (nadir of $8.3 \pm 1.6\%$ HbA_{1c} was reached at 12 weeks), followed by a gradual increase of glucose levels thereafter, despite uptitration of the dose. The HbA_{1c} values at 36 weeks and onwards were not significantly different from baseline (8.7 ± 1.6 vs $9.0 \pm 1.4\%$, respectively). In contrast, for triglitazone the maximum decrease of HbA_{1c} occurred later, at 24 weeks, but the achieved lowering of HbA_{1c} was sustained throughout the observation of 96 weeks[76]. In addition, as may be expected from the improvement of insulin sensitivity, triglycerides were lowered and high-density lipoprotein (HDL)-cholesterol increased with troglitazone: 3.15 ± 3.91 vs 2.14 ± 1.38 mmol/l and 1.02 ± 0.32 vs 1.18 ± 0.33 mmol/l, for triglycerides and HDL-cholesterol at baseline and 48 weeks, respectively. This improvement of the characteristic 'diabetic' dyslipidaemia was accompanied by a small but significant rise of low-density lipoprotein (LDL)-cholesterol: 3.48 ± 0.92 to 3.77 ± 0.98 mmol/l at 48 weeks. The rise in LDL-cholesterol has also been observed with other interventions, especially use of fish oil and fibrates[72,77-79]. It is interesting that fibrates and fatty acids also act via the PPARγ and the PPARδ receptors, respectively[72]. The rise in LDL has been ascribed to a higher metabolic rate of the triglyceride-enriched lipoprotein particles by lipoprotein lipase, resulting in a higher flux to LDL. The LDL size is also of importance; small, dense, LDL particles have now been recognized as a component of the insulin resistance syndrome and have been demonstrated as being associated with an elevated cardiovascular disease risk[80]. It is obvious that further studies are required to elucidate the effects of thiazolidinediones on lipoprotein metabolism. As troglitazone also has antioxidant properties, this may lower the propensity of LDL to be oxidized[81]. These earlier observations are supported by recent studies in people at high risk of developing diabetes, e.g. women with IGT and a history of gestational diabetes mellitus, demonstrating an improvement of insulin sensitivity with troglitazone[82,83].

In published studies, no change in body weight has been reported, which in itself is remarkable because one would expect an increase in body weight with improvement of insulin sensitivity. These favourable early observations have led to the initial inclusion of troglitazone as one of the intervention arms in the large multicenter Diabetes Prevention Programme in the US[59]. It is designed to compare various interventions: intensive lifestyle and metformin or troglitazone with minimal lifestyle only in 4000 subjects, with a follow-up of 3–6 years (see Table 16.1). So far, the most serious side-effect from the use of troglitazone is a disturbance of liver function. Although mild liver injury occurred in 1.9% of participants in controlled trials, the US Food and Drug Administration has received five post-marketing cases of severe liver disease resulting in death or liver transplantation. This has led to withdrawal of troglitazone in the UK and in the aforementioned Diabetes Prevention Programme in the US.

LOWERING OF THE BURDEN OF THE β CELL

β-Cell dysfunction is now recognized as an important contributing factor in the development of glucose intolerance[11–14]. The most characteristic defect is the failure of the β cell to respond adequately with a first-phase insulin response to a glucose stimulus. Mitrakou et al.[11] showed an inverse association between the 30-min post-oral glucose-challenge insulin levels and the 2-hour blood glucose values, again demonstrating the pivotal role of the first-phase insulin response in maintaining glucose tolerance. Therefore, it has been suggested, but not yet demonstrated, that insulin supplementation, by lowering the demands on the islets, may retard the progressive loss of the insulin-secretory capacity. Two separate ways of insulin supplementation may be considered, either with an insulin preparation with a prolonged action, to enhance the basal insulin levels or alternatively, with a very short-acting insulin (insulin analogues, nasal insulin) to mimic the first-phase insulin secretion. These different approaches are, from a research point of view, of great interest, but no data are as yet available.

OTHER POTENTIAL APPROACHES

Serotonin Reuptake Inhibitors

Examples of these drugs are (dex)fenfluramine and fluoxetine. These drugs have been shown to be capable of inducing weight loss in overweight subjects[84,85]. The weight reduction resulting from dexfenfluramin was accompanied by some improvement of metabolic control and insulin sensitivity[86]. Very recent reports have suggested that these anorectic drugs, and especially the use of the combination of dexfenfluramine and phentermine, are associated with the occurrence of valvular heart disease and primary pulmonary hypertension[87-89]. For this reason, these drugs are no longer suitable options for prevention strategies in obese subjects at high risk for the development of type 2 diabetes, despite the considerable risks of type 2 diabetes itself and the enhanced risk of cardiovascular disease[90].

Leptin

Obesity is an enormous and ever-increasing problem in developed countries. For this reason, it is understandable that leptin, the satiety factor released by adipose tissue, has gained enormous interest[91]. The growing understanding about the role and mode of action of leptin in the regulation of body weight has led to the interesting speculation that the thrifty gene, the underlying cause of obesity and insulin resistance, may be synonymous with the leptin receptor[92]. Loss of sensitivity could result in overfeeding in times of plenty, allowing survival in periods of shortage. However, in Westernized societies, the loss of leptin sensitivity would inevitably lead to obesity and, in those who are genetically predisposed, to diabetes. Administration of exogenous leptin should thus increase the leptin levels needed to enhance satiety, to lower appetite and to increase thermogenesis, thus reversing the detrimental course to diabetes. This therapeutic intervention is of great interest and attractive because of its physiological nature and targeted approach.

This optimistic forecast can be seriously tempered if the leptin injections result in a reset of the hypothalamic 'leptinstat' to a higher level, rendering the leptin administration ineffective[91].

The road to the development of leptin as a therapeutic agent is still very long, and even longer for chronic use in high-risk subjects.

β_3-Adrenergic Agents

Studies in various animal models have convincingly demonstrated that β agonists can modify body fat content and body weight without necessarily influencing nutrient intake[93,94]. Sympathetic nerve activity is an important regulator of energy expenditure in brown fat. In obese rodents, impaired brown fat tissue function has been demonstrated. Therefore, the search for a specific human β_3-adrenergic agonist has been intensified. One key question is whether β_3-selective agonists will also be effective in populations at high risk of developing diabetes. If proved to be metabolically effective, these agonists may improve insulin sensitivity and thus delay the onset of diabetes. So far, the utility of the tested β-agonists that are less selective is extremely limited because of side-effects[94]. Theoretically, this class of drugs is of great interest and the main potential advantages are the modes of action and the ease of administration. However, as described for leptin, first the physiological role in humans of this class of agents still needs to be clarified; second, the side-effects need to be investigated. It may be speculated that these drugs, if they prove to be efficacious, will gain a prominent role in the treatment of obese patients after a lifestyle intervention. As these drugs may prevent the lowering of energy expenditure, as normally seen with restriction of energy intake, it will be less difficult to adjust to a new lifestyle and may also reduce the side-effects of weight loss, in particular feeling cold and less energetic. Admittedly, it is highly speculative, but it may illustrate that this class of potential drugs is of great interest for an important proportion of the Western population.

ONGOING STUDIES

Several trials have now been initiated to answer the intriguing question of whether it is feasible to stop the development of diabetes in high-risk populations. Most studies have defined high risk as the glucose intolerance state (IGT) and some have relied upon slightly raised fasting blood glucose levels[65,96]. The major characteristics of these studies are summarized in Table 16.1.

CONCLUSIONS

The estimated major increase in the incidence of diabetes worldwide makes it imperative to consider all possible ways of reducing the burden of diabetes and its related complications in a serious way.

It is widely accepted that just pinpointing the required changes in lifestyle, i.e. eating less saturated fat, together with more exercise, will not be the solution. In fact, the changes in lifestyle observed worldwide, and particularly in developing countries, will certainly result in a tremendous increase in obesity, diabetes and cardiovascular disease[96]. It is difficult to imagine that societies converting from a rural to a more Westernized urban lifestyle will avoid this gloomy prediction. We therefore have to consider other possible interventions as outlined in Table 16.2. It may rightfully be argued that most, if not all, of the drug interventions are merely early treatments of the diabetic condition. This may be true for the well-known oral hypoglycaemic agents, but it is not necessarily true for the newer drugs that still are in the 'pipeline'. Drugs that directly affect the pathogenic mechanism, in particular insulin sensitivity or energy expenditure, and which predispose the person to obesity and glucose intolerance (e.g. leptin, β_3-adrenergic agents), are of more specific interest in this respect. Admittedly, because of the high costs associated with any drug treatment, large-scale interventions are not a realistic alternative in developing countries, which are facing the greatest increase in the incidence of cardiovascular disease and diabetes. Therefore, it remains essential to consider targeted lifestyle interventions at the population level; the aim is to lower the obesity rate by proper nutritional advice to the (very) young population[97]. Drug intervention is only feasible when it is focused at specifically defined, high-risk groups of subjects in whom a fair trial with lifestyle intervention has not resulted in the required change in either body weight or glucose tolerance. These groups can be readily characterized as suggested by the American Diabetes Association[10] (Table 16.3). It is hoped that the ongoing trials will identify an efficacious drug for treatment of the identified high-risk population in order to avoid the devastating consequences of type 2 diabetes.

Table 16.2. Drugs that may be used for the prevention of type 2 diabetes and their main mode of action

Main mode of action	Drugs	Route of administration	Availability
Stimulation of insulin secretion	Sulphonylurea	Oral	+
	GLP-1	i.v. Buccal?	Clinical studies
	Non-sulphonylurea Repaglinide A4166	Oral	Clinical studies
	Antioxidants?	Intravenous/oral	+
Inhibition of hepatic glucose production	Biguanides	Oral	+
Retardation of intestinal glucose absorption	α-Glucosidase inhibitors	Oral	
	Acarbose		+
	Miglitol		Clinical studies
	Pramlintide	Subcutaneous	Clinical studies
Enhancers of insulin sensitivity	Thiazolidinediones	Oral	+
'Lowering of the β-cell strain'	Insulin	Subcutaneous	+
Weight reduction	Serotonin reuptake inhibitors	Oral	Withdrawn
	Leptin	Subcutaneous	Early preclinical studies
	β_3-Adrenergic agents	Oral	–

Table 16.3. Factors associated with a high risk of developing type 2 diabetes

Obesity (BMI > 27 kg/m^2)
A first-degree relative with diabetes
Member of a high-risk ethnic population
Woman who has delivered a baby weighing >4.5 kg or who has had previous gestational diabetes mellitus
Hypertension (>140/90 mmHg)
Dyslipidaemia, characterized by low HDL-cholesterol levels (<0.9 mmol/l) and/or trigliceride levels >3 mmol/l
Previous IGT

REFERENCES

1. King H, Rewers M, WHO Ad Hoc Diabetes Reporting Group: Global estimates for prevalence of diabetes mellitus and impaired glucose tolerance in adults. *Diabetes Care* 1993; **16**:157.
2. Harris MI, Hadden WC, Knowler WC, Bennett PH. Prevalence of diabetes and impaired glucose tolerance and plasma glucose levels in the US population. *Diabetes* 1987; **36**:5234–37.
3. Mooy JM, Grootenhuis PA, de Vries H et al. Prevalence and determinants of glucose intolerance in a Dutch Caucasian population: the Hoorn Study. *Diabetes Care* 1995: **18**:1270–3.
4. Haffner SM, Stern MP, Hazuda HP, Mitchell BD, Patterson JK. Cardiovascular risk factors in confirmed prediabetic individuals. Does the clock for coronary heart disease start ticking before the onset of clinical diabetes? *JAMA* 1990; **263**:2893–8.
5. Fontbonne A, Eschwege E, Cambien F et al. Hypertriglyceridaemia is a risk factor of coronary heart disease in subjects with impaired glucose tolerance or diabetes: results from the 11 year follow-up of the Paris Prospective Study. *Diabetologia* 1989; **32**:300–4.
6. Lehto S, Rönnemaa T, Haffner SM, Pyörälä K, Kalio V, Laakso M. Dyslipidemia and hyperglycemia predict coronary heart disease events in middle aged patients with NIDDM. *Diabetes* 1997; **46**:1354–9.
7. Heine RJ, Mooy JM. Impaired glucose tolerance and unidentified diabetes. *Postgrad Med J* 1996; **72**:67–71.
8. Harris MI, Klein RF, Welborn TA, Knuiman MW. Onset of NIDDM occurs at least 4–7 years before clinical diagnosis. *Diabetes Care* 1992; **15**:815–19.
9. De Sonnaville JJJ, Bouma M, Colly LP, Devillé W, Wijkel D, Heine RJ. Sustained good glycaemic control in NIDDM patients by implementation of structured care in general practice: 2 yr follow up study. *Diabetologia* 1997; **20**:1870–73.
10. Expert committee on the diagnosis and classification of diabetes mellitus. Report on the Expert Committee on the Diagnosis and Classification of Diabetes Mellitus. *Diabetes Care* 1997; **20**:1183–97.
11. Mitrakou A, Kelley D, Mokan M et al. Role of reduced suppression of glucose production and diminished early insulin release in impaired glucose tolerance. *N Engl J Med* 1992; **326**:22–9.
12. Davis MJ, Rayman G, Grenfell A, Gray IP, Day JL, Hales CN. Loss of the first phase insulin response to intravenous glucose in subjects with persistent impaired glucose tolerance. *Diabetic Med* 1994; **11**:432–6.
13. Davis MJ, Rayman G, Gray IP, Day JL, Hales CN. Insulin deficiency and increased plasma concentration of intact and 32/33 split proinsulin in subjects with impaired glucose tolerance. *Diabetic Med* 1993; **10**:31–20.
14. Saad MF, Knowler WC, Pettitt DJ et al. A two step model for development of non insulin dependent diabetes. *Am J Med* 1991; **90**:229–35.
15. Mykkänen L, Haffner SM, Kuusisto J, Pyörälä K, Hales CN, Laakso M. Serum proinsulin levels are disproportionately increased in elderly prediabetic subjects. *Diabetologia* 1995; **38**:1176–82.
16. Nijpels G, Popp-Snijders C, Kostense PJ, Bouter LM, Heine RJ. Fasting proinsulin and 2 h post load glucose levels predict the conversion to NIDDM in subjects with impaired glucose tolerance: the Hoorn Study. *Diabetologia* 1996; **39**:113–18.
17. Haffner SM, Gonzales C, Mykkänen L, Stern M. Total immunoreactive proinsulin, immunoreactive insulin and specific insulin in relation to conversion to NIDDM: the Mexico City Diabetes Study. *Diabetologia* 1997; **40**:830–7.

18. Edelstein SL, Knowler WC, Bain RP et al. Predictors of progression from impaired glucose tolerance to NIDDM. An analysis of 6 prospective studies. *Diabetes* 1997; **46**:701–10.
19. Gerich JE. Oral hypoglycaemic agents. *N Engl J Med* 1980; **321**:1232–45.
20. Sartor G, Scherstén B, Carlström S, Melander A, Norden A, Persson G. Ten year follow-up of subjects with impaired glucose tolerance: prevention of diabetes by tolbutamide and diet regulation. *Diabetes* 1980; **29**:41–9.
21. Keen H, Jarrett RJ, McCartney P. The 10 year follow up of the Bedford Study (1962–72): glucose tolerance and diabetes. *Diabetologia* 1982; **22**:73–8.
22. Melander A. Oral antidiabetic drugs: an overview. *Diabetic Med* 1996: **13**: S143–7.
23. Alberti KGMM. The clinical relevance of impaired glucose tolerance. *Diabetic Med* 1996; **13**:927–37.
24. Knowler WC, Sartor G, Melander A, Schersten B. Glucose tolerance and mortality, including a substudy of tolbutamide treatment. *Diabetologia* 1997: **40**:680–6.
25. University Group Diabetes Program: a study of the effects of hyperglycemic agents on vascular complications in patients with adult-onset diabetes. *Diabetes* 1970; **19**(suppl 2): 747–830.
26. Ratzman KP, Witt S, Schulz B. The effect of long term glibenclamide treatment on glucose tolerance, insulin secretion and serum lipids in subjects with impaired glucose tolerance. *Diabetic Med* 1983; **9**:87–93.
27. Smits P, Thien T. Cardiovascular effects of sulphonylurea derivatives. Implications for the treatment of NIDDM? *Diabetologia* 1995; **38**:116–21.
28. Heine RJ. Role of sulphonylureas in non insulin dependent diabetes mellitus – 'the cons'. *Horm Metab Res* 1996; **28**:522–6.
29. Bijlstra PJ, Lutterman JA, Russel FGM, Thien T, Smits P. Interaction of sulphonylurea derivatives with vascular ATP sensitive potassium channels in humans. *Diabetologia* 1996; **39**:1083–90.
30. Van der Wal PS, Draeger KE, Van Iperen AM, Martini C, Aarsen M, Heine RJ. Beta cell response to oral glimepiride administration during and following a hyperglycaemic clamp in NIDDM patients. *Diabetic Med* 1997; **14**:556–63.
31. Schneider DJ, Nordt ThK, Sobel DE. Stimulation by proinsulin of expression of plasminogen activator inhibitor type 1 in endothelial cells. *Diabetes* 1992; **41**: 890–5.
32. Leibowitz G, Cerassi E. Sulphonylurea treatment of NIDDM patients with cardiovascular disease: a mixed blessing? *Diabetologia* 1996; **39**:503–14.
33. Holst JJ. GLP-1 in NIDDM. *Diabetic Med* 1996; **13**:S156–60.
34. Nauck MA, Kleine N, Orskov C, Holst JJ, Willms B, Creutzfeldt W. Normalisation of fasting hyperglycaemia by exogenous glucagon-like peptide 1 (7–36 amide) in type 2 (non insulin dependent) diabetic patients. *Diabetologia* 1993; **36**:741–4.
35. Gutniak MK, Linde B, Holst JJ, Efendic S. Subcutaneous injection of the incretin hormone glucagon-like peptide 1 abolishes postprandial glycemia in NIDDM. *Diabetes Care* 1994; **17**:1039–44.
36. Rachman J, Barrow BA, Levy JC, Turner RC. Near-normalisation of diurnal glucose concentrations by continuous administration of glucagon-like peptide 1 (GLP-1) in subjects with NIDDM. *Diabetologia* 1997; **40**:205–11.
37. Rachman J, Gribble FM, Barrow BA, Levy JC, Buchanan KD, Turner RC. Normalization of insulin response to glucose by overnight infusion of glucagon-like peptide 1 (7–36) amide in patients with NIDDM. *Diabetes* 1996; **45**: 1524–30.

38. Nauck MA, Wollschlager D, Werner J et al. Effects of subcutaneous glucagon-like peptide 1 (GLP-1 (7–36 amide)) in patients with NIDDM. *Diabetologia* 1996; **39**:1546–53.
39. Gutniak MK, Larsson H, Heiber S, Juneskans OT, Holst JJ, Ahren B. Potential therapeutic levels of glucagon-like peptide 1 achieved in humans by a buccal tablet. *Diabetes Care* 1996; **19**:843–8.
40. Kikuchi M. Modulation of insulin secretion in non-insulin dependent diabetes mellitus by two novel oral hypoglycaemic agents, NN 623 and A 4166. *Diabetic Med* 1996; **13**:S151–5.
41. Akiyoshi M, Kakei M, Nakazaki M et al. A new hypoglycaemic agent, A-4166, inhibits ATP-sensitive potassium channels in rat pancreatic β cells. *Am J Physiol* 1995; **268**:E185–93.
42. Wolff SP, Jiang ZY, Hunt JV. Protein glycation and oxidative stress in diabetes mellitus and aging. *Free Radic Biol Med* 1991: **10**:339–52.
43. Stahl W, Sies H. Antioxidant defense: vitamins E and C and carotenoids. *Diabetes* 1997; **46**(suppl 2): S14–18.
44. Rimm EB, Stampfer MJ, Ascherio A, Giovannucci E, Colditz GA, Willett WC. Vitamin E consumption and the risk of coronary heart disease in men. *N Engl J Med* 1997; **328**:1450–6.
45. Flagg EW, Coates RJ, Greenberg RS. Epidemiology studies of antioxidant and cancer in humans. *J Am Coll Nutr* 1995; **14**:419–26.
46. Rapola JM, Virtamo J, Ripatti S et al. Randomized trial of alpha-tocopherol and beta-carotene supplements on incidence of major coronary events in men with previous myocardial infarction. *Lancet* 1997; **349**:1715–20.
47. Khamaisi M, Potashnik R, Barnee E. et al. Effect of lipoic acid on glucose homeostasis and muscle glucose transporters in diabetic rats. *Pharmacol Res* 1995; **31S**:85.
48. Paolisso G, Giugliano D, Pizza G et al. Glutathione infusion potentiates glucose-induced insulin secretion in aged patients with impaired glucose tolerance. *Diabetes Care* 1992; **15**:1–7.
49. Vijayalingam S, Parthiban A, Shanmugasundaram KR, Mohan V. Abnormal antioxidant status in impaired glucose tolerance and non insulin dependent diabetes mellitus. *Diabetic Med* 1996; **13**:715–19.
50. Stumvoll M, Nurijhan N, Perriello G, Dailey G, Gerich JE. Metabolic effects of metformin in non insulin dependent diabetes mellitus. *N Engl J Med* 1995; **333**:550–4.
51. Bailey CJ, Turner RC. Metformin. *N Engl J Med* 1996; **334**:574–9.
52. Bailey CJ. Biguanides and NIDDM. *Diabetes Care* 1992; **15**:755–72.
53. UK Prospective Diabetes Study (UKPDS) Group. Effect of intensive blood-glucose control with metformin on complications in overweight patients with Type 2 diabetes. *Lancet* 1998; **352**:854–65.
54. DeFronzo RA, Goodman AM. Multicenter Metformin Study Group. Efficacy of metformin in patients with non-insulin dependent diabetes mellitus. *N Engl J Med* 1995; **333**:541–9.
55. Nagi DK, Mohammed Ali V, Yudkin JS. Effect of metformin on intact proinsulin and des 31,32 proinsulin concentrations in subjects with non insulin dependent (type 2) diabetes mellitus. *Diabetic Med* 1996; **13**:753–7.
56. Nagi DK, Yudkin JS. Effects of metformin on insulin resistance, risk factors for cardiovascular disease, and plasminogen activator inhibitor in NIDDM subjects: a study of two ethnic groups. *Diabetes Care* 1993; **16**:621–9.
57. Galloway JA, Hooper SA, Spradling CT, Howey DC, Frank BH, Bowsher RR. Biosynthetic human proinsulin: review of chemistry, in vitro and in vivo recep-

tor binding, animal and human pharmacology studies, and clinical trial experience. *Diabetes Care* 1992; **15**:666–92.

58. Jarrett RJ, Keen H, Fuller JH, McCartney P. Treatment of borderline diabetes: controlled trial using carbohydrate restriction and phenformin. *BMJ* 1977; **2**: 861–5.
59. Fujimoto WY for the DPP Research Group. A national multicenter study to learn whether type 2 diabetes can be prevented: the diabetes prevention programme. *Clin Diabetes* 1997; **15**:13–15.
60. Fontbonne A, Charles MA, Juhan-Vague I et al. The effects of metformin on the metabolic abnormalities associated with upper-body fat distribution. BIGPRO Study Group. *Diabetes Care* 1996; **19**:920–6.
61. Yki-Järvinen H. Glucose toxicity. *Endocrine Rev* 1992; **13**:415–31.
62. Chiasson J-L, Josse RG, Hunt JA et al. The efficacy of acarbose in the treatment of patients with non-insulin dependent diabetes mellitus. *Ann Intern Med* 1994; **121**:928–35.
63. Chiasson JL, Josse RG, Leiter LA et al. The effect of acarbose on insulin sensitivity in subjects with impaired glucose tolerance. *Diabetes Care* 1996; **19**:1190–3.
64. Johnson AB, Taylor R. Does suppression of postprandial blood glucose excursions by the alpha-glucosidase inhibitor miglitol improve insulin sensitivity in diet-treated type 2 diabetic patients? *Diabetes Care* 1996; **19**:559–63.
65. Chiasson J-L. Possible therapeutic approaches to impaired glucose tolerance. *IDF Bull* 1996; **41**:16–20.
66. Cooper GJS, Willis AS, Clark A, Turner RC, Sim RB, Reid KB. Purification and characterization of a peptide from amyloid-rich pancreas of type 2 diabetic patients. *Proc Natl Acad Sci USA* 1987; **84**:8628–32.
67. Young AA, Gedulin B, Vine W, Percy A, Rink TJ. Gastric emptying is accelerated in diabetic BB rats and is slowed by subcutaneous injection of amylin. *Diabetologia* 1995; **38**:642–8.
68. Macdonald IA. Amylin and the gastrointestinal tract. *Diabetic Med* 1997; **14**: S24–8.
69. Westermark P, Engstrom U, Johnson KH, Westermark GT, Betsholtz C. Islet amyloid polypeptide. Pinpointing amino acid residues linked to amyloid fibril formation. *Proc Natl Acad Sci USA* 1990; **87**:5036–40.
70. Thompson RG, Gottlieb A, Organ K, Koda J, Kisicki J, Kolterman OG. Pramlintide: a human amylin analogue reduced postprandial plasma glucose, insulin, and C-peptide concentrations in patients with type 2 diabetes. *Diabetic Med* 1997; **14**:547–55.
71. Thompson R, Pearson L, Schoenfeld S, Kolterman O. Pramlintide, an analogue of human amylin, improves glycaemic control in patients with type 2 diabetes requiring insulin. *Diabetes* 1997; **40**:30A.
72. Saltiel AR, Olefsky JM. Thiazolidinediones in the treatment of insulin resistance and type II diabetes. *Diabetes* 1996; **45**:1661–9.
73. Nolan JJ, Ludvik B, Beerdsen P, Joyce M, Olefsky J. Improvement in glucose tolerance and insulin resistance in obese subjects treated with troglitazone. *N Engl J Med* 1994; **331**:1188–93.
74. Fujita T, Sugiyana Y, Taketomi S et al. Reduction of insulin resistance in obese and/or diabetic animals by 3[-4-(1 methylcyclohexylmethoxy) benzyl-thiazolidine-2,4 dione (ADD-3870,U63287, ciglitazone), a new antidiabetic agent. *Diabetes* 1983; **32**:804–10.
75. Ghazzi MN, Perez JE, Antonucci TK et al. Cardiac and glycemic benefits of troglitazone treatment in NIDDM. *Diabetes* 1997; **46**:433–9.

76. Driscoll J, Ghazzi M, Perez J, Huang S, Whitcomb R. A 96 week follow up on cardiac safety in patients with type 2 diabetes treated with troglitazone. *Diabetes* 1997; **46**(suppl):574A.
77. Howard BV. Pathogenesis of diabetic dyslipidaemia. *Diabetes Rev* 1995; **3**: 423–32.
78. Heine RJ. Dietary fish oil and insulin action in humans. *Ann NY Acad Sci* 1993; **683**:110–21.
79. Vinik AI, Colwell JA. Effects of gemfibrozil on triglyceride levels in patients with NIDDM. *Diabetes Care* 1993; **16**:37–44.
80. Stampfer MJ, Krauss RM, MA J et al. A prospective study of triglyceride levels, low density lipoprotein particle diameter, and risk of myocardial infarction. *JAMA* 1996; **276**:882–8.
81. Cominacini L, Garbin U, Pastorino M et al. Effects of troglitazone on in vitro oxidation of LDL and HDL induced by copper ions and endothelial cells. *Diabetologia* 1997; **40**:165–72.
82. Henry RR. Effects of troglitazone on insulin sensitivity. *Diabetic Med* 1996; **13**(suppl 6): S148–50.
83. Berkowitz K, Peters R, Kjos SL et al. Effect of troglitazone on insulin sensitivity and pancreatic beta cell function in women at high risk for NIDDM. *Diabetes* 1996; **45**:1572–9.
84. Weintraub M, Harday JD, Mushlin AI, Lockwood DH. A double-blind clinical trial in weight control: use of fenfluramine and phentermine alone and in combination. *Arch Intern Med* 1984; **144**:1143–8.
85. Davis R, Faulds D. Dexfenfluramine. An updated review of its therapeutic use in the management of obesity. *Drugs* 1996; **52**:696–724.
86. Scheen AJ, Paolisso G, Salvatore T, Lefèbvre PJ. Improvement of insulin-induced glucose disposal in obese patients with NIDDM after 1 week treatment with *d*-fenfluramin. *Diabetes Care* 1991; **14**:325–32.
87. Connolly HM, Crary JL, McGoon MD et al. Valvular heart disease associated with fenfluramine: phentermine. *N Engl J Med* 1997; **337**:581–8.
88. Mark EJ, Pataloa ED, Chang HT, Evans RJ, Kessler SC. Fatal pulmonary hypertension associated with short-term use of fenfluramine and phentermine. *N Engl J Med* 1997; **337**:602–6.
89. Curfman GD. Diet pills Redux. *N Engl J Med* 1997; **337**:629–30.
90. Everhart JE, Pettitt DJ, Bennett PH, Knowler WC. Duration of obesity increases the incidence of NIDDM. *Diabetes* 1992; **41**:234–40.
91. Caro JF, Sinha MK, Kolaczynski JW, Zhang Pei Li, Considine RV. Leptin: the tale of an obesity gene. *Diabetes* 1996; **45**:1455–62.
92. Zimmet P, Alberti KGMM. Leptin: is it important in diabetes? *Diabetic Med* 1996; **13**:501–3.
93. Lowell BB, Flier JS. Brown adipose tissue, beta 3 adrenergic receptors, and obesity. *Ann Rev Med* 1997; **48**:307–16.
94. Yen TT. Beta agonists as antiobesity, antidiabetic and nutrient partitioning agents. *Obesity Res* 1995; **3**(suppl 4): 531–6S.
95. Knowler WC, Narayan KMV, Hanson RL et al. Preventing non insulin dependent diabetes mellitus. *Diabetes* 1995; **44**:483–8.
96. Laurier D, Guiget M, Chau NP et al. Prevalence of obesity: a comparative survey in France, the United Kingdom and the US. *Int J Obesity* 1992; **16**:565–72.
97. Uusitupa MI. Early lifestyle intervention in patients with non-insulin-dependent diabetes mellitus and impaired glucose tolerance. *Ann Med* 1996; **28**:445–9.

17

Non-diabetic Relatives: Characteristics and Opportunities for Intervention

M. WALKER

Human Diabetes and Metabolism Research Centre, School of Clinical Medical Sciences, The Medical School, Newcastle upon Tyne NE2 4HH, UK

There has been immense interest in the phenotypic characterization of non-diabetic first-degree relatives of patients with type 2 diabetes; this followed the now well-established observation that such relatives are at increased risk of progressing to diabetes. There are four main parts to this chapter: (1) review of the extent of the risk to non-diabetic relatives; (2) review of the phenotypic characteristics; (3) consideration of the risk factors that predict the development of type 2 diabetes; and (4) discussion of potential screening and intervention strategies.

RISK IN NON-DIABETIC RELATIVES

The evidence that unaffected relatives are at increased risk of developing type 2 diabetes has accrued from studies that span the last three decades. The very early studies are not reviewed here because they have been previously considered[1-3] and suffer from the general problem of failing to distinguish between type 1 and type 2 diabetes. Keen and Track[4] attempted to distinguish between the two types by determining the risks for relatives of diabetic patients diagnosed before and after the age of 35 years. The study included 1149 non-diabetic relatives of 735 Caucasian diabetic patients and 514 age-

Type 2 Diabetes: Prediction and Prevention. Edited by Graham A. Hitman

sex-matched control subjects. Importantly, the prevalence of diabetes in relatives and control subjects was established both by reporting and by direct measurement of glucose tolerance. Overall, this study showed that first-degree relatives of patients with type 2 diabetes have an approximately threefold increased prevalence of this type compared with the similar age- and sex-matched control subjects. Kobberling and Tillil[5] also studied Caucasian diabetic patients, but used more specific definitions for type 1 and type 2 diabetes, based on the age of onset and clinical features of insulin and non-insulin dependence. They determined the age-corrected risk for non-diabetic relatives of the patients with type 2 diabetes, which effectively provides an overall risk based on the assumption that survival will be to the age of 80 years. The calculated rates for age-corrected prevalence were 38% and 32% for sibs and offspring, respectively, and were threefold higher than the values for non-diabetic controls. However, the age-corrected prevalence rate for the parents of patients with type 2 diabetes was lower at 21%, although this might have reflected problems of ascertainment. Indeed an important deficiency of this study is that identification of non-diabetic relatives was by history alone, so that undiagnosed but affected relatives were missed. Beaty and colleagues[6] studied Caucasians and found that the number of siblings with type 2 diabetes had a much greater influence on the risk of developing diabetes than the parental history of type 2 diabetes. They proposed that this differential risk between non-diabetic relatives might reflect environmental influences that were stronger within a generation than between generations.

The increased risk of type 2 diabetes in non-diabetic, first-degree relatives has also been observed in other populations of different ethnic backgrounds. Even though the prevalence of type 2 diabetes is very high in the general Pima Indian[7] and Mexican–American[8] populations, there is still an important familial effect in both of these groups. In the Pima Indian population, the risk of developing diabetes was increased 2.3 and 3.9 times in the offspring who had one and two affected parents, respectively, when compared with offspring who had two non-diabetic parents[9]. Mitchell and colleagues studies 375 relatives of 29 Mexican–American pedigrees of type 2 diabetes and found that its prevalence was increased 2.0 and 1.3 times in the first- and second-degree non-diabetic relatives, respectively, of the type 2 diabetic probands[10]. It was interesting that the risk was much greater for relatives of patients who had early onset type 2 diabetes, compared with those who had relatives with late-onset diabetes; this might reflect an increased genetic load. Support for this comes from a study in which subjects with early onset type 2 diabetes (aged 25–40 years) invariably had two parents with abnormal glucose tolerance, and it was proposed that the offspring with type 2 diabetes received a 'double dose' of genetic risk from the affected parents[11]. This could explain the increased risk of diabetes in the offspring of two affected parents observed in other populations[9,12].

TWIN STUDIES

All of the studies mentioned above have focused on first-degree relatives who will share a proportion of the genetic load with the type 2 diabetic proband. As monozygotic twins share identical genetic information, the concordance rate for type 2 diabetes has been examined as a means of assessing the contribution of genetic factors in its aetiology. Several key studies are mentioned briefly. Barnett and colleagues[13] assessed 200 monozygotic twin pairs in which at least one of the pair had either type 1 or type 2 diabetes. Of those with type 2 diabetes, 48 of the 53 (91%) twin pairs were concordant for diabetes, suggesting a major genetic effect. However, the design of the study suggested that ascertainment bias was likely to have overestimated the concordance rate, and hence the genetic influence type 2 diabetes. This was circumvented in a subsequent study in which 250 monozygotic twin pairs were recruited irrespective of the presence or absence of diabetes[14]. Although less than the rates reported by Barnettt and colleagues, the concordance rate for type 2 diabetes was nevertheless increased at 58%, compared with the expected background prevalence. Of more importance, of the 15 discordant monozygotic twin pairs, only one remained discordant for type 2 diabetes after follow-up of 10 years, indicating the very high risk in the genetically identical siblings. A recent study has, however, suggested that the increased risk of type 2 diabetes in monozygotic twins may be partly related to a shared low birthweight secondary to fetal undernutrition. This is based on the observation that birthweight was significantly lower in the diabetic twin in a series of 14 twin pairs discordant for type 2 diabetes[15]. The analysis was complicated by the fact that seven of the non-diabetic twins actually had abnormal glucose tolerance in the form of impaired glucose tolerance (IGT), and indeed, six of the eight twin pairs concordant for abnormal glucose tolerance had the largest differences in birthweight. The potential impact of low birthweight on the risk of type 2 diabetes in monozygotic twin pairs therefore requires clarification. Finally, although studies of monozygotic twins have highlighted the importance of genetic factors, the magnitude of this effect remains unclear. Concordance rates of less than 100% indicate that environmental factors are still important. However, as shown by Newman and colleagues[14], the true genetic influence can be fully recognized only by conducting longitudinal studies.

PHENOTYPIC CHARACTERISTICS

It is well known that type 2 diabetes is a complex metabolic condition. Decreased insulin secretion and impaired insulin action on the liver, muscle and adipose tissue lead to hyperglycaemia and abnormalities of lipid metabolism, which include raised circulating levels of non-esterified fatty acids and tryglycerides. These metabolic changes, in turn, exert secondary effects on the defects of insulin secretion and insulin action as reviewed elsewhere[16,17]. Thus, there is very little hope of discerning the primary metabolic effects that predate the development of type 2 diabetes by studying patients with frank diabetes. It is for this reason that non-diabetic, but at-risk, first-degree relatives of patients with type 2 diabetes have been studied in order to limit the confounding secondary metabolic effects of raised circulating glucose and lipid levels. The study of these relatives therefore allows the possibility of identifying early metabolic defects that might point to the underlying genetic abnormalities, and also provides the opportunity to develop prevention strategies.

Metabolic studies have been conducted in non-diabetic, first-degree relatives for many years, and the findings have recently been reviewed by Pimenta and colleagues[18]. It is clear that a number of important points need to be considered when interpreting the metabolic data of such studies. First, metabolic differences between relatives and control subjects could arise as a result of poor matching of the level of glucose tolerance and the degree and distribution of body fat, which will influence insulin action and insulin secretion independently. Importantly, we and others have shown that subjects with IGT have evidence of both decreased insulin secretion and decreased insulin action independent of a family history of diabetes[19]. Second, the importance of certain metabolic defects seems to differ between different ethnic groups. Third, until very recently insulin levels were determined by radioimmunoassay and cross-reactivity with proinsulin-like molecules made overestimation of the true insulin levels a potential problem. This is particularly important because circulating insulin levels are frequently used as a surrogate index of insulin sensitivity, although the recent availability of specific hormone assays has reduced the errors in insulin measurements. Finally, different forms of metabolic tests have been used to measure insulin secretion and action in different studies.

ASSESSMENT OF INSULIN SECRETION AND RESISTANCE

A large number of studies have been conducted in non-diabetic relatives of Caucasian patients with type 2 diabetes. O'Rahilly and colleagues[20] examined 154 non-diabetic relatives and examined insulin secretion and insulin sensitivity using the CIGMA (continuous infusion of glucose with model assessment) test. Although they found that the relatives had impaired insulin secretion, this was not the case for those who had normal glucose tolerance, suggesting that the abnormalities of insulin secretion may have been secondary to IGT. In two subsequent large studies[21,22] hyperinsulinaemia independent of adiposity was a key finding in normal glucose-tolerant (NGT) relatives. The elevated insulin levels were interpreted as reflecting insulin resistance as the early metabolic defect, although it is worth noting that in both studies the NGT relatives had higher glucose levels than the corresponding control subjects; in addition radioimmunoassays were used to measure the insulin levels. Eriksson and colleagues[23] used the euglycaemic and hyperglycaemic clamps to measure directly insulin sensitivity and insulin secretion, respectively. They found that the IGT relatives had both decreased insulin secretion and decreased insulin sensitivity, whereas the only abnormality in the NGT relatives was a decrease in insulin sensitivity. However, the same methods were subsequently used by Pimenta and colleagues[18], although they went to great lengths to match the NGT relatives and control subject groups for age, sex, body mass index (BMI) and waist : hip ratio. In contrast to Eriksson and colleagues, they found that the relatives had decreased insulin secretion but normal insulin sensitivity. To produce the best match for potentially confounding factors, we individually pair-matched 100 NGT relatives and control subjects on the basis of age, sex, BMI and waist : hip ratio[24]. Hormone levels were measured by specific enzyme immunoassays. We found that C-peptide levels were decreased in keeping with decreased insulin secretion, whereas the HOMA index was increased, indicating decreased basal insulin sensitivity (Table 17.1). It was interesting that this combination of decreased insulin secretion and decreased insulin sensitivity has also been reported in other studies of NGT relatives, although using different techniques[25,26].

In summary, it is clear that, even when metabolic studies are conducted in non-diabetic relatives from a specific ethnic group, no single, consistent defect emerges. The variability between studies may in part reflect differences in methodologies and study designs, but also a true heterogeneity between the different study populations even though they are of the same ethnic background. It is appreciated that metabolic heterogeneity is a feature of established type 2 diabetes, with some patients having a principal defect of insulin secretion whereas others have a major abnormality of insulin action. It is quite possible therefore that such heterogeneity exists in the non-diabetic relatives, and this predates the development of diabetes and reflects underlying aetiological heterogeneity.

Similar metabolic studies have been conducted in the relatives of other ethnic backgrounds. The Pima Indians are a relatively homogeneous and well-characterized population in which the unaffected relatives have a principal defect of insulin action[27] Insulin resistance is also the key feature of non-diabetic relatives of south Asian extraction[28,29], although a recent report on Mexican–American relatives indicates both decreased insulin secretion and decreased insulin action[30], similar to the findings in Caucasians. Thus, metabolic abnormalities have been described in non-diabetic relatives drawn from a range of different ethnic backgrounds.

Table 17.1. Metabolic measurements for 100 pair-matched normal glucose tolerance relatives and control subjects (pair-matching was based on age, sex, waist : hip ratio and BMI)

Measure	Relatives	Control subjects	SD	p value
Age (years)	38	39	4	NS
BMI (kg/m^2)	26.0	25.8	1.7	NS
WHR	0.82	0.82	0.01	NS
HOMA (index)	2.1	1.8	1.3	0.03
Blood glucose (mmol/l)				
Fasting	4.5	4.6	0.8	NS
30 min	7.6	7.4	1.8	NS
120 min	4.7	4.6	1.4	NS
C-peptide (pmol/l)				
Fasting	442	516	262	0.01
30 min	1712	2082	1071	0.0003
120 min	4060	5280	1200	0.005
Insulin (pmol/l)				
Fasting	64	56	37	0.05
30 min	529	496	387	NS
120 min	265	246	289	NS
Intact proinsulin (pmol/l)				
Fasting	4	4	4	NS
30 min	10	11	9	NS
120 min	18	21	19	NS
Total proinsulin (pmol/l)				
Fasting	11	11	9	NS
30 min	48	48	43	NS
120 min	67	69	71	NS
C-peptide/insulin molar ratio				
Fasting	7.8	11.0	7.8	0.0002
30 min	3.5	5.0	2.1	0.0001
120 min	7.7	10.8	6.6	0.0001

All data are presented as the respective means and the SD of the differences. Reproduced with the permission of Springer-Verlag, Berlin, from Humphriss et al.[24]
WHR, waist : hip ratio.

CHARACTERIZATION OF THE INSULIN RESISTANCE

Despite a number of detailed and well-designed studies, the biochemical and molecular basis for the decreased insulin sensitivity in non-diabetic relatives has not been determined. Interestingly, in both Pima Indian and Caucasian populations, it has been shown that decreased insulin sensitivity exhibits familial clustering[31,32]. Lilloja and colleagues[31] determined insulin sensitivity using the hyperinsulinaemic clamp in 116 non-diabetic siblings from 45 Pima families with type 2 diabetes. They determined the mean M value (index of insulin sensitivity) for each family and plotted them from the least to the most insulin-sensitive family (Figure 17.1). They were able to show that the variability between families was significantly greater than that within families, and that the familial effect accounted for about 34% of the variance of insulin sensitivity independent of body adiposity. The inference from these studies is, therefore, that important familial effects influence insulin sensitivity, although it is not possible to determine whether such effects are the result of environmental and/or gene effects. Nevertheless we have preliminary data that support the premise that genetic factors influence the level of insulin sensitivity in at-risk relatives and their families with type 2 diabetes. Human skeletal muscle has been cultured after muscle biopsy in insulin-resistant relatives of families with type 2 diabetes and insulin-sensitive control subjects with no family history of diabetes. Insulin-stimulated glycogen synthesis was found to be decreased in the cultured muscle cells from some relatives[33], indicating a persistent in vitro defect of insulin action.

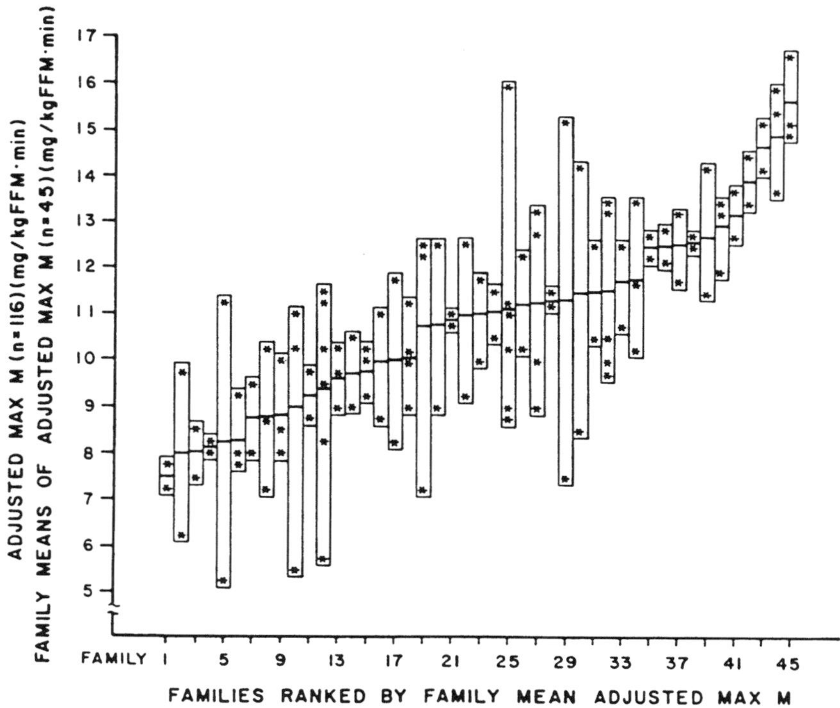

Figure 17.1. Glucose uptake (M_{max}), adjusted for age, sex and obesity, is shown for each non-diabetic relative. Relatives (*) are grouped by family (open bars) and families ranked according to mean adjusted M_{max} (horizontal lines). (Reproduced, with the permission of the American Diabetes Association, from Lillioja et al.[31]).

Using a combination of the hyperinsulinaemic clamp and indirect calorimetry, it has been shown that non-diabetic relatives of families with type 2 diabetes have decreased insulin-stimulated, non-oxidative glucose disposal[23,24]; this in turn, is thought to reflect primarily glucose disposal as glycogen[35]. In support, it was subsequently shown that glycogen synthase activity was decreased in muscle biopsy samples from non-diabetic relatives[36], although Rothman and colleagues[34] also showed, using nuclear magnetic resonance, that muscle glucose-6-phosphate levels were decreased in NGT relatives which indicated a proximal defect of glucose transport and/or phosphorylation. They initially proposed that the decreased glycogen synthesis could be secondary to this proximal defect. To explore this further, the same group studied the effect of exercise on the metabolic defects[37], and showed that this normalized the defect in glucose-6-phosphate levels, but that the rate of insulin-stimulated glycogen synthesis remained low. It was therefore established that the decreased muscle glycogen synthesis in the relatives was not secondary to the proximal defective glucose-6-phosphate metabolism, and indeed it pointed to an independent and possibly primary defect. Other factors are also likely to contribute to the decreased insulin sensitivity in non-diabetic relatives. Exercise capacity, as determined by Vo_2 max (maximum oxygen consumption) was found to be decreased in NGT relatives and closely correlated with the index of insulin sensitivity[25]. No clear explanation was found for this relationship and it did not appear to reflect an abnormality of muscle blood flow.

CHARACTERIZATION OF THE INSULIN-SECRETORY DEFECT

Studies have also attempted to characterize the pancreatic β-cell defect observed in non-diabetic relatives. Pulsatile insulin secretion was found to be deranged in Caucasian non-diabetic relatives, and it was suggested that this might point to a primary metabolic defect[38]. However, the relatives were heavier and less glucose tolerant than the corresponding control subjects, so it was never established whether the altered β-cell function resulted from an inherited defect or was secondary to the potential confounding metabolic and anthropometric changes. With the development of specific hormone assays; it has emerged that circulating proinsulin levels are increased in patients with type 2 diabetes[39,40]. In a recent review[41], it was found that the hyperproinsulinaemia could result from a number of possible mechanisms, although it could be a marker for a specific pancreatic β-cell defect. This possibility has been explored further by measuring specific hormone levels in non-diabetic relatives. We compared 154 non-diabetic relatives of families with two living patients with type 2 diabetes, who are of north European extraction, and 154 non-diabetic control subjects with no family history of diabetes[24]. Fasting total and intact proinsulin levels were raised in the relatives, although subgroup analysis of 100 pair-matched NGT relatives and control subjects showed that the increase was secondary to differences in adiposity and glucose tolerance (see Table 17.1). We did not therefore find any abnormalities of proinsulin levels in NGT relatives, which is in keeping with other recent reports[42,43]. However, a small increase in split-proinsulin levels has been reported by Gelding and colleagues in NGT relatives after an intravenous glucose tolerance test[44], whereas total proinsulin levels were found to be increased in Mexican–American offspring[45]. Thus, the current balance of evidence suggests that NGT relatives have normal proinsulin levels, although subtle defects may be present in certain ethnic groups and in response to some specific stimuli.

CHARACTERIZATION OF CARDIOVASCULAR RISK FACTORS

The discussion so far has focused on the defects of insulin secretion and action in relation to carbohydrate metabolism. However, other metabolic and anthropometric abnormalities have been described in non-diabetic relatives, which might be important determinants for the development of diabetes. An intriguing observation relates to body weight. Both we and others found that the non-diabetic relatives were heavier than the age- and sex-matched control subjects with no family history of diabetes[21,24]. A simple and obvious explanation is sample bias, particularly as lean and health control subjects may be more likely to volunteer for studies that involve the assessment of cardiovascular risk. This seems unlikely, however, in our study because the controls were randomly selected from the local population and, if anything, tended to be slightly heavier than the background population when stratified for age[46]. Further support for the observation comes from the San Antonio Heart Study in which parental history of diabetes was ascertained after recruitment into the study[45]. The offspring of patients with type 2 diabetes were significantly heavier than those subjects who had no parental history of diabetes.

If real, the increased body weight in the relatives could be caused by several potential mechanisms. It may reflect shared lifestyle factors, such as eating behaviour and attitudes to physical activity, or genetic influences that regulate such factors as body fat distribution, appetite and thermogenesis. Leptin deficiency produces abnormalities of appetite regulation and obesity[47], although we and others found increased rather than decreased leptin levels in relatives of families with type 2 diabetes[48,49]. Moreover, the increased levels were secondary to the metabolic features of the relatives and did not reflect a primary familial effect. Finally, hyperinsulinaemia has been reported in some studies and could promote increased body weight simply through a sustained anabolic stimulus.

The clustering of certain cardiovascular risk factors within individuals was highlighted by Reaven and is generally described as Reaven's syndrome or the metabolic syndrome[50]. Many patients with type 2 diabetes have features of the metabolic syndrome, which is typified by a marked decrease in insulin sensitivity and secondary hyperinsulinaemia. We therefore examined the six key features of the metabolic syndrome as originally defined by Reaven (abnormal glucose tolerance, hypertension, decreased high-density lipoprotein [HDL] cholesterol, increased triglyceride levels, obesity and decreased insulin sensitivity) in our 154 non-diabetic relatives and 154 control subjects[51]. Overall, the prevalence of these cardiovascular factors was markedly increased in the relatives, whereas others have shown familial clustering in keeping with an inherited basis[52]. These findings prompted us to examine in greater detail the lipid profiles in the non-diabetic relatives. Lipoprotein (a) [Lp(a)] is a particularly strong predictor for cardiovascular disease and is under strong genetic control[53]. However, we found no differences between our relatives and control subjects in Lp(a) concentration and phenotypes. Other abnormalities of lipid metabolism have been reported in non-diabetic relatives and include decreased sensitivity of free fatty acid metabolism to insulin in both the basal[54] and the insulin-stimulated[55] states. This indicates that the decreased insulin sensitivity in the non-diabetic relatives is not restricted to carbohydrate metabolism. Thus, the overall impression from these observations is that the relatives have multiple metabolic defects and an increased cardiovascular risk which is well established before the development of frank diabetes.

PREDICTORS FOR THE DEVELOPMENT OF TYPE 2 DIABETES IN RELATIVES

A number of important risk factors for the development of type 2 diabetes have been identified from general population studies and are considered in detail in other chapters. The purpose of this section is to focus on those factors that have been studied in the non-diabetic relatives of families with type 2 diabetes. A problem with this approach is that there have been only a small number of longitudinal follow-up studies in such relatives.

Probably one of the most comprehensive studies is based at the Joslin Clinic. Martin and colleagues[56] studied 155 NGT offspring of two Caucasian parents with type 2 diabetes. The offspring underwent a frequent sampled intravenous glucose tolerance test with Minimal Model assessment at baseline; they were then followed up over a period of 6–25 years. The intravenous glucose tolerance test was used to determine acute insulin secretion, whole-body insulin sensitivity (S_I), and glucose effectiveness (S_G), which is an index of the ability of glucose to promote its own clearance under basal insulin levels[57]. Of the original 155 relatives, 25 developed type 2 diabetes over the follow-up period. The key baseline predictors for the development of type 2 diabetes were decreased insulin sensitivity (low S_I) and a decreased glucose effectiveness (low S_G); these effects were independent and additive (Figure 17.2). Although the relatives who developed diabetes were heavier at baseline than those who did not develop it, body weight was not an important predictor in the multiple logistic model. This may be because the principal effect of increased adiposity is to decrease insulin sensitivity, and so the effect of increased body weight was represented as a predictor in the decreased insulin sensitivity. Somewhat surprisingly, decreased insulin secretion was not a predictor for the subsequent development of diabetes.

The same group recently conducted a similar analysis of 29 offspring with (IGT). As before, decreased insulin sensitivity was a key predictor for the progression from IGT to type 2 diabetes, but a decreased insulin secretion rather than a decreased glucose effectiveness was the other independent predictor[58]. This apparent disparity between the two follow-up studies may be the result of the fact that the IGT subgroup studied was not representative of all of the relatives. Certainly, it is recognized that some relatives progress rapidly from normal glucose tolerance to frank diabetes, and it may be that the relatives with IGT followed a less dramatic path in terms of metabolic decompensation. Nevertheless, it is clear from both studies that decreased insulin sensitivity is a major predictor for the development of type 2 diabetes. Unfortunately, what the studies did not show is how the metabolic defects detected at baseline changed with time and influenced the ultimate development of diabetes.

A similar longitudinal study has been reported in the Pima Indian population. Young offspring aged between 5 and 19 years underwent baseline

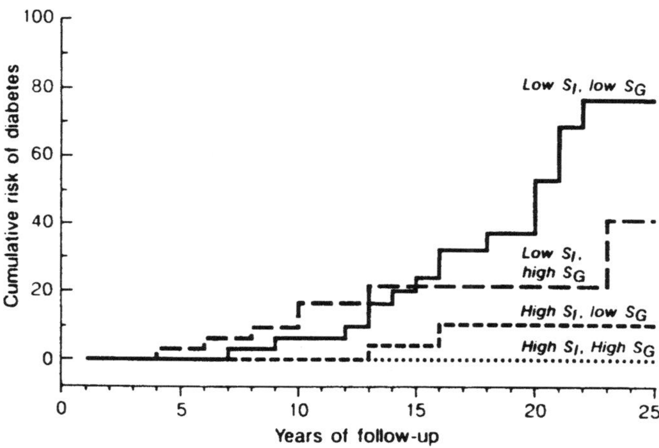

Figure 17.2. Cumulative risk of type 2 diabetes according to insulin sensitivity (S_I) and glucose effectiveness (S_G) at study entry. (Reproduced, with the permission of *The Lancet*, from Martin et al.[57])

assessment and follow-up[59]. Of the 1120 offspring with at least one diabetic parent, 9% had developed type 2 diabetes over an 8-year follow-up period. The baseline predictors were: increased body weight; increased 2-hour blood glucose concentration after an oral glucose tolerance test (OGTT); and increased fasting insulin concentration, which as mentioned above is a surrogate index for insulin sensitivity. Thus decreased insulin sensitivity is an important predictor for the development of diabetes in relatives of different ethnic backgrounds. Somewhat intriguingly, the same group subsequently reported that the risk of developing type 2 diabetes was high in the offspring of parents who had diabetes plus diabetic nephropathy, when compared with offspring whose parents had diabetes alone[60]. Again, there is no pointer to whether this reflects shared environmental and/or genetic factors.

A great deal of interest has been generated by the observed link between low birthweight and increased prevalence of abnormal glucose tolerance in adulthood[61]. The mechanisms underlying this relationship have not been defined, but it has been proposed that fetal undernutrition, leading to long-term programming of tissue function into adult life, may play a critical role[62]. Cook and colleagues[63] examined the relationship between birthweight and metabolic variables in first-degree relatives of families with type 2 diabetes. The relatives had a range of glucose tolerance, from NGT through to type 2 diabetes. Although a significant relationship was identified between low birthweight and decreased pancreatic β-cell function, there was no significant difference in mean birthweight between the NGT and type 2 diabetic relatives. Thus, although low birthweight might contribute to a decrease in β-cell function and the development of diabetes, its influence on the prevalence of type 2 diabetes appears to be obscured by the effects of other aetiological factors.

Other influences have been examined in relation to the risk of non-diabetic relatives developing diabetes. Several studies have reported that the risk to the unaffected offspring is greater if the mother had diabetes rather than the father[64–66]. In other words, there is an excess maternal transmission that might reflect genetic influences such as abnormalities of the maternally transmitted mitochondrial DNA[67], and/or abnormalities of intrauterine environment and fetal development. It has recently been reported that pancreatic β-cell function was more severely impaired in the offspring of mothers with type 2 diabetes compared with the offspring with this type of father[68]. This lends support to a maternal influence on the risk of developing diabetes in unaffected offspring

POTENTIAL COMPENSATORY MECHANISMS

The discussion has so far focused entirely on factors that positively promote the development of diabetes in at-risk relatives. However, there is another aspect of risk that requires consideration. As previously described, we showed that NGT relatives had evidence of both decreased insulin secretion and decreased insulin sensitivity when compared with NGT control subjects who were carefully pair-matched for age, sex, waist : hip ratio and BMI[24]. The obvious question then arises as to how NGT is maintained in these relatives in the presence of the dual metabolic abnormalities. We found that the relatives had a decreased C-peptide : insulin ratio, in keeping with decreased insulin clearance (see Table 17.1) and proposed that this would serve to counteract the other adverse metabolic defects by maintaining peripheral insulin levels. Henricksen and colleagues[26] similarly reported both decreased insulin secretion and decreased insulin action in NGT relatives, although they found that the relatives had increased glucose effectiveness when compared with the control subjects. An increase in glucose-mediated glucose disposal would also help to preserve NGT in the relatives. We therefore propose that the risk of NGT relatives developing diabetes is determined by a balance between (1) the compensatory mechanisms that serve to maintain normal glucose tolerance and (2) those factors that adversely influence insulin secretion and action, and thereby actively promote the development of diabetes. It is interesting to recall that decreased glucose effectiveness was one of the factors that predicted the progression to type 2 diabetes in the NGT offspring[56]. These considerations naturally have important implications for the prevention of diabetes in at-risk relatives, and we need to think carefully about strategies that will maintain potential compensatory mechanisms as well as prevent the influence of adverse factors.

PREVENTION: SHOULD NON-DIABETIC RELATIVES BE SCREENED?

The evidence reviewed in the preceding sections has allowed us to consider this important question. Several points have been established:

1. Non-diabetic first-degree relatives of patients with type 2 diabetes who have two- to threefold increased risk of developing type 2 diabetes compared with subjects who have no family history of diabetes.
2. Defects of insulin secretion and action, and increased prevalence of cardiovascular risk factors, are important findings in the non-diabetic relatives.
3. Decreased insulin sensitivity is an important predictor for the development of type 2 diabetes.
4. The points listed above apply to relatives of different ethnic extraction.

On this basis, there is compelling support for the development and implementation of strategies that will decrease the risk of non-diabetic relatives developing diabetes. However, although the risk of developing type 2 diabetes is increased in non-diabetic relatives as a group, when compared with control subjects who have no family history of diabetes, we know that the majority of such relatives will in fact never progress to diabetes. How can the relatives destined to develop type 2 diabetes be identified? Genetic markets are beginning to emerge that allow the identification of at-risk relatives. As discussed in detail in Chapter 6, the gene mutations that cause MODY1, -2 and -3 (maturity-onset diabetes of the young) are being defined; this allows non-diabetic but genetically susceptible relatives of affected pedigrees to be identified for the purposes of prevention. Maternally inherited diabetes and deafness (MIDD) is another subtype of type 2 diabetes that is linked to the A to G substitution at position 3243 of the mitochondrial $tRNA^{Leu(UUR)}$ gene[67]. Again, this allows non-diabetic but at-risk relatives of affected pedigrees to be identified. However, MODY and MIDD account for only a small part of type 2 diabetes, and there are as yet no genetic markers for the screening of the non-diabetic relatives of most patients with type 2 diabetes.

As previously reviewed, a common finding from the longitudinal studies of non-diabetic relatives was that decreased insulin sensitivity was a key predictor for the development of type 2 diabetes. In this regard, we have a potential metabolic marker for the identification of at-risk relatives, although several important considerations prevail. First, decreased insulin sensitivity is just one of several metabolic determinants and, indeed, in the study of Martin and colleagues[56] relatives with both decreased insulin sensitivity and decreased glucose effectiveness had the greatest risk of developing type 2 diabetes. In other words, it is not a specific marker.

Second, insulin sensitivity is difficult to measure in the clinical setting, and surrogate measures such as fasting insulin levels are imprecise. Nevertheless, it is clear that decreased insulin sensitivity is a major determinant and this almost certainly reflects an important aetiological role. Thus, it is a widely held belief that decreased insulin sensitivity contributes to the development of type 2 diabetes by applying a sustained secretory demand on to the susceptible pancreatic β-cells. Although no study to date has shown that an increase in insulin sensitivity decreases the progression to type 2 diabetes in non-diabetic relatives, there is indirect evidence that suggests that this is likely to be true.

POSSIBLE INTERVENTIONS

Insulin sensitivity is a complex state and is influenced by the interplay of many factors. Obesity is an important cause of decreased insulin sensitivity[69], and this is of particular relevance because, as reviewed earlier, non-diabetic relatives have been found to be heavier than control subjects with no family history of diabetes. However, not only the amount but also the distribution of body fat are important, with decreased insulin sensitivity being more of a marker in subjects who have central as opposed to peripheral adiposity[70]. Physical inactivity is linked to decreased insulin sensitivity[71] and, as described above, exercise results in a substantial improvement in skeletal muscle and whole-body insulin sensitivity. Other determinants include dietary composition, birthweight and genetic factors. It will be immediately apparent that only a proportion of these factors will be amenable to modification as part of an intervention strategy for the prevention of diabetes. The impact of exercise and the treatment of obesity in the prevention of type 2 diabetes is dealt with in detail in Chapters 11 and 15, respectively, although the experience in relatives, albeit rather limited is reviewed here. A comparatively small study examined the effects of calorie restriction and calorie plus dietary fat restriction in obese non-diabetic women of families with type 2 diabetes[72]. Both dietary interventions resulted in a significant weight loss of 7 kg over a 4-month period, which was accompanied by a decrease in fasting blood glucose and total cholesterol levels. However, with longer follow-up this degree of weight loss was not sustained and the metabolic benefits were no longer apparent. Unfortunately, the study did not examine the effect of such diets on insulin sensitivity itself and clearly was not designed to look at the effects of dietary intervention on the long-term development of type 2 diabetes.

Several studies have provided useful information in relation to exercise in at-risk relatives. Shulman and colleagues[37] showed that a programme of exercise resulted in the same comparable improvement in insulin sensitivity in relatives and control subjects (42% v 38% compared to baseline), but because insulin-stimulated glycogen disposal remained impaired in the relatives the exercise failed to normalize insulin sensitivity[37]. The relationship between exercise and the risk of developing type 2 diabetes was examined in a large cohort of American women[73]. Exercise was assessed by questionnaire, and it was shown that the risk of developing diabetes was significantly decreased in those women who took one or more bouts of vigorous exercise per week, when compared with those who took no exercise at all. Importantly, the benefits were the same for women who had a positive family history of diabetes in comparison to those women with no family history of diabetes.

A similar study in a large cohort of men found that exercise decreased the risk of developing type 2 diabetes, but interestingly the benefits were greater in those men classified as high risk on the basis of being obese and having hypertension and a positive family history of type 2 diabetes[74]. Thus, exercise does improve insulin sensitivity and decreases the risk of developing diabetes in at-risk relatives. It will be quite apparent that decreased body fat and exercise, as a means of improving insulin sensitivity, can be achieved through lifestyle modification. This is comparatively cheap and safe, and provides additional health benefits, although it may not be an option for all individuals. Nevertheless, because of these qualities it can be recommended to all non-diabetic relatives irrespective of their individual risk of developing type 2 diabetes. This is not the same for other possible intervention strategies. Pharmacological agents such as the thiazolidinediones are now available which specifically improve insulin sensitivity[75], and therefore present a strong case for inclusion in prevention strategies. However, there are clear cost and safety implications, particularly as the long-term effects of these agents on insulin sensitivity remain to be established. Further work is therefore required to determine the effects of such agents on type 2 diabetes risk reduction in non-diabetic relatives. A stronger case might be made for using such agents in those subtypes of type 2 diabetes in which genetically at-risk relatives can be clearly identified.

The current state of knowledge therefore leads to a recommendation for lifestyle changes that improve insulin sensitivity for all non-diabetic relatives, knowing that these interventions will also improve cardiovascular risk. However, we need to know more about the compensatory mechanisms and specific metabolic defects, and to have access to markers that accurately identify the relatives who will develop diabetes, in order to apply more potent and targeted prevention strategies in the future.

REFERENCES

1. Cook J, Turner R. Family studies: perspectives on the genetic and environmental determinants of non-insulin dependent diabetes mellitus. In: Leslie RDG ed. *Causes of Diabetes*. Chichester: Wiley, 1993: 219–47.
2. Ganda OP, Soeldner SS. Genetic, acquired, and related factors in the etiology of diabetes mellitus. *Arch Intern Med* 1977; **137**:461–9.
3. Pierce M, Keen H, Bradley C. Risk of diabetes in offspring of parents with non-insulin dependent diabetes. *Diabetic Med* 1995; **12**:6–13.
4. Keen H, Track NS. Age of onset and inheritance of diabetes: The importance of examining relatives. *Diabetologia* 1968; **4**:317–21.
5. Köbberling J, Tillil H. *Empirical Risk Figures for First Degree Relatives of Non-insulin Dependent Diabetics*. London: Academic Press, 1982; 201–9.
6. Beaty TH, Neel JV, Fajans SS. Identifying risk factors for diabetes in first degree relatives of non-insulin dependent diabetic patients. *Am Epidemiol* 1982; **115**:380–97.
7. Knowler WC, Bennett PH, Hamman RF, Miller M. Diabetes incidence and prevalence in Pima Indians: A 19-fold greater incidence than in Rochester, Minnesota. *Am J Epidemiol* 1978; **108**:497–505.
8. Mitchell BD, Stern MP, Haffner SM, Hazuda HP, Patterson JK. Risk factors for cardiovascular mortality in Mexican Americans and non-Hispanic whites: the San Antonio Heart Study. *Am J Epidemiol* 1990; **131**:423–33.
9. Knowler WC, Petititt DJ, Savage PJ, Bennett PH. Diabetes incidence in Pima Indians: Contributions of obesity and parental diabetes. *Am J Epidemiol* 1981; **113**:144–56.
10. Mitchell DB, Kammerer CM, Reinhart LJ, Stern MP. NIDDM in Mexican American families. *Diabetes Care* 1994; **17**:567–73.

11. O'Rahilly S, Spivey RS, Holman RR, Nugent Z, Clark A, Turner RC. Type II diabetes of early onset: A distinct clinical and genetic syndrome? *BMJ* 1987; **294**:923–8.
12. Viswanathan M, Mohan V, Snehalatha C, Ramachandran A. High prevalence of Type 2 (non insulin dependent) diabetes among the offspring of conjugal type 2 parents in India. *Diabetologia* 1985; **28**:907–10.
13. Barnett AH, Eff C, Leslie RDG, Pyke DA. Diabetes in identical twins: a study of 200 pairs. *Diabetologia* 1981; **20**:87–93.
14. Newman B, Selby JV, King MC, Slemenda C, Fabsitz R, Friedman GD. Concordance for type 2 (non-insulin-dependent) diabetes mellitus in male twins. *Diabetologia* 1987; **30**:763–8.
15. Poulsen P, Vaag AA, Kyvik KO, Moller Jensen D, Beck-Nielsen H. Low birth weight is associated with NIDDM in discordant monozygotic and dizygotic twin pairs. *Diabetologia* 1997; **40**:439–46.
16. Boden G. Role of fatty acids in the pathogenesis of insulin resistance and NIDDM. *Diabetes* 1996; **45**:3–10.
17. Yki-Jävinen H. Glucose toxicity. *Endocrine Rev* 1992; **13**:415–31.
18. Pimenta W, Korytkowski M, Mitrakou A et al. Pancreatic beta-cell dysfunction as the primary genetic lesion in NIDDM. *JAMA* 1995; **273**:1855–61.
19. Walker M, Berrish TS, Stewart MW, Humphriss DB, Barriocanal L, Alberti KGMM. Metabolic heterogeneity in impaired glucose tolerance. *Metabolism* 1997; **46**:914–17.
20. O'Rahilly SP, Rudenski AS, Burnett MA et al. Beta-cell dysfunction, rather than insulin insensitivity, is the primary defect in familial type 2 diabetes. *Lancet* 1986; **ii**:360–4.
21. Warram JH, Martin BC, Krolewski AS, Soeldner JS, Kahn CR. Slow glucose removal rate and hyperinsulinemia precede the development of type II diabetes in the offspring of diabetic parents. *Ann Intern Med* 1990; **113**:909–15.
22. Elbein SC, Maxwell TM, Schumacher MC. Insulin and glucose levels and prevalence of glucose intolerance in pedigrees with multiple diabetic siblings. *Diabetes* 1991; **40**:1024–32.
23. Erikksson J, Franssila-Kallunki A, Ekstrand A et al. Early metabolic defects in persons at increased risk for non-insulin-dependent diabetes mellitus. *N Engl J Med* 1989; **321**:337–43.
24. Humphriss DB, Stewart MW, Berish TS et al. Multiple metabolic abnormalities in normal glucose tolerant relatives of NIDDM families. *Diabetologia* 1997; **40**:1185–90.
25. Nyholm B, Mengel A, Nielsen S et al. Insulin resistance in relatives of NIDDM patients: the role of physical fitness and muscle metabolism. *Diabetologia* 1996; **39**:813–22.
26. Henriksen JE, Alford F., Handberg A et al. Increased glucose effectiveness in normoglycaemic but insulin resistant relatives of patients with non-insulin dependent diabetes mellitus. *J Clin Invest* 1994; **94**:1196–204.
27. Aronoff SL, Bennett PH, Gorden P, Rushforth N, Miller M. Unexplained hyperinsulinemia in normal and 'prediabetic' Pima Indians compared with normal Caucasians. *Diabetes* 1977; **26**:827–40.
28. Gelding SV, Niththyananthan R, Chan SP et al. Insulin sensitivity in non-diabetic relatives of patients with non-insulin-dependent diabetes from two ethnic groups. *Clin Endocrinol* 1994; **40**:55–62.
29. Ramachandran A, Snehalatha C, Mohan V, Bhattarcharya PK, Viswanathan M. Decreased insulin sensitivity in offspring whose parents both have type 2 diabetes. *Diabetic Med* 1990; **7**:331–4.

30. Haffner SM, Miettinen H, Stern MP. Secretion and resistance in nondiabetic Mexican Americans and non-Hispanic Whites with a parental history of diabetes. *J Clin Endocrinol Metab* 1996; **81**:1846–51.
31. Lillioja S, Mott DM, Zawadzki JK et al. In vivo insulin action is familial characteristic in nondiabetic Pima Indians. *Diabetes* 1987; **36**:1329–35.
32. Martin BC, Warram JH, Rosner B, Rich SS, Soeldner JS, Krolewski AS. Familial clustering of insulin sensitivity. *Diabetes* 1992; **41**:850–4.
33. Hurel SJ, Wells AM, Barriocanal L et al. Metabolic defects present in cultured myoblasts from first degree insulin resistant relatives of patients with NIDDM. *Diabetic Med* 1996; **13** (suppl 2): 528.
34. Rothman DL, Shulman RG, Shulman GI. P nuclear magnetic resonance measurements of muscle glucose-6-phosphate. *J Clin Invest* 1992; **89**:1069–75.
35. Bogardus C, Lillioja S, Stone K, Mott D. Correlation between muscle glycogen synthase activity and in vivo insulin action in man. *J Clin Invest* 1984; **73**: 1185–90.
36. Vaag A, Henriksen JE, Beck-Nielsen H. Decreased insulin activation of glycogen synthase in skeletal muscles in young nonobese Caucasian first-degree relatives of patients with non-insulin-dependent diabetes mellitus. *J Clin Invest* 1992; **89**:782–8.
37. Perseghin G, Price TB, Petersen KF et al. Increased glucose transport-phosphorylation and muscle glycogen synthesis after exercise training in insulin-resistant subjects. *N Engl J Med* 1996; **335**:1357–62.
38. O'Rahilly S, Turner RC, Matthews DR. Impaired pulsatile secretion of insulin in relatives of patients with non-insulin-dependent diabetes. *N Engl J Med* 1988; **318**:1225–30.
39. Temple RC, Carrington CA, Luzio CD et al. Insulin deficiency in non-insulin dependent diabetes. *Lancet* 1989; **i**:293–5
40. Ward WK, LaCava EC, Paquette TL, Beard JC, Wallum BJ, Porte D Jr. Disproportionate elevation of immunoreactive proinsulin in type 2 (non-insulin-dependent) diabetes mellitus and in experimental insulin resistance. *Diabetologia* 1987; **30**:698–702.
41. Rhodes CJ, Alarcon C. What beta-cell defect could lead to hyperproinsulinaemia in NIDDM? *Diabetes* 1994; **43**:511–17.
42. Birkeland KI, Torjesen PA, Erikson J, Vaaler S, Groop L. Hyperproinsulinaemia of type II diabetes is not present before the development of hyperglycaemia. *Diabetes Care* 1994; **17**:1307–10.
43. Beer SF, O'Rahilly S, Spivey RS, Hales CN, Turner RC. Plasma proinsulin in first-degree relatives of type 2 diabetic patients. *Diabetes Res* 1990; **14**:51–4.
44. Gelding SV, Andres C, Nithtyananthan R, Gray IP, Mather H, Johnston DG. Increased secretion of 32,33 split proinsulin after intravenous glucose in glucose-tolerant first-degree relatives of patients with non-insulin dependent diabetes of European, but not Asian, origin. *Clin Endocrinol* 1995; **42**:255–64.
45. Haffner SM, Stern MP, Miettinen H, Gingerich R, Bowsher RR. Higher proinsulin and specific insulin are both associated with a parental history of diabetes in non-diabetic Mexican–American subjects. *Diabetes* 1995; **44**:1156–60.
46. Harrington B, White M, Foy C, Raybould S, Harland J. *Health and Lifestyles in Newcastle*. Newcastle upon Tyne: Newcastle Health Authority and Department of Epidemiology and Public Health, 1993.
47. Caro JF, Sinha MK, Kolaczynski JW, Zhang PL, Considine RV. Leptin: the tale of an obesity gene. *Diabetes* 1996; **45**:1455–62.
48. Walker M, Ashworth LA, Stewart MW et al. Leptin levels in non-diabetic relatives of NIDDM families. *Diabetic Med* 1997; **14** (suppl 1): 526.

49. Nyholm B, Fisker S, Lund S, Moller N, Schmitz O. Increased circulating leptin concentrations in insulin-resistant first-degree relatives of patients with non-insulin-dependent diabetes mellitus: relationship to body composition and insulin sensitivity but not to family history of non-insulin dependent diabetes mellitus. *Eur J Endocrinol* 1997; **136**:173–9.
50. Reaven GM. Role of insulin resistance in human disease. *Diabetes* 1988; **37**:1595-607.
51. Stewart MW, Humphriss DB, Berrish TS et al. Features of Syndrome X in first-degree relatives of NIDDM patients. *Diabetes Care* 1995; **18**:1020–2.
52. Levy JC, Barrow BA, Lever DE, Morris RJ, Turner RC. Familial association and λs for diabetes, obesity, high triglycerides and low HDL-cholesterol in sibs of NIDDM patients. *Diabetes* 1997; **46**:136A.
53. Rhoads GG, Dahlen G, Berg K, Morton NE, Dannenberg AL. Lp(a) lipoprotein as a risk factor for myocardial infarction. *Am J Med Assoc* 1986; **256**:2540–4.
54. Perseghin G, Ghosh S, Gerow K, Shulman GI. Metabolic defects in lean non-diabetic offspring of NIDDM parents. *Diabetes* 1997; **46**:1001–9.
55. Gulli GT, Ferrannini E, Stern M, Haffner S, DeFronzo RA. The metabolic profile of NIDDM is fully established in glucose-tolerant offspring of two Mexican–American NIDDM parents. *Diabetes* 1992; **41**:1575–86.
56. Martin BC, Warram JH, Krolewski AS, Bergman RN, Soeldner JS, Kahn CR. Role of glucose and insulin resistance in development of type 2 diabetes mellitus: results of a 25-year follow-up study. *Lancet* 1992; **340**:925–9.
57. Ader M, Ni T-C, Bergman RN. Glucose effectiveness assessed under dynamic and steady state conditions: comparability of uptake versus production components. *J Clin Invest* 1997; **99**:1187–99.
58. Warram JH, Sigal RJ, Martin BC, Krolewski AS, Soeldner JS. Natural history of impaired glucose tolerance: Follow-up at Joslin Clinic. *Diabetic Med* 1996; **13**:540–5.
59. McCance DR, Pettitt DJ, Hanson RL, Jacobsson LTH, Bennett PH, Knowler WC. Glucose, insulin concentrations and obesity in childhood and adolescence as predictors of NIDDM. *Diabetologia* 1994; **37**:617–23.
60. McCance DR, Hanson RL, Pettitt DJ et al. Diabetic nephropathy: a risk factor for diabetes mellitus in offspring. *Diabetologia* 1995; **38**:221–6.
61. Phillips DIW, Barker DJP. The thrifty phenotype hypothesis. In: Leslie RDG, ed. *Causes of Diabetes*. Chichester: Wiley, 1993; 291–303.
62. Phillips DIW. Insulin resistance as a programmed response to fetal undernutrition. *Diabetologia* 1996; **39**:1119–22.
63. Cook JTE, Levy JC, Page, RCL, Shaw JAG, Hattersley AT, Turner RC. Association of low birth weight with B cell function in the adult first degree relatives of non-insulin dependent diabetic subjects. *BMJ* 1993; **306**:302–6.
64. Alcolado JC, Alcolado R. Importance of maternal history of non-insulin dependent diabetic patients. *BMJ* 1991; **302**:1178–80.
65. Lin RS, Lee WC, Lee YT, Chou P, Fu CC. Maternal role in type 2 diabetes mellitus: indirect evidence for a mitochondrial inheritance. *Int J Epidemiol* 1994; **23**:886–90.
66. Mitchell BD, Kammerer CM, Stern MP, Macluer JW. Is there an excess in maternal transmission of NIDDM? *Diabetologia* 1995; **38**:314–17.
67. Daly M, Turnbull D, Walker M. Mitochondrial DNA and diabetes. In: Marshall SM, Hone PD, Rizza RA, eds. *The Diabetes Annual/10* Amsterdam: Elsevier Science; 1996; 37–50.
68. Kasperska-Czvzyk T, Jedynasty K, Bowsher RR et al. Difference in the influence of maternal and paternal NIDDM on pancreatic beta-cell activity and blood

lipids in normoglycaemic non-diabetic adult offspring. *Diabetologia* 1996**; 39**: 831–37.

69. Bonadonna RC, Groop LC, Kraemer N, Ferrannini E, Del Prato S, DeFronzo RA. Obesity and insulin resistance in humans: A dose response study. *Metabolism* 1990; **39** 452–9.
70. Kissebah AH. Insulin resistance in visceral obesity. *Int J Obesity* 1991; **15** (suppl 2): 109–15.
71. Sato Y, Iguchi A, Sakamoto N. Biochemical determination of training effects using insulin clamp technique. *Horm Metab Res* 1984; **16**:483–6.
72. Pascale RW, Wing RR, Butler BA, Mullen M, Bononi P. Effects of a behavioral weight loss program stressing calorie restriction versus calorie plus fat restriction in obese individuals with NIDDM or a family history of diabetes. *Diabetes Care* 1995; **18**:1241–8.
73. Manson JE, Rimm EB, Stampfer MJ et al. Physical activity and incidence of non-insulin-dependent diabetes mellitus in women. *Lancet* 1991; **338**:774–8.
74. Helmrich SP, Ragland DR, Leung RW, Paffenbarger RS. Physical activity and reduced occurrence of non-insulin-dependent diabetes mellitus. *N Engl J Med* 1991; **325**:147–52.
75. Saltiel AR, Olefsky JM. Thiazolidinediones in the treatment of insulin resistance and type II diabetes. *Diabetes* 1996; **45**:1661–9.

Part E

Future Development

18

Problems Specific to Developing Countries and the Effects of Westernization

A. RAMACHANDRAN AND C. SNEHALATHA
Diabetes Research Centre, 4 Main Road, Royapuram, Madras 600 013, India

The importance of well-planned epidemiological studies on diabetes has been recognized in the past two decades. The literature on the epidemiology of type 2 diabetes is therefore increasing, rapidly indicating several interesting variations based on geographical, ethnic and socioeconomic factors. The general trend shows that the prevalence is on the increase, especially in developing countries[1-5]. In some countries that are becoming rapidly industrialized and urbanized, there is an apparent increasing trend in the prevalence of diabetes and its associated complications[1-10]. Repeated cross-sectional and sequential studies would throw more light on the natural history of the disease and also on the factors influencing diabetogenesis. The widespread interest in the epidemiology of type 2 diabetes has been sparked by several factors, such as (1) its increasing prevalence in most countries, especially in the developing countries where most of the world's population live; (2) the association of type 2 diabetes with other risk factors for cardiovascular disease (CVD), which is also emerging as a public health problem in many nations[11]; and (3) the high morbidity and mortality caused by the long-term vascular complications specific to diabetes, such as nephropathy, retinopathy and peripheral vascular disease[5,12].

RISING PREVALENCE OF TYPE 2 DIABETES

Reports from several countries, such as the UK[13-15], Fiji[16,17], Singapore[18,19], South Africa[20,21], Mauritius[5,7], Trinidad[22,23] and Tanzania[24], showed that

Type 2 Diabetes: Prediction and Prevention. Edited by Graham A. Hitman

migrant south Asian Indians have a high prevalence of diabetes compared with the co-inhabitants of other ethnicity of those countries (Tables 18.1 and 18.2). There were no identifiable risk factors in the south Asians that could explain the higher prevalence of diabetes. More detailed studies have pointed out a high genetic predisposition as the basic cause for this high prevalence.

Settlement in affluent conditions results in lifestyle changes, including changes in diet and physical activity that are sufficient to unmask the genetic tendency of diabetes. In the past two decades, the consequences of the Westernization phenomenon apparent in the migrant south Asians is becoming manifest in the homelands as well, with increasing urbanization and industrialization. The rising trends in the prevalence of type 2 diabetes reported from several such nations, including India, is shown in Table 18.3[19–35]. In China, where the prevalence of diabetes was previously considered to be very low, the recent large epidemiological study showed that 3.1% of the population aged 20–74 years had diabetes[35]. In those aged over 60 years, 10.1% were diabetic.

RISK FACTORS

All the studies mentioned above have shown that the rising trend in the prevalence of type 2 diabetes could be attributed to the following risk factors:

- genetic inheritance
- insulin resistance (syndrome X)
- obesity and central adiposity
- urbanization with adoption of Western lifestyle: unhealthy dietary habits and sedentary lifestyle.

The interaction of diet, obesity and physical activity is complex, and adoption of an affluent lifestyle, within the country or abroad, is associated with changes in all three factors, each of which has an immense influence on the development of diabetes.

GENETIC COMPONENT IN THE AETIOLOGY OF TYPE 2 DIABETES

Type 2 diabetes is a multifactorial disease with an equally strong genetic and environmental etiology. The familial nature of the disorder was recognized even by the ancient physicians of India. However, even after intensive and multiprobed attempts by several well-known geneticists, the genetic basis of type 2 diabetes is still elusive[36]. Simmons et al., in the study of the south

Table 18.1. Prevalence of diabetes in migrant Asian Indians compared with other ethnic groups

Year	Author	Town/Country	Prevalence (%)						
			Caucasians*	Africans*	Melanesians*	Malays	Chinese	Creoles	Indians*
1958	Wright et al[22]	Trinidad		1.4					1.7
1986	Beckles et al[23]	Trinidad	4.3, 10.2	8.2, 14.8					21.6
1967	Cassidy[16]	Fiji			0.6				5.7
1983	Zimmet et al[17]	Fiji			3.5, 7.1 (U) (R)				12.9, 11.0 (U) (R)
1969	Marine et al[20]	South Africa		3.6		6.6			10.4
1975	Cheah et al[19]	Singapore				2.4	1.6		6.1
1988	McKeigue et al[21]	East London	10, 4.0						23.0
1989	Simmons et al[15]	Coventry, UK	2.8, 4.3						11.2, 8.9
1989	Dowse et al[7]	Mauritius					11.5	10.4	12.6
1989	Swai et al[24]	Tanzania		1.9					7.1
1992	Cheah and Thai[19]	Singapore				9.3	8.0		12.8
		Malaysia				3.0	4.9		16.0
1994	Omar et al[21]	South Africa							13.0

* Male, female.

Table 18.2. Rising prevalence of type 2 diabetes in migrant Indians

		Age (years)	Diabetes (%) Male	Female	Total
Trinidad[22,23]					
	1958	> 14	2.3	1.0	1.7
	1968	All ages	2.5	2.3	4.5
	1986	(36–69)			21.6
South Africa[20,21]					
	1969	> 15			10.4
	1985	≥ 15			11.1
	1994	≥ 15	15.0	10.4	13.0
Fiji[16,17]					
	1967				5.7
	1983		12.9	11.0	
Singapore[18,19]					
	1975	All ages	8.1	3.1	6.1
	1984		13.4	5.1	8.9
	1992				12.8

Asians in Coventry in the UK, noted that all the five communities studied, namely Punjabi Sikhs, Punjabi Hindus, Gujarati Muslims, Gujarati Hindus and Pakistani Muslims, had a higher prevalence of diabetes (8.9–16.0% in men and 7.5–20.4% in women) than Caucasians despite their known dietary, cultural and socioeconomic differences[37]. This suggested a strong genetic predisposition to diabetes in all the Asian communities, although environmental factors might have been necessary for the expression of the disorder.

Epidemiological evidence for a strong genetic component in the aetiology of type 2 diabetes is large and comes from different sources.

FAMILIAL AGGREGATION OF DIABETES

Asian Indians have a strong familial aggregation of diabetes with a higher prevalence of diabetes among their first-degree relatives and a vertical transmission through two or more generations. It was found that 45% of Indians, compared with 38% of Caucasians, have a positive family history of diabetes[38]. A recent analysis of family history in the patients with type 2 diabetes who attended the Diabetes Research Centre, Madras, India showed that 54% of the probands had a parent with known diabetes and, in an additional 22.8%, siblings had diabetes[39]. It was also noticed by Viswanathan et al.[39] that the prevalence of diabetes increased with an increasing family history of diabetes. They noted that the prevalence of diabetes among the offspring with one diabetic parent was 36%, which increased to 54% when there was also a positive family history of diabetes on the non-diabetic parental side[40]. The prevalence rate (62%) and the risk

Table 18.3. Prevalence of type 2 diabetes in South-East Asia

Country	Year	Urban (%)	Rural (%)
India	1972[25]	2.3	
	1975[26]	3.0	1.3
	1988[27]	5.0	
	1992[28]	8.2	2.4
	1997[3]	11.6	
Singapore[18,19]			
Chinese	1987	4.0	
	1992	8.0	
Malays	1984	7.6	
	1992	8.2	2.8
Migrant Indians	1984	8.9	
	1992	12.8	
Philippines	1992	8.4–12.0	3.8–9.7
Malaysia	1984	7.6	
	1992[19]	9.3	
	1994[a]		12.2
Thailand	1971	2.5	
	1986	6.0	6.0
	1989[35]		6.7
Sri Lanka	1994[29]	5.0	
	1995[30]	8.1	
Pakistan	1995[31]	16.2 (M) 11.7 (F)	
Bangladesh	1995[32]		2.2
	1997[33]	4.5	
South Korea	1995[34]	7.2	
China	1986[35]	1.6	
	1997	3.1	
Vietnam	1992[b]	2.5	0.55

[a]Personal communication (Khalid BAK, Singapore).
[b]Personal communication (Mai Then Trach, Vietnam).

(73%) increase further when both parents have diabetes. The increasing risk of diabetes with increasing familial aggregation was put forward by Steinberg in 1959, and the phenomenon of anticipation reported by him was also borne out by our results[41]. The offspring of diabetic parents were noted to develop the disease at least a decade earlier than their parents.

In a survey in a south Indian population, we noted that 43% of the diabetic patients had a first-degree family history of diabetes[28]. It has been observed that, in Asian Indians, Pima Indians and Nauruans, the onset of diabetes is mostly between 40 and 50 years, unlike in Caucasians[4], with the effect of the phenomenon of anticipation, the age at onset could be even lower in many. Therefore, morbidity resulting from the long-term complications of diabetes would occur at a very young age. Familial aggregation was found to be high in several other populations, such as the Nauruans[5], Pima Indians[42],

Hispanics, Mexican–Americans[43] and Australian Aborigines[5]. Excess maternal transmission of type 2 diabetes has been reported in several Caucasian populations[44-46], although two studies in south Asian families did not show excessive maternal transmission[39,47]. Two other studies in non-Caucasian populations also did not notice sex-specific transmission of type 2 diabetes, namely in south Asian migrants in Manchester (the UK)[48] and in Mexican–Americans[49].

GENETIC SUSCEPTIBILITY IN ETHNIC GROUPS

Certain ethnic populations show a high prevalence of type 2 diabetes. Zimmet[2] has classified populations based on the degree of susceptibility to type 2 diabetes (Table 18.4). It is also interesting to note the wide differences in the prevalence of the disease in different ethnic groups who live in the same geographical regions and environmental conditions. Indians in Fiji[17] and Singapore[19] are shown to have higher prevalence of type 2 diabetes compared with the host population; the Pima Indians[42], Mexican–Americans and Hispanics[43] are found to have higher rates compared with Caucasians in the USA. This disparity in the prevalence of diabetes in different ethnic groups points to their greater genetic susceptibility to type 2 diabetes, which is unmasked by environmental influences[2,36,50]. A high frequency of diabetes in separate ethnic populations, when exposed to changing environment, provides strong evidence for the presence of a genetic trait, which in the past could have been of selective advantage, as first proposed by Neel as the 'thrifty genotype hypothesis[51].

INBREEDING OF POPULATIONS

Several genetic disorders are prevalent in highly inbred populations. High prevalence of diabetes in small islands, such as Nauru, Mauritius, Fiji and Malta, are attributed partly to the close inbreeding of the populations[10]. A

Table 18.4. Genetic susceptibility to type 2 diabetes in various ethnic groups[2]

Genetic susceptibility		
Low	Moderate	High
White	Africans	Native Americans
Melanesians (non-Austronesian)	Chinese	Micronesians
	Melanesian (Polynesian admixture)	Polynesians
Inuits		Asian Indians
Others	Japanese	Australian Aborigines
		Mexican–Americans
		Hispanics

study in Nauruans[52] and another in Pima Indians showed that foreign admixture produced relatively lower prevalence of type 2 diabetes in comparison to the inbred population[53]. South Indians also have a high rate of consanguinity which is probably a cause of the rising prevalence of diabetes in this population, both in India and in the Tamil Indian community in South Africa[10]. Dravidians in south India are mostly inbred with very little admixture of castes, unlike the north Indian population, which is an admixture of several races. Prevalence of diabetes was found to be high in Parsees in north-western India and in tribal populations in Orissa, providing evidence for higher genetic susceptibility in inbred populations[10].

AUTOSOMAL DOMINANT INHERITANCE OF DIABETES

Autosomal dominant inheritance of type 2 diabetes, with vertical transmission of the disease through at least three generations, is quite frequent in Indians, Nauruans and Pima Indians, who also have a high prevalence of the disease. Among the south Asians, we and others have reported younger age at onset of the disease compared with the Western population[54]. The other major problem is the high prevalence of type 2 diabetes in the young. This phenomenon and the prevalence of this form of diabetes probably suggest the strong influence of genetic loading in unmasking diabetes early in life[55]. In India, although macrovascular complications are infrequent in type 2 diabetes in the young, the specific microvascular complications are as common as in classic type 2 diabetes[56].

Nutrition *in utero*

Barker has hypothesized that fetal and childhood malnutrition, by programming metabolism, predisposes to chronic diseases in adulthood such as hypertension, coronary heart disease and type 2 diabetes[57]. A 'thrifty phenotype' has been proposed, in which inadequate fetal nutrition programs development of insulin resistance in adulthood. There is ample evidence in favour of this hypothesis as a major determinant of type 2 diabetes in Caucasians[58,59]. It may well be that such a phenomenon is more relevant in those developing countries where malnutrition is a major health problem. However, there have been no data to substantiate this[4]. There have been only very few studies from India which showed some evidence for a link between malnutrition *in utero* and a high prevalence of insulin resistance[60].

INSULIN RESISTANCE

Insulin resistance and β-cell deficiency are the two major pathogenic factors in diabetes. Several studies suggest that insulin resistance is the primary event that leads to abnormalities in glucose metabolism and that it is present long before the metabolic abnormalities become manifested[61]. Insulin resistance and hyperinsulinaemia are more common in populations such as Asian Indians[3], Afro-Caribbeans, Hispanics and Native Americans than in Caucasians[62–65].

Comparison of south Asians and Caucasians by several groups of researchers has shown that the former have a higher insulin response, both at fasting levels and in response to glucose[36,66–68]. Similar reports have been published comparing other ethnic groups in South Africa, Fiji and Singapore[2,69].

Epidemiological studies in southern India have highlighted that normoglycaemic Indians with ideal body mass also have hyperinsulinaemic responses, when compared with the reported values in Caucasians[62,66]. Measurement of insulin resistance by the euglycaemic clamp method[70] or by measurement of the index of insulin-mediated glucose metabolism, K_{ITT} during an insulin tolerance test (ITT)[71] also show direct evidence for higher insulin-resistant state in south Asians. More recently, studies from India[72] and the UK[68] have shown that the hyperinsulinaemic responses in the Asian Indians are the result of higher concentrations of specific insulin and not of increased secretion of proinsulin or its split products. Hyperinsulinaemia and lower insulin sensitivity have been reported in normoglycaemic offspring of diabetic parents, from south India[71,73].

OBESITY

The relationship between obesity and type 2 diabetes is complex and confounded by many heterogeneous factors. Although varied observations have been reported in studies examining the role of obesity in the pathogenesis of type 2 diabetes, it is generally agreed that obesity definitely contributes to the unmasking of the disease in a genetically prone individual.

The 1980 WHO Expert Committee on Diabetes concluded that the most powerful risk factor for type 2 diabetes is obesity[12]. Most of the studies discussed earlier had shown body mass index (BMI) to be a positively associated risk factor for diabetes and impaired glucose tolerance (IGT). In populations such as the Pima Indians, Nauruans and Mexican–Americans, the rates of obesity are high[5,2]. It was also shown by Collins and associates[74] that the dramatic increase in the prevalence of type 2 diabetes in Western Samoa had also occurred with an associated increase in obesity, the mean BMI exceeding 30 kg/m^2 in both sexes. Increase in obesity was greater in the rural areas, which paralleled the escalation in the prevalence of type 2 diabetes. Generation differences were observed in the association of BMI with the risk of type 2 diabetes. In our studies, BMI had been found to be a strong predictive factor of type 2 diabetes in women, in contrast to its marginal significance in men[28]. In recent studies, the relationship of body weight to diabetes appeared to be related to regional distribution of adiposity.

In all the studies in southern Indians, BMI has been strongly associated with glucose intolerance, although the mean BMI has been much below the obesity level, in both the urban and the rural populations[3,28]. This suggested that increase in body weight, although within the ideal levels of body mass, could increase the risk of diabetes. The cut-off values for ideal body weight that are applicable to Western populations might not hold good in the generally lean Asian Indians. Moreover, insulin resistance, which was found to be a characteristic feature of Asian Indians, despite their lean body mass, could be adversely affected by even small increments in body mass. The high prevalence of type 2 diabetes in Indians in India or in Fiji, Singapore, Malaysia and South Africa, and in Asian Indians in the UK, compared with respective co-inhabitants, was not a result of the high BMI[10,75].

CENTRAL OBESITY

McKeigue et al.[15] noted that the Afro-Caribbeans who had high prevalence of type 2 diabetes, similar to that in Asian Indians, did not have hyperinsulinaemic responses or central obesity, unlike Asian Indians[15]. They resembled Caucasians in these features. These findings were also confirmed in the UK Prospective Diabetes Study (UKPDS)[67]. Thus, variations in risk factors for diabetes are evident in different ethnic groups.

In several ethnic populations, including the relatively non-obese south Indian population, the android pattern of body fat, typified by more upper-body adiposity measured as waist:hip ratio (WHR) was found to be a greater risk factor for type 2 diabetes than general obesity. Similar observations on obesity have been made by Shelgikar et al.[76] from Maharashtra, India, who found that the WHR was significantly greater in subjects with IGT and diabetes compared with that in non-diabetic subjects of the same sex. A comparison of the WHR in non-diabetic Asian Indians and the Mexican–Americans showed that, although the former had a much lower BMI, they had a WHR comparable to that of the Mexican–Americans who were obese[77]. The risk conferred by increasing BMI and WHR were high in both populations when compared with the white population. Hyperinsulinaemia and adverse upper-body adiposity coexist in Mexican–Americans and Asian Indians, but the former population is generally obese whereas the latter is non-obese. It is likely that the presence of upper-body adiposity, in the absence of overall obesity, is an index of insulin resistance and the risk conferred by this could rise further if the rate of obesity increases in the Asian Indians. Table 18.5 shows a comparison of BMI and WHR in Asian Indians and Mexican–Americans.

Table 18.5. Comparison of age-adjusted BMI and WHR (mean ± SD) in Asian Indians and Mexican–Americans

	BMI		WHR	
	Asian Indians	Mexican–Americans	Asian Indians	Mexican–Americans
Men	21.9 ± 4.0	27.7 ± 4.3*	0.91 ± 0.07	0.92 ± 0.07
Women	22.3 ± 4.7	27.9 ± 6.2*	0.83 ± 0.09	0.82 ± 0.08

* $p < 0.001$.

A cluster of risk factors has been demonstrated to be associated with central obesity[78,79], including glucose intolerance, obesity, hyperinsulinaemia, hypertriglyceridaemia and hypertension; all are important risk factors for ischaemic heart disease. Recent studies comparing body fat topography in migrant Asians with that in Caucasians also found a higher WHR in migrant Asians despite comparable BMI values, and showed an association of WHR with hyperglycaemia, plasma insulin concentrations, blood lipids and coronary heart disease[15,67,80]. The WHR correlated with glucose intolerance in Mauritius Indians independent of the BMI[2]. There is no evidence, however, that the differences in body fat distribution can explain the higher prevalence of type 2 diabetes in migrant Asians compared with other races.

Recently, a population study conducted in urban south India showed that there was a high prevalence of the clustering cardiovascular risk factors, namely, central adiposity, obesity, hyperinsulinaemia, dyslipidaemia, hypertension and glucose intolerance in the adults aged 40 years or older[81]. Isolated prevalence of individual components was lower and combinations of one or more of them occurred more frequently (1.5–4 times) than expected by chance.

McKeigue et al.[80] reviewing the reports of coronary heart disease (CHD) in migrant Asian Indians, found that they had higher prevalence of CHD compared with indigenous populations in Fiji, the UK and Singapore. Conventional risk factors, such as cholesterol, cigarette smoking or hypertension, could not explain the higher prevalence of CHD in Indians, and it was suggested that the insulin resistance syndrome might have an important aetiological role for the same. Clustering of the components of insulin resistance was also demonstrated in the Mauritian population, including the Indian migrants[79].

IMPACT OF URBANIZATION

The wide urban–rural difference in the prevalence of type 2 diabetes in southern India provides strong evidence for the impact of urbanization on its prevalence[28]. The two populations studied belonged to the same ethnic group and differed only in the socioeconomic background and lifestyle. It was also interesting to note that the prevalence of IGT was similar (8.7% and

7.5% in urban and rural, respectively) in the two groups, despite a fourfold higher prevalence of diabetes in the urban areas (2.4% in rural and 8.2% in urban areas), probably indicating a common genetic basis for the disease. The favourable environmental conditions probably protected the rural population from diabetes. A study in Orissa state in India, and a multicentric study by the Indian Council of Medical Research, have also shown that the prevalence of diabetes is higher in urban areas compared with rural areas[82]. Urban–rural differences in the prevalence of type 2 diabetes have been evident in several countries (see Tables 18.1 and 18.3).

Epidemiological data from Mauritius, showing a remarkably similar prevalence of IGT and type 2 diabetes in Hindu Indians (12.4% and 16.2%), Muslim Indians (13.3% and 15.3%), Creoles (10.4% and 17.5%) and Chinese (11.9% and 16.6%) probably indicate that the genetic predisposition is high even in the Chinese population, who have low rates of diabetes in mainland China[7]. A similar situation is also evident in the Chinese migrants in Singapore[19]. With the change of lifestyle, environmental influences unmask diabetes in a large number of migrants. Effects of modernization are evident in Africans in America[83] and Mauritius[7]. Joffe and Seftel[6] have also reported that the urban black population of South Africa show escalating incidence of type 2 diabetes, with an age-adjusted prevalence approaching 7%[6]. This is higher than the prevalence in the white population. Similar reports have been published in urban South Africans[21], in Tunisia[84] and in Sudan[85].

A follow-up survey conducted in the Pacific Island population of Western Samoa, over a 13-year period (1978–1991) has been yet another example of dramatic change brought about by urbanization in the prevalence of type 2 diabetes[74]. One urban and two rural representative areas were studied; in the urban area (Apia), the prevalence increased from 8.1% to 9.5% in men and from 8.2% to 13.4% in women. In the rural Poutasi area, a dramatic increase from 0.1% to 5.3% was seen in men and only 5.4% to 5.6% in women. In the other rural area (Tuasivi), the increases were 2.3% to 7.0% in men and 4.4% to 7.5% in women. The rural areas now had access to goods and services that were previously available in the urban (area) only, which resulted in definite lifestyle changes in these areas. Therefore, the impact of urbanization on the prevalence of type 2 diabetes has been most marked in such rural areas.

WESTERNIZATION OF LIFESTYLE

The impact of Westernization or modernization on the prevalence of glucose intolerance has been apparent in several populations in developing countries, and also in migrant populations in developed countries. Examples have been the Nauruans, some Native Americans, Mexican–Americans, the multiethnic community in Mauritius and the Australian Aborigines[2]. Some of the

Native Americans and the Australian Aborigines have been hunter–gatherers and the other populations were mainly agriculturists. Even populations such as the Japanese and Chinese, who were previously believed to have been protected against type 2 diabetes, developed high rates of diabetes when they migrated to Westernized communities or adopted affluent lifestyles. As mentioned by Stern[86], the vast literature on the impact of Westernization on migrants from various developing countries demarcates the Caucasian populations as being relatively resistant to the diabetogenic impact of Westernization. The difference between the Caucasians and the Westernized migrants may be largely attributed to the genetic susceptibility of the latter for type 2 diabetes, because the environmental conditions are mostly similar.

Studies by O'Dea and colleagues[87-89] on the Australian Aborigines have elegantly demonstrated the impact of Westernization on the prevalence of obesity, diabetes and cardiovascular disease. The study of the aboriginal groups that continue to live in the traditional lifestyle had helped to yield information about their diet and lifestyle, and therefore analysis of the change that had caused the metabolic abnormalities. A temporary revision of the Westernization of Aborigines to the traditional style was also studied, providing information on the dietary composition, eating patterns, food preferences and physical activity level[89].

DIET

Lifestyle and food habits that have been advantageous for survival of human populations at the time when they were hunter–gatherers or agriculturists have given way to modernization, leading to more consumption of energy, refined carbohydrates and fats, and also the expenditure minimal physical activity. Thus, the energy balance has tilted towards conservation of energy as depot fat, which is rarely utilized. West[90] reported that the prevalence of diabetes was low in countries in which high-carbohydrate diets were consumed; these included most of the Afro-Asian countries[90]. A high-carbohydrate diet, as several studies have shown, produces high insulin sensitivity. However, this occurs mostly with complex carbohydrates and soluble food fibre. Changes in food habits have crept in with Westernization and changes in lifestyle. The hunter–gatherer had food sources from a wide variety of wild animals and uncultivated plant food and honey, yielding food rich in protein, vitamins and dietary fibre, low in sodium, but rich in potassium, magnesium and calcium[89]. It had complex carbohydrates and low fat, and low-energy density. The food procurement was an energy-intensive process. Seasonal fluctuations, and drought or flood, were frequent causes of food deprivation. Similar situations could have occurred in other hunter–gatherers such as the Pima Indians, and also among the peasant agricultural labourers of the Asian Indian communities. Food sources of agriculturists were from cultivated crops, mainly cereals and vegetables, and from meat and milk from domesticated animals. The 'thrifty genotype' may have operated to favour survival under conditions of food deprivation, which was common. Feasting at times of plenty with conversion of excess energy into depot fat would have facilitated their survival.

The Western diet, rich in energy and low in fibre, promotes weight gain and insulin resistance, even in the low-risk populations such as Caucasians. The mechanisms responsible for this might operate more strongly in the high-risk populations, who already have insulin resistance. Evidence from several epidemiological studies supports the hypothesis that the high-fat/low-carbohydrate diet prevalent in Westernized societies contributes to the excess obesity and type 2 diabets in those societies. In the San Luis Valley Diabetes Study, Marshall and coworkers[91] have clearly shown that fat consumption significantly predicts risks of type 2 diabetes in subjects with IGT after controlling for obesity, plasma glucose and insulin level. Both the quantity and the quality of food are important. Excess calorie consumption leads to obesity and, qualitatively, specific nutrients have an influence on fat disposition, glucose oxidation, insulin sensitivity and overall metabolic balance[10]. Flat[92] has shown that dietary interventions to produce sustained weight loss are most likely to be successful with limited fat intake, especially fat of the saturated type. Inclusion of refined carbohydrates, devoid of plant fibres, and use of liberal amounts of fats to improve the flavour and consistency of cooked food have been the consequences of modernization. The present decade has also seen remarkable changes in food habits, with a large proportion changing over to the fast food culture for convenience. Unhealthy nutritional habits, sedentary lifestyle and coping with the day-to-day stresses of life have been the prices paid for modernization or urbanization.

Excessive energy intake itself promotes insulin resistance in humans even before significant weight gains[93]. High-fat diets produce insulin resistance by increased fatty acid oxidation, by decreased suppression of hepatic glucose production and by decreased glucose disposal via insulin-mediated pathways.

SEDENTARY LIFESTYLE AND PHYSICAL ACTIVITY

Availability of food in plenty around the year and modern living conditions have led to a sedentary lifestyle in most urban areas. The sequelae of such 'modernization' are evident in the periurban population of south India studied recently (unpublished observations). Although most of the population are still engaged in manual labour, more amenities in the form of household gadgets, easy accessibility of water and day-to-day requirements have become available. The prevalence of diabetes in this population has doubled compared with that in the rural population, who are still living in the traditional style. As shown in Table 18.6, decreasing physical activity has been a major determinant of the rising prevalence of diabetes in the periurban population, compared with the urban and rural populations. It is likely that the effect of physical activity is most markedly seen in people in a transitional stage of lifestyle.

Bjorntorp et al.[94] showed that physically trained insulin-resistant obese subjects could decrease their plasma insulin levels by about 50%, without decreasing body fat. In the Mauritius study, it was noted that the physically active men had significantly lower serum insulin levels than the inactive men[7]. The importance of exercise-induced improvement of insulin sensitivity has great importance in both the management and the prevention of type 2 diabetes and also of coronary heart disease. Even in populations such as the Pima Indians, who have a high prevalence of diabetes and also a high genetic susceptibility, an association between obesity and physical activity is evident[95].

Several cross-sectional studies in the Pacific, Polynesian and Micronesian populations give strong support to an association between prevalence of type 2 diabetes and physical activity, because there was a lower prevalence of type 2 diabetes in physically active men. The association was independent of age, obesity and urban living[2]. The strong association of physical inactivity and diabetes was brought out well in our recent study of the periurban population of southern India. Similarly, O'Dea and colleagues had noted a strong association between the two parameters in Australian Aborigines[87–89]. These studies suggested that the impact of physical inactivity was manifested more markedly in populations who had been accustomed initially to heavy physical activity[87–89]. Recently Schultz and Weidensee[96] demonstrated the protective effect of physical activity in the Mixtec Indian men of Mexico, who had a genetic predisposition to diabetes. Among them, women who were sedentary had a higher prevalence of diabetes.

Studies in Caucasians[97] and Chinese[98] show that progression of IGT to diabetes can be prevented by increased physical activity, which may protect against development of type 2 diabetes both directly or through its effects on

Table 18.6. Influence of decreasing physical activity corrected for age, sex and BMI, on development of diabetes comparison in urban, periurban and rural south Indians.

	Rural		Periurban		Rural	
Physical activity	OR	*p*	OR	*p*	OR	*p*
Moderate	1.26	0.46	9.7	0.03	0.83	0.74
Light	1.03	0.94	9.5	0.03	0.63	0.58
Sedentary	1.03	0.92	18.6	0.007	2.17	0.27

OR, odds ratio.
Heavy used as standard.

obesity and fat metabolism. Figure 18.1 summarizes the impact of Westernization of societies. It shows the slow change over in the mechanisms that could have resulted in survival adaptation to adverse mechanisms that produce environmental maladaptation.

IMPAIRED GLUCOSE TOLERANCE

Impaired glucose tolerance was classified as an entity that was different from diabetes because long-term follow-up studies showed that a large proportion of people with IGT may remain as such or revert to normal tolerance. Moreover, the presence of microvascular complications such as retinopathy, a hallmark of diabets mellitus, was negligible in subjects with IGT[99].

The ratio of the prevalence of IGT/diabetes varies in different populations and is usually around 1. A study by Swai et al[24] in Tanzania showed a very high prevalence rate of 21.5% of IGT among the Indians there. The study

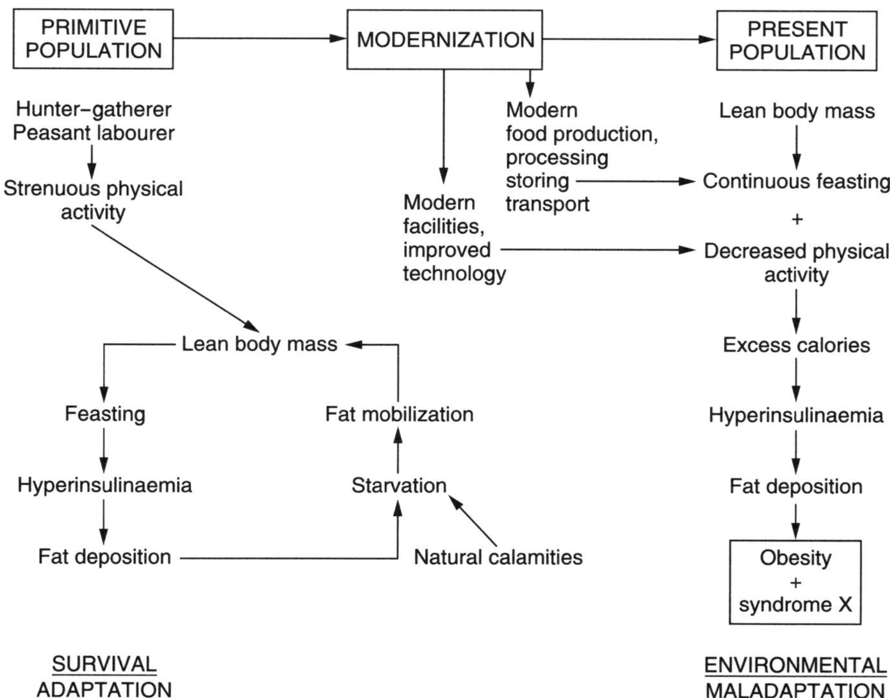

Figure 18.1. Impact of modernization.

from Mauritius also described a high prevalence of IGT in Indians and other ethnic groups, and this was believed to be a reflection of the recent type 2 diabetes epidemic[7].

An important observation made in the Madras survey of diabetes was that although the prevalence of diabetes was four times lower in the rural population, the prevalence of IGT was almost similar in both populations[28] (8.7% and 7.8% in the urban and rural areas, respectively). This observation of a high prevalence of IGT assumes great significance in view of our earlier observation that about 35% of the subjects with IGT become diabetic during a mean period of 5 years[100]. A similar observation has been made in several other populations[101]. Furthermore, it has also been shown that subjects with IGT carry a high cardiovascular risk. With increasing urbanization, there would be a higher conversion rate from IGT to diabetes and the prevalence of diabetes is expected to rise in the future. A high prevalence of IGT has been reported in all the recent epidemiological studies form various developing nations, such as India[3] (8.7%), Pakistan[31] (14.2% in women, 8.2% in men), Bangladesh[33] (15.7%), South Korea[34] (8.9%) and urban South Africa[21] (7%). Even in certain races, such as Africans in the Cameroons (urban and rural), where the prevalence of diabetes is still low (<1.6%), the prevalence of IGT appears to be increasing[102].

MAGNITUDE OF THE PROBLEM

According to the statistics currently available, the prevalence of diabetes is increasing in many developing countries[2-5,103]. Almost half the population in most of these countries are under 20 years old. The average life expectancy has improved considerably in India over the years[104], and similar trends are seen in other developing nations. We must, therefore, anticipate that there will be a huge increase in the number of people with diabetes.

Based on the increasing prevalence of type 2 diabetes seen in urban southern India[3,27,28], it is estimated that, by AD 2000, India is likely to have approximately 33 million people with diabetes (Table 18.7) (Figure 18.2). These figures are similar to the estimates projected by Zimmet[105]. By extra-

Table 18.7. Estimated burden of diabetes by AD 2000 in adult Indian $\geq$ 20 years

	1990	1995	2000
Prevalence (%) of type 2 diabetes			
Urban	8.2	11.6	14.7
Rural	2.4	2.4	2.4
Number			
Diabetic (millions)	22	28	33

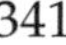

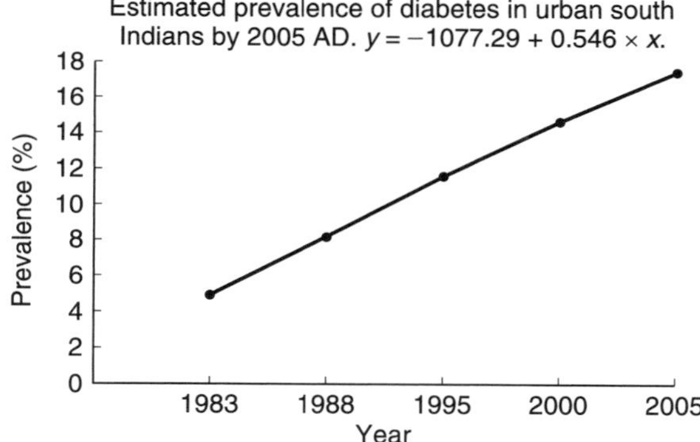

Figure 18.2 Estimated prevalence of diabetes in urban south Indians by AD 2005.

polation of the data available from our centre, it is estimated that the prevalence of type 2 diabetes in the adult urban population will be 17.4% by AD 2005

SCOPE FOR PREVENTION OF DIABETES

Primary prevention of type 2 diabetes is the urgent need of any nation, more so in the developing countries. There is evidence from many parts of the world that the prevention of type 2 diabetes is a reality[105–109]. Identification of high-risk individuals on the basis of their familial background of diabetes, and implementation of dietary modifications and physical activity with constant motivation and supervision, have shown encouraging results. A recent study from south India has shown that reduction in body weight by the above measures helps to prevent type 2 diabetes even in people who are not overweight[109] (Table 18.8). The studies in Asian Indians, Pima Indians, Nauruans, Australian Aborigines and Japanese and Americans[9] show that the major precipitating factor for development of diabetes has been a change in lifestyle as a result of modernization. It is also evident that weight loss,

Table 18.8. Effect of change in body weight on glucose tolerance

Body weight at follow-up	n	Diabetic[a] (%)	NGT[b] (%)
No change	69	7.2	37.7
Decreased	82	8.5	29.3
Increased	111	22.5	25.2

[a]Trend $\chi^2 = 9.4$; $p = 0.002$.
[b]$\chi^2 = 3.04$; $p = 0.08$
Period of follow-up 8 ± 4.2 years.

low-fat diet and increased physical activity will improve insulin sensitivity and, thereby, can be used as the means of achieving primary prevention of diabetes in the high-risk group. Recently, pharmacological interventions have also been tried in cases of IGT in China and the results have been encouraging[98].

Measures that help to prevent diabetes are beneficial in reducing the risk of other components of insulin resistance syndrome, namely, hypertension and hyperinsulinaemia. Therefore, primary prevention of diabetes should be the primary goal of the epidemiologists in the field.

REFERENCES

1. King H, Rewers M, on behalf of the WHO Ad Hoc Diabetes Reporting Group. Global estimates for prevalence of diabetes mellitus and impaired glucose tolerance in adults. *Diabetes Care* 1993; **16**:157–76.
2. Zimmet PZ. Challenges in diabetes epidemiology. From west to the rest. *Diabetes Care* 1992; **15**:232–52.
3. Ramachandran A, Snehalatha C, Latha E, Vijay V, Viswanathan M. Rising prevalence of NIDDM in urban population in India. *Diabetologia* 1997; **40**:232–7.
4. Valle T, Tuomilehto J, Eriksson J. Epidemiology of NIDDM in Europids. Alberti KGMM, Zimmet P, DeFronzo RA, Keen H (eds). In: *International Textbook of Diabetes Mellitus*, 2nd edn. 1997: 1–12.
5. Zimmet PZ. The Epidemiology of diabetes mellitus and related conditions. In: Alberti KGMM, Krall LP, eds. *The Diabetes Annual No. 6*. Amsterdam: Elsevier Science: 1991.
6. Joffle BI, Sefetel. Diabetes Mellitus the black communities of South Africa. *J Intern Med* 1994; **235**:137–42.
7. Dowse GK, Gareeboo H, Zimmet P, Alberti KGMM, Tuomilehto J, Fareed D. The high prevalence of non insulin dependent diabetes and impaired glucose tolerance in Indians, Creole and Chinese Mauritians. *Diabetes* 1990; **39**:390–6.
8. Ramachandran A, Snehalatha C. NIDDM in India and Indians: is it increasing? *IDF Bull* 1995; **40**:27–9.
9. Fujimoto WY. The growing prevalence of non insulin dependent diabetes in migrant Asian population and its implications for Asia. *Diab Res Clin Pract* 1991; **15**:167–84.
10. Ramaiya KL, Kodali VRR, Alberti KGMM. Epidemiology of diabetes in Asians of the Indian Sub continent. *Diabetes Metab Rev* 1990; **6**: 125–46.
11. Stern MP. Perspectives in diabetes – diabetes and cardiovascular disease. The 'Common Soil Hypothesis'. *Diabetes* 1995; **44**:369–74.
12. WHO Expert committee. *Diabetes Mellitus, 2nd Report. WHO Technical Report Series 646.* Geneva: WHO, 1980.
13. Mather HM, Keen H. The Southall diabetes survey: prevalence of known diabetes in Asians and Europeans. *BMJ* 1985; **291**:1081–4.
14. Simmons D, Williams DRR, Powell MJ. Prevalence of diabetes in a predominantly Asian community: preliminary findings of the Coventry diabetes study. *BMJ* 1989; **298**:18–21.

15. McKeigue PM, Pierpoint T, Ferrie JE, Marmot MG. Relationship of glucose intolerance and hyperinsulinaemia to body fat pattern in south Asians and Europeans. *Diabetologia* 1992; **35**:785–91.
16. Cassidy JT. Diabetes in Fiji. *NZ Med J* 1967; **66**:167–72.
17. Zimmet P, Taylor R, Ram P et al. Prevalence of diabetes and impaired glucose tolerance in the biracial (Melanesian and Indian) population of Fiji: a rural urban comparison. *Am J Epidemiol* 1983; **118**:673–88.
18. Thai Ac, Yeo PPB, Lun KC et al. Changing prevalence of diabetes in Singapore over a 10 year period. *J Med Assoc Thailand* 1987; **70**(suppl 2): 63–87.
19. Chea JS, Thai AC. Epidemiology of non insulin dependent diabetes mellitus (NIDDM). In: *ASEAN Proceedings of the 7th Congress of the ASEAN Federation of Endocrine Societies*, 1993; S641: 58.
20. Marine N, Vinik AI, Edelstein I, Jackson WPU. Diabetes, hyperglycaemia and glycosuria among Indians, Malays and Africans (Bantu) in Cape Town, South Africa. *Diabetes* 1969; **18**:840–57.
21. Omar MAK, Seedat MA, Dyer RB et al. South African Indians show high prevalence of NIDDM and bimodality in plasma glucose distribution patterns. *Diabetes Care* 1994; **17**:70–3.
22. Wright HB, Taylor B. The incidence of diabetes in a sample of the adult population in south Trinidad. *West Indian Med J* 1958; **7**:123–33.
23. Beckles GLA, Miller GJ, Kirkwood BR, Alexis SD, Carson DC, Byam NTA. High total and cardiovascular mortality in adults of Indian descent in Trinidad unexplained by major coronary risk factors. *Lancet* 1986; **i**:1298–300.
24. Swai ABM, McLarty D, Sherrif F et al. Diabetes and impaired glucose tolerance in an Asian community in Tanzania. *Diabetes Res Clin Pract* 1990; **8**:227–34.
25. Ahuja MMS, Sivaji L, Garg VK, Mitroo P. Prevalence of diabetes in northern Indian (Delhi area). *Horm Metab Res* 1974; **4**:321–4.
26. Gupta OP, Joshi MH, Dave SK. Prevalence of diabetes in India. *Adv Metab Dis* 1978; **9**:147–65.
27. Ramachandran A, Jali MV, Mohan V, Snehalatha C, Viswanathan M. High prevalence of diabetes in an urban population in South India. *BMJ* 1988; **297**:587–90.
28. Ramachandran A, Snehalatha C, Daisy Dharmaraj, Viswanathan M. Prevalence of glucose intolerance in Asian Indians: urban-rural difference and significance of upper body adiposity. *Diabetes Care* 1992; **15**:1348–55.
29. Fernando DJS, Siribaddana S, De Silva D. Impaired glucose tolerance and diabetes mellitus in a suburban Sri Lankan community. *Postgrad Med J* 1994; **70**:347–49.
30. Samarage SM. Some epidemiological aspects of non-insulin dependent diabetes mellitus in a defined population in the Kalutara district of Sr Lanka. Thesis of Doctor of Medicine, University of Colombo, June 1995.
31. Shera AS, Rafique G, Kwaja IA, Ara J, Baqai A, King H. Pakistan National Diabetes Survey: Prevalence of glucose intolerance and associated factors in Shikarpur, Sindh province. *Diabetic Med* 1995; **12**:1116–21.
32. Sayeed MA, Banu A, Khan AR, Hussain MZ. Prevalence of diabetes and hypertension in a rural population of Bangladesh. *Diabetes Care* 1995; **18**:555–8.
33. Sayeed MA, Hussain MZ, Banu A, Rumi MAK, Khan AKA. Prevalence of diabetes in a suburban population of Bangladesh. *Diabetes Res Clin Pract* 1997; **34**:149–55.

34. Park Y, Lee H, Koh CS, Min H, Yoo K, Kim Y, Shin Y. Prevalence of diabetes and IGT in Yonchon country, South Korea. *Diabetes Care* 1995; **18**:545–8.
35. Ke-An Wang et al. Chinese academy of preventive medicine-epidemiological characteristics of diabetes mellitus in China. *Diabetologia* 1997; **40** (suppl 1) (A193): 755.
36. Hitman GA, McCarthy MI, Mohan V, Viswanathan M. The genetics of non-insulin dependent diabetes mellitus in South India: An overview. Special section: Molecular genetics and genetic epidemiology of cardiovascular disease and diabetes. *Ann Med* 1992; **24**:491–7.
37. Simmons D, Williams DRR, Powell MJ. Prevalence of diabetes in different regional and religious south Asian communities in Coventry. *Diabetic Med* 1992; **9**:428–31.
38. Mohan V, Sharp PS, Aber V, Mather HM, Kohner EM. Family histories of Asian Indian and European NIDDM patients. *Pract Diabetes* 1986; **3**:254–6.
39. Viswanathan M, McCarthy MI, Snehalatha C, Hitman GA, Ramachandran A: Familial aggregation of Type 2 (non-insulin-dependent) diabetes mellitus in south India: absence of excess maternal transmission. *Diabetic Med* 1996; **13**:232–7.
40. Ramachandran A, Mohan V, Snehalatha C, Viswanathan M. Prevalence of non-insulin dependent diabetes mellitus in Asian Indian families with single diabetic parent. *Diabetes Res Clin Pract* 1988; **4**:241–5.
41. Steinberg AG. The genetics of diabetes: a review. *Ann NY Acad Sci* 1959; **82**:197–207.
42. Knowler WC, Bennett PH, Petit PJ, Savage PJ. Diabetes incidence in Pima Indians, contributions of obesity and parental diabetes. *Am J Epidemiol* 1981; **113**:115–6.
43. Haffner SM, Stern MP, Mitchel BD, Hazuda HP, Patterson JK. Incidence of type II diabetes in Mexican Americans predicted by fasting insulin and glucose levels obesity and body fat distribution. *Diabetes* 1990; **39**:283–8.
44. Alcolado JC, Alcolado R. Importance of maternal history of non-insulin dependent diabetic patients. *BMJ* 1991; **302**:1178–80.
45. Thomas F, Balkau B, Vauzelle-Kervroedan F, Papox L, The codiab–Inserm–Zeneca Study Group. Maternal effect and familial aggregation in NIDDM. The CODIAB Study. *Diabetes* 1994; **43**:63–7.
46. Dorner G, Mohnike A, Steindel E. On possible genetic and epigenetic modes of diabetes transmission. *Endokrinologie* 1975; **66**:225–7.
47. McCarthy MI, Cassell P, Tran T et al. Evaluation of the importance of maternal history of diabetes and of mitochondrial variation in the development of NIDDM. *Diabetic Med* 1996; **13**:420–8.
48. Young CA, Kumar S, Young MJ, Boulton AJM. Excess maternal history of diabetes in White Caucasian and Afro origin Type 2 diabetic patients suggests dominant maternal factors in disease transmission (Abstract). *Diabetic Med* 1994; **11**(suppl): p 121.
49. Mitchell BD, Valdez R, Hazuda HP, Haffner SM, Monterrosa A, Stern MP. Differences in the prevalence of diabetes and impaired glucose tolerance according to maternal or paternal history of diabetes. *Diabetes Care* 1993; **16**:1262–7.
50. Hazuda HP, Haffner SM, Stern MP, Eifler CW. Effects of acculturation and socio-economic status on obesity and diabetes in Mexican Americans: the San Antonio Heart Study. *Am J Epidemiol* 1988; **128**:1289–301.
51. Neel JV. Diabetes Mellitus: a 'thrifty' genotype rendered detrimental by 'progress'? *Am J Hum Genet* 1962; **14**:353–62.

52. Serjeantsen SW, Owerbach D, Zimmet P, Nerup J, Thomas K. Genetic of diabetes in Nauru: effects of foreign admixture, HLA antigens and the insulin genelinked polymorphism. *Diabetologia* 1983; 25:13–17.
53. Gardner LI, Stern MP, Haffner SM, Gaskill SP, Hazuda HP, Relethford JH. Prevalence of diabetes in Mexican Americans: relationship to percent of gene pool derived from native American sources. *Diabetes* 1984; **33**:86–92.
54. Mohan V, Ramachandran A, Viswanathan M. Tropical Diabetes. In: Alberti KGMM, Krall LP eds. *Diabetes Annual No. 2* Amsterdam: Elsevier Science Publishers, 1986, 30–8.
55. Mohan V, Ramachandran A, Snehalatha C, Rema Mohan, Bharani G, Viswanathan M. High prevalence of maturity onset diabetes of the young (MODY) among Indians. *Diabetes Care* 1985; **8**:371–4.
56. Ramachandran A, Mohan V, Snehalatha C et al. Clinical features of diabetes in the young as seen at a diabetes centre in south India. *Diab Res Clin Pract* 1988; **4**:117–25.
57. Barker DJ, Hales CN, Fall CH, Osmond C, Phipps K, Clark PM. Type 2 (non insulin dependent) diabetes mellitus, hypertension and hyper dyslipideamia syndrome X): relation to reduced foetal growth. *Diabetologia* 1993; **36**:62–7.
58. Lithell OH, McKeigue PM, Berglund L, Mohsen R, Lithell UB, Leon DA. Relation of size at birth to non-insulin dependent diabetes and insulin concentrations in men aged 50–60 years. *BMJ* 1996; **312**:406–10.
59. McCance DR, Pettitt DJ, Hanson RL, Jacobson LTH, Knowler WC, Bennett PH. Birth weight and non-insulin dependent diabets: thrifty genotype, thrifty phenotype or surviving small body genotype? *BMJ* 1994; **308**:942–5.
60. Yajnik CS, Fall CHD, Vaidya U et al. Fetal growth and glucose and insulin Metabolism in four-year-old Indian Children. *Diabetes Med* 1995; **12**:330–6.
61. DeFronzo RA, Bonadonna RC, Ferrannini E. Pathogenesis of NIDDM: a balanced overview. *Diabetes Care* 1992; **15**:318–68.
62. Snehalatha C, Ramachandran A, Vijay V, Viswanathan M. Differences in plasma insulin responses in urban and rural Indians: a study in southern Indians. *Diabetic Med* 1994; **11**:445–8.
63. Nabulsi AA, Folsom AR, Hesis G et al. Fasting hyperinsulinemia and cardiovascular risk factors in nondiabetic adults: stronger associations in lean versus obese subjects. *Metabolism* 1995; **44**:914–22.
64. Boyko EJ, Keane EM, Marshall JA, Hamman RF. Higher insulin and C-peptide concentrations in Hispanic population at high risk for NIDDM: San Luis Valley Diabetes Study. *Diabetes* 1991; **40**:509–15.
65. Aronoff SL, Bennett PH, Gorden P, Rushforth N, Miller M. Unexplained hyperinsulinemia in normal and 'prediabetic' Pima Indians compared with Caucasians: an example of racial differences in insulin secretion. *Diabetes* 1977; **26**:827–40.
66. Mohan V, Sharp PS, Cloke HR, Burrin JM, Schumer B, Kohner EM. Serum immunoreactive insulin responses to a glucose load in Asian Indian and European type 2 (non-insulin dependent) diabetic patient and control subjects. *Diabetologia* 1986; **29**:235–7.
67. UK Prospective Diabetes Study Group. UK Prospective Diabetes Study XII. Differences between Asian, Afro-Caribbean and White Caucasian type 2 diabetic patients at diagnosis of diabetes. *Diabetic Med* 1994; **11**:670–7.
68. Nagi DK, Jain SK, Mohammed Ali V, Yudkin JS, Walji S. Hyperinsulinemia in nondiabetic Asian subjects using specific assays for insulin, intact proinsulin, and Des 31,32-proinsulin. *Diabetes Care* 1996; **19**:39–42.

69. Omar MAK, Asmal AC. Insulin responses to oral glucose in young African and Indian non-insulin dependent diabets mellitus patients. *Natal Trop Geog Med* 1983; **35**:59–64.
70. Sharp PS, Mohan V, Levy JC, Mather HM, Kohner EM. Insulin resistance in patients of Asian Indians European origin with non-insulin dependent diabets. *Horm Metab Res* 1987; **19**:84–5.
71. Ramachandran A, Snehalatha C, Mohan V, Bhattarcharya PK, Viswanathan M. Decreased insulin sensitivity in offspring whose parents both have type 2 diabetes. *Diabetic Med* 1990; **7**:331–4.
72. Snehalatha C, Ramachandran A, Satyavani K, Vijay V, Haffner SM. Specific insulin and proinsulin concentration in non-diabetic South Indians. *Metabolism* 1998; **47**: 230–33.
73. Ramachandran A, Snehalatha C, Mohan V, Viswanathan M. Development of carbohydrate intolerance in offspring of Asian Indian conjugal type 2 diabetic parents. *Diab Res Clinic Pract* 1990; **8**:269–73.
74. Collins VR, Aloaina FL, Dowse GK, Spark RA, Toelupe AM, Zimmet PZ. Increasing prevalence of NIDDM in the pacific island population of Western Samoa over a 13 year period. *Diabetes Care* 1994: **17**:288–96.
75. Ahuja M. Vicissitudes of epidemiological studies of diabetes mellitus. *J All India Inst Med Sci* 1976; **2**:5–13.
76. Shelgikar KM, Jockaday TDR, Yajnik CS. Central rather than generalized obesity is related to hyperglycaemia in Asian Indian subjects. *Diabetic Med* 1991; **8**:712–17.
77. Ramachandran A, Snehalatha C, Vijay V, Viswanathan M. Haffner SM. Risk of NIDDM conferred by obesity and central adiposity in different ethnic groups – A comparative analysis between Asian Indians, Mexicans Americans and Whites. *Diab Res Clin Pract* 1997; **36**:121–5.
78. Defronzo RA, Ferrannini E. Insulin resistance: A multifaceted syndrome responsible for NIDDM, obesity, hypertension, dyslipidemia, and atheroslerotic cardiovascular disease, *Diabetes Care* 1991; **14**:173–94.
79. Zimmet PZ, Collins VR, Dowse GK et al. Is hyperinsulinaemia a central characteristic of a chronic cardiovascular risk factor clustering syndrome? Mixed findings in Asian Indian, Creole and Chinese Mauritians. *Diabetic Med* 1994; **11** 388–96.
80. McKeigue PM, Bela shah, Marmot MG. Relation of central obesity and insulin resistance with high diabetes prevalence and cardiovascular risk in South Asians, *Lancet* 1991; **337**:382–6.
81. Ramachandran A, Snehalatha C, Latha E, Satyavani K, Vijay V. Clustering of cardiovascular risk factors in urban Asian Indians. *Diabetes Care* 1998; **21**: 967–71.
82. Tripathy BB, Panda NC, Tej SC, Sahoo GN, Kar BK. Survey for detection of glycosuria, hyperglycemia and diabetes mellitus in urban and rural areas of Cuttack district. *J Assoc Physicians India* 1971; **19**:681–92.
83. Osei K, Schuster DP. Ethnic differences in secretion sensitivity, and hepatic extraction of insulin in Black and White Americans. *Diabetic Med* 1994; **11**: 755–62.
84. Papoz L, Ben Khalifa F, Eschwege E, Ban Ayed H. Diabetes mellitus in Tunisia: descriptions in urban and rural populations. *Int J Epidemiol* 1989; **17**:419–22.
85. Elbagir MN, Kadam IMS, Eltom MA, Berne C, Elmahadi EMA. A population-based study of the prevalence of diabetes and impaired glucose tolerance in Adults in Northern Sudan. *Diabetes Care* 1996; **19**:1126–8.

86. Stern MP. Primary prevention of type II diabetes mellitus. *Diabetes Care* 1991; **14**:399–410.
87. O'Dea K. Obesity and diabetes in 'the land of milk and honey'. *Diabetes Metab Rev* 1992; **8**:373–88.
88. O'Dea K. Westernisation, insulin resistance and diabetes in Australian aborigines. *Med J Aust* 1991; **155**:258–64.
89. O'Dea K. Marked improvement in carbohydrate and lipid metabolism in diabetic Australian aborigines after temporary reversion to traditional lifestyle. *Diabetes* 1984; **33**:596–603.
90. West KM. *Epidemiology of Diabetes and its Vascular Lesions*. New York: Elsevier, 1978: 1–10.
91. Marshall JA, Hoag, S, Shetterly S, Hamman RF. Dietary fat predicts conversion from impaired glucose tolerance to NIDDM. The San Luis Valley Diabetes Study. *Diabetes Care* 1994; **17**:50–6.
92. Flat JP. The biochemistry of energy expenditure. In Bray GA, ed. *Recent Advances in Obesity Research*: II Proceedings of the 2nd International Congress on Obesity (Westport, CT: Technomic Publishing) 1978; 211–28.
93. Bazelmans J, Nestel PJ, O'Dea K, Esler MD. Blunted norepinephrine responsiveness to changing energy states in obese subjects. *Metabolism* 1985; **34**: 154–60.
94. Bjorntorp P, De Jounge K, Sjostrom L, Sullivan L. The effect of physical training on insulin reduction in obesity. *Metabolism* 1970; **19**:631–8.
95. Kriska AM, La Porte RE, Pettitt DJ et al. The association of physical activity with obesity, fat distribution and glucose tolerance in Pima Indians. *Diabetolgia* 1993; **36**:863–9.
96. Schultz LO, Weidensee RC. Glucose tolerance and physical activity in a Mexican indigenous population. *Diabetes Care* 1995; **18**:1274–6.
97. Eriksson KF, Lindgarde F. Prevention of type 2 (non-insulin-dependent) diabetes mellitus by diet and physical exercise: the six-year Malmo feasibility study. *Diabetologia* 1991; **34**:891–8
98. Pan X, Li G, Hu Y, Bennett PH, Howard BV. Effect of dietary and/or exercise interventions on incidence of diabetes in subjects with IGT: the Da-Qing IGT and Diabetes Study. Abstract presented at the International Diabetes Federation Congress, Kobe, Japan, November 1994.
99. WHO Study Group. *Diabetes Mellitus Technical Report Series no. 727*. Geneva: World Health Organization, 1985.
100. Ramachandran A, Snehalatha C, Naik RAS, Mohan V, Shobana R, Viswanathan M. Significance of impaired glucose tolerance in an Asian Indian population: A follow up study. *Diab Res Clin Pract* 1986; 2:173–8.
101. Alberti KGMM. The clinical implications of impaired glucose tolerance. *Diabetic Med* 1996; 13:927–37.
102. Mbanya JCN, Ngogang J, Salah JN, Minkoulou E, Balkau B. Prevalence of NIDDM and impaired glucose tolerance in a rural and an urban population in Cameroon. *Diabetologia* 1997; **40**:824–9.
103. King H, Aubert RE, Herman WH. Global burden of diabetes 1995–2025. Prevalence, numerical estimates, and projection. *Diabetes Care* 1998, **21**: 1414–31.
104. Ministry of Health and Family Welfare. *Year book 1982–83. Family Welfare programme in India*. New Delhi Government of India, 1984, 1.
105. Zimmel P. Diabetes care and prevention: Around the world in 80 ways. *IDF Bull* 1991; **36**:29–32.

106. Knowler WC, Narayan KMV, Hanson RL et al. Preventing noninsulin dependent diabets. *Diabetes* 1995; **44**:483–8.
107. Zimmet P. Primary prevention of diabetes mellitus. *Diabetes Care* 1988; **112**:258–62.
108. Stern MP. Kelly West Lecture: Primary prevention of type II diabetes mellitus. *Diabetes Care* 1991; **41**:399–410.
109. Viswanathan M, Snehalatha C, Vijay V, Vidyavathi P, Indu J, Ramachandran A. Reduction in body weight helps to delay the onset of diabetes even in non obese with strong family history of the disease. *Diabetes Res Clin Pract* 1997; 35:107–12.

19

Genetic Counselling and Ethical Aspects

P. BEALES

Division of Medical and Molecular Genetics, Guy's Hospital, London SE1 9RT, UK

The key aim of the Human Genome Project, namely the sequencing of the complete human genome, is now in sight. The next step involving the identification of the 100 000 or so human genes is already under way. The project itself aims to advance knowledge about the human genome rather than to identify genetic disease. However, it is this latter function that forms the bulk of associated genome research. Clearly, the estimated 5000 single gene disorders mapped to date represent a small proportion of all genes. The next millennium will be concerned with the function of genes as well as their interactions with each other and the environment. Such findings will help us to understand how variations lead to susceptibility to common diseases. As more and more single and susceptibility genes are mapped, the pressure to utilize this information in medical practice becomes much greater. With this come many potential dangers that should be addressed before they overtake us in the ensuing commercial race. In this chapter, the bases of genetic counselling and screening are described, and some of the ethical issues surrounding them discussed.

GENETIC COUNSELLING: PRINCIPLES AND PRACTICE

Francis Galton, Charles Darwin's cousin, first described the concept and purpose of eugenics. He proposed the improvement of humanity by altering its genetic composition through the encouragement of breeding by those presumed to have desirable genes (positive eugenics) and the

Type 2 Diabetes: Prediction and Prevention. Edited by Graham A. Hitman

discouragement of breeding in those presumed to have undesirable genes (negative eugenics). The abuse of genetics by war-time Germany, and many despotic regimes since, has brought eugenics into disrepute. One of the functions of genetic counselling, on the other hand, serves to inform individuals and their families of the risks of carrying disease genes, thereby giving them the opportunity to exercise reproductive choice. The first genetic counselling clinics were opened in the USA, in Michigan in 1940. The first such clinic to open in the UK did so in 1946 at the Hospital for Sick Children in Great Ormond Street, London.

Kelly[1] provides a concise definition of genetic counselling: '... an educational process that seeks to assist affected and/or at risk individuals to understand the nature of the genetic disorder, its transmission and the options open to them in management and family planning'.

Genetic counselling requires accurate genetic knowledge, adequate time and the ability to communicate. The main components in imparting advice[2]

- A correct diagnosis
- The estimation of genetic risk (family history and pedigree construction)
- The provision of information about existence of risk and any options for avoiding it or managing it once the disease appears
- Accessibility for long-term contact (at-risk individuals may need genetic advice on several occasions in their lives).

The World Health Organization has stated that everyone who suspects a personal genetic risk of serious disease or malformation should have access to genetic counselling[2]. In the delivery of genetic counselling the autonomy of the consultand is paramount; he or she has the right to complete information and the utmost confidentiality must be maintained[3]. It is generally agreed that genetic counselling should be 'non-directive'. This implies that the consultand should be helped to reach his or her own decision based on the facts given and not coloured by the beliefs of the counsellor.

In general, recessive conditions carry less psychological side-effects when compared with dominantly X-linked inherited disorders[2]. This is because carriers either are unaware of their status or usually have little or no personal risk. Moreover, the overall risk to offspring depends on the carrier status of their partner. In contrast, a dominantly inherited disorder such as Huntington's disease presents many ethical and social problems that were not necessarily foreseen before the advent of presymptomatic testing. The main reasons for these arise because of the absence of effective treatment and the late onset of disease, often after reproductive choices have already been made. As a consequence, the uptake of presymptomatic testing has been low and is often requested only to assist in reproductive planning or for a perceived benefit to existing children[4].

Another highly contentious area is the testing of mentally handicapped individuals for fragile X syndrome. The psychological impact on carrier females is only just coming to light, where the reproductive risk is independent of the partner.

With the pace of technology, it is fast becoming apparent that specialist genetic centres alone cannot provide complete care for many conditions. In the next century, genetic counselling will need to be integrated into existing health services, including antenatal, family planning and primary care[2]. In many countries, this is already a reality and is a cost-effective method of delivery, provided that the health care worker is adequately trained and/or supported by specialist genetic councillors.

RISK ESTIMATION IN NON-MENDELIAN DISORDERS

Although genetic counselling for mendelian traits is no less complex than for non-mendelian traits, the estimation of risk is often more straightforward in the former. Mendelian risks are usually simple estimates based on the mode of inheritance (e.g. 50% risk to offspring in autosomal dominant conditions and 25% risk to offspring for carrier parents of an autosomal recessive gene), but can be modified by other factors. The relative or final risk can then be calculated using Bayes' theorem (a good account is given by Young[5]).

Multifactorial conditions are the result of a number of additive influences, some of which are polygenetic and others environmental. The mode of inheritance is not usually apparent but may be influenced by the degree of contribution of a major gene. The beginning of the next century will be marked by the identification of such susceptibility genes, in particular their relative contributions and interactions.

Multifactorial disorders differ from single gene disorders in a number of aspects, summarized in Table 19.1[6].

RISK ESTIMATION IN MULTIFACTORIAL DISORDERS

Several mathematical models to determine the risk to relatives of a given polygenic disorder have been formulated. Thankfully, the results of these models are largely similar and can be applied to conditions in which there are few existing risk data (Table 19.2). To calculate these recurrence risks one needs to know:

1. The frequency of the disorder
2. Some idea of the heritability
3. Types of affected relative, e.g. parents or siblings.

Table 19.1. Summary of fundamental differences between single gene and multifactorial disorders

1. Increased risk is greatest among closest relatives and decreases rapidly with distance of relationship
2. The risk of recurrence depends on the incidence of the disorder; A useful approximation when specific figures are not available is that the maximum risk to first-degree relatives is approximately the square-root of the incidence
3. As inheritance is non-mendelian, the risk for siblings is comparable to that for offspring
4. Where there is an unequal sex incidence, the risk is higher for relatives of a patient of the sex in which the condition is less common
5. The risk may be greater when the disorder is more severe; the greater severity reflects greater liability
6. The risk is increased when multiple family members are affected; this results from the concentration of genetic liability in the family and is in contrast to the mendelian situation where the number of affected members is irrelevant; the influence of more distant relatives is less easy to determine

Adapted from Harper[6]

Although there are many targeted common disorders such as asthma, obesity, schizophrenia and osteoporosis, three common, but complex diseases have been selected for further discussion: diabetes, coronary atherosclerosis and cancer.

DIABETES

The subdivision of diabetes mellitus into insulin-dependent (type 1) and non-insulin-dependent (type 2) forms, has clearly helped define the genetic aetiology. However, apart from the rare maturity-onset diabetes in the young (MODY) form which appears to follow autosomal dominant inherit-

Table 19.2. Recurrence risks (%) in multifactorial inheritance

		Affected parents								
		0 Affected sibs			1 Affected sibs			2 Affected sibs		
Population frequency (%)	Heritability (%)	0	1	2	0	1	2	0	1	2
1	80	1	6.5	14.2	8.3	18.5	27.8	40.9	46.6	51.6
	50	1	3.9	8.4	4.3	9.3	15.1	14.6	20.6	26.3
	20	1	2	3.3	2.0	3.3	4.8	3.7	5.3	7.1
0.1	80	0.1	2.5	8.2	2.9	9.8	17.9	31.7	37.4	42.4
	50	0.1	1.0	3.2	1.0	3.4	6.9	6.6	10.9	15.3
	20	0.1	0.3	0.7	0.3	0.7	1.3	0.8	1.4	2.3

After Harper[6]. Based on Smith[59]

ance, the inheritance of diabetes mellitus itself is not known[7]. Risk estimates have therefore been based on large numbers of observations (Table 19.3)[6,8]. There is considerable risk of perinatal mortality in children born to diabetic mothers. The rate appears to be related to the average blood glucose level during the third trimester. One study has shown that a mean glucose level of less than 5.5 mmol/l (< 100 mg/dl) was associated with a 3.8% perinatal mortality, compared with 23.6% when the mean glucose was more than 8.3 mmol/l (150 mg/dl)[9]. Couples also need to be counselled about the risk of congenital malformation. Again there is a direct relationship to the severity of diabetes with women who have type 1 diabetes being at greatest risk (five to six times) and those with gestational diabetics having virtually no excess risk compared with non-diabetics[10,11]. In contrast to perinatal mortality, poor control in the preconceptual period and early first trimester (4–7 weeks) confers the greatest risks[10]. The spectrum of malformation is wide ranging, affecting the skeletal system, central nervous system, and the renal and cardiovascular systems[10,12]. Table 19.4 lists some of the most commonly described malformations.

Counselling for patients with diabetes needs to begin well before pregnancy. In the same way as folic acid supplements must be taken before conception to alter the risk of neural tube defects, good glycaemic control needs to be implemented before conception and throughout the pregnancy[13]. Ideally, a team approach to care throughout pregnancy should be offered. Prenatal diagnosis of most structural defects can now be made by early and serial, detailed ultrasonography. Maternal serum α-fetoprotein (AFP) levels must be interpreted against specific tables adjusted for those with diabetes[14].

CORONARY ATHEROSCLEROSIS

Coronary atherosclerosis (CAD) has a multifactorial aetiology. The causative factors vary between individuals and families. The genetic contribution can be divided into two classes:

1. Familial hypercholesterolaemia (FH) which accounts for about 15% of CAD
2. Polygenic factors.

Familial aggregation has been noted for many years[15,16]. One population study compared CAD mortality in the first-degree relatives of 121 men and 96 women with premature CAD (deaths in men < 55 years, deaths in women < 65 years). Male relatives of male index cases had a five fold increase in mortality rate, compared with the general population, and a sevenfold increase in mortality if the index case was a woman[17]. Female relatives of male cases had a 2.5-fold increased risk compared with the general population risk (Table 19.5). Familial studies in a Finnish population

Table 19.3. Recurrence risk estimates in diabetes mellitus

Disease	General population risk	Sib of isolated case	Sib, no shared HLA haplotype	Sib, 2 or more shared HLA haplotypes	Sib and another first-degree relative affected	Offspring of isolated case	Monozygous co-twin affected
IDDM	1 in 500	1 in 14	1 in 100	1 in 6	1 in 6	1 in 25	1 in 3
NIDDM	1–5%	1 in 10	NA	NA	1 in 5	1 in 10	1 in 2

Based on Vadheim et al.[60].

Table 19.4. Some of the congenital malformations seen in children born to diabetic mothers

Caudal regression (sacral agenesis)
Situs inversus
Renal anomalies (agenesis, cystic dysplasia, duplication)
Neural tube defects (spina bifida, hydrocephalus, anencephaly)
Cardiovascular (transposition of great vessels, VSD, ASD)
Anal atresia

ASD, atrial septal defect; VSD, ventricular septal defect.

revealed a 3.5-fold risk for CAD in brothers of men with CAD and a twofold risk in their sisters. Furthermore, there were similarities between brothers in the type and severity of CAD within the family[18-20].

Heritability has been estimated as high as 0.67[21]. The concordance rates for monozygotic (MZ) and dizygotic (DZ) twins vary from study to study, with up to 66% for MZ and 25% for DZ in one Norwegian study[22]. As CAD is a composite phenotype, a reductionist approach to genetic aetiology has been pursued. Thus, investigation of the genetics of the underlying risk factors is now under way. The greatest of these is hyperlipidaemia which can be further divided into cholesterol, apolipoproteins (apo-B, apo-E) and lipid-related genes [Lp(a); LDL receptor and lipoprotein lipase, lecithin cholesterol acyltransferase][23]. Other genetic risk factors include hypertension (and the underlying genes involved), diabetes, obesity and genes affecting thrombogenesis, thrombolysis and fibrinolysis (e.g. elevated fibrinogen levels).

In counselling, the presence of premature coronary heart disease with hyperlipidaemia should always prompt screening in other family members. Familial combined hyperlipidaemia and FH should be excluded first of all. Gene inheritance is autosomal dominant with 50% risks to offspring and siblings. However, the risks of developing heart disease are less than 50%, particularly in females (Table 19.6)[24]. The gene frequency of FH is estimated at one in 500 but may be as high as one in 100 in some populations (Afrikaners)[25]. The disease is caused by mutations (> 200) in the low-density lipoprotein (LDL) receptor gene on 19p13.2–p13.12[26] and occasionally in the

Table 19.5. Mortality risks from CAD in relatives of patients with CAD

	First-degree relative	
	Male	Female
Male index case	1/12	1/36
Female index case	1/10	1/12

Table 19.6. Age-related risks of developing heart disease in familial hypercholesterolaemia

Age (years)	Men (%)	Women (%)
30	5	0
30–39	24	0
40–49	51	12
50–59	85	57
60–69	100	74

apo-B gene. As a result, both receptor-absent and receptor-defective mutants occur, leading to abnormalities of cholesterol internalization. Heterozygotes develop tendinous xanthomas, corneal arcus and coronary artery disease; the last usually becoming evident in the fourth or fifth decade. The rare homozygotes develop these features in childhood.

Until the relative contributions of susceptibility genes for CAD are worked out, only empirical risks for non-FH disease can be given to people seeking advice.

CANCER GENETICS AND COUNSELLING

Genetics has contributed enormously to our understanding of the pathogenesis, susceptibility and prognosis of many cancers. Although most cancers are sporadic, all of them result from genetic alterations in the normal control of cellular growth and proliferation. However, up to 10% of cancers are familial as a consequence of germline mutations. There are two categories of cancer-related gene: tumour suppressors and oncogenes. As a general rule, tumour-suppressor genes behave in a recessive manner in as far as both alleles need to be inactivated to deem the cell cancerous (Knudson's 'two-hit' hypothesis). In contrast, oncogenes act dominantly at the cellular level, with only one allele mutation being required for cell transformation. Familial cancer predisposition is usually inherited in an autosomal dominant manner and is caused by mutations in tumour-suppressor genes; however, most familial cancers have reduced penetrance which is probably a reflection of the need for other environmental or genetic influences. Over 100 such genes have been mapped with some 20–30 hereditary disorder genes cloned[27]. Some of the most studied cancer genes are listed in Table 19.7.

How can this knowledge be utilized effectively? In the case of breast cancer, for example, the overall female population risk in the UK is one in 12 (one in nine in the USA) and accounts for some 30% of all cancers in women. However, 5–10% of breast cancers are inherited, with approximately 45% of these being attributed to the *BRCA-1* gene and 35% to the *BRCA-2* gene. As a consequence, there is a two- to threefold increase in risk of breast

Table 19.7. Well-characterized cancer genes

Gene	Disease
RB1 (13q14)	Retinoblastoma
Mismatch repair genes (*MSH2* (2p16), *MLH1* (3p21), *PMS1* (2q32), *PMS2* (7p22)	Hereditary non-polyposis colorectal cancer (HNPCC), endometrial cancer, stomach cancer
APC (5q21)	Familial adenomatous polyposis (FAP)
TP53 (17p13.1)	Breast cancer, sarcoma, brain tumour (Li–Fraumeni syndrome)
RET (10q11)	Medullary thyroid cancer, phaeochromocytoma (MEN type 2)
BRCA-1 (17q21)	Breast, ovarian, prostate, colon cancer
BRCA-2 (13q12-13)	Breast (males as well), ovarian, pancreas, prostate cancer
P16 (9p21)	Melanoma, pancreas, oesophagus, bladder cancer

cancer among first-degree relatives of patients with premenopausal breast cancer, especially if the patient is young (< 35 years). In those families identified as being at high risk (first-degree relative with breast cancer aged < 50 years or a relative with bilateral breast cancer), predictive testing for *BRCA-1* is now becoming a viable option[28]. If a woman carries a mutation in *BRCA-1* or *BRCA-2*, then the risk of developing breast cancer by the age of 70 years is 85% (65% in the contralateral breast)[29,30]. There are also additional lifetime risks of developing ovarian cancer (40–60% for *BRCA-1*; 10–15% for *BRCA-2*), breast cancer in men (5–10% with *BRCA-2*), prostate cancer (threefold risk with *BRCA-1*) and colon cancer (fourfold risk for either sex)[31]. Genetic counselling is complicated by the technical difficulties encountered in detection of the vast number of mutations in *BRCA-1* that have already been described (> 200)[32]. Once identified, such at-risk people need to be entered into an approved surveillance programme. The screening options available for high-risk women are mammography, but this is controversial in the young, or measurement of CA125 (ovarian tumour marker). Preventive options include prophylactic bilateral mastectomy (subcutaneous/total) and/or oophorectomy. The efficacy of surgical operation and technique has yet to be evaluated and there is still a risk (albeit reduced) of cancer arising in any remaining tissue. Most advocates agree that removal of over 95% of tissue will drastically reduce the risk. Nevertheless, many women have already had preventive mastectomy and many more have contemplated it. One study has shown that of 100 women undergoing subcutaneous mastectomy, none developed cancer over a mean follow-up period of 5 years[33]. A second study followed 1500 women who had subcutaneous mastectomy for 22 years, and only one developed breast cancer[34]. This is in contrast to a third study of 1500 women followed for 9 years of whom six developed cancer[35].

SCREENING

We must distinguish between genetic and non-genetic screening as there are fundamental differences. Non-genetic screening programmes usually benefit the individual, for example screening for breast and cervical cancer, hypertension or diabetes. In contrast, there may be little direct benefit to an individual in knowing his or her carrier status; the main benefits are usually to the subsequent generations by providing reproductive choice.

The vast majority of existing genetic screening programmes are connected with autosomal recessive conditions. Autosomal recessive genes are common in the population but are of course largely silent in the heterozygous state. However, in certain populations the gene frequency is particularly high and thus the incidence of disease in homozygotes is significant (e.g. β-thalassaemia in the Mediterranean region and sickle-cell disease in west Africa). Population screening would at first appear to be a beneficial course of action but could actually do more harm than good if not properly implemented[36].

Screening serves to determine which people within a defined population may be more susceptible to a particular disorder than the screened population. Once identified, these individuals can then undergo detailed diagnostic investigation and treatment. For example, in Down's syndrome screening, the defined population consists of pregnant women of 35 years plus. A test is applied (such as nuchal translucency) which, if found to be above a predetermined threshold, suggests that there is a higher risk of Down's syndrome (or other trisomies) relative to the general population; in this case pregnant women less than 35 years old[37,38]. Further investigations may be offered, such as amniocentesis, in which a diagnosis is sought and a course of action then decided upon.

It is important to design a screening programme carefully or it will be worthless. The ideal screening test must be:

- simple to administer and perform
- safe
- ethically, culturally and socially acceptable
- repeatable
- both sensitive and specific with a high predictive value (see below)
- cost-effective.

For the screening programme to be successful, the target disease must:

- be common, severe or both
- be an important health concern to the community
- have a defined natural history
- be readily diagnosed
- have a known prevalence and incidence
- be preventable
- in the case of genetic disorders, provide acceptable reproductive choice (identification of carriers).

The effectiveness of a screening test can be measured by two parameters: its 'specificity' and its 'sensitivity'. The specificity is the proportion of unaffected people who have a negative result on screening. In other words, it is the proportion of true negative screening tests to negative diagnostic tests.

On the other hand, sensitivity is the proportion of affected people with a positive result on screening, i.e. it is the proportion of true positive screening tests to positive diagnostic tests. This provides the detection rate of the programme.

Of those with a positive screening test, the proportion who really have the disease gives the test its 'predictive value' (or the proportion of true positive screening tests to all positive screening tests). The predictive value will be high if screening is applied to a small high-risk population with a high disease prevalence, rather than to a broad population with low disease prevalence. However, screening specificity and sensitivity remain the same regardless of the prevalence. Moreover, sensitivity may be reduced by genetic heterogeneity in that a single test does not pick up all or most of the mutations.

The most successful screening programmes target the high-risk subpopulation and have a high uptake of the test. The greatest compliance appears to be by those people who already have an affected family member.

In Cypriots, the carrier rate of β-thalassaemia is 17% and in Cyprus itself the health costs of treating homozygotes were previously enormous. In fact, the Greek–Cypriot Orthodox church now encourages couples to be tested for carrier status before marriage, and this has subsequently had a profound effect in reducing the disease incidence by 95%[39]. The first screening programme for Tay-Sachs disease was instituted in 1971 in California, using an outreach approach in the high-risk Jewish community[40]. By 1986, the programme had extended to over 50 US cities and 350 000 individuals had been screened. As a consequence, the incidence of Tay–Sachs disease fell by 70–85%. The greatest uptake was in at-risk adolescents offered screening in school and demonstrates that testing of at-risk people well before they are likely to reproduce can be effective[41].

Many more difficulties lie ahead with more complex diseases such as breast cancer. The issues surrounding family and personal risk of developing this common cancer have already been discussed. The national breast screening programme has been implemented to identify those at general risk (one in 12) of breast cancer and is available only to those over 50 years of age. As more information becomes available, we must provide means of identifying those at higher than population risk. Family history is one identifiable risk; however, this depends on another family member presenting with the disease. At present there is no easy or reliable screening test for the *BRCA* genes. Recently, one group has been shown to be at increased risk of disease as a result of higher gene mutation frequency. One per cent of Ashkenazi Jews have been shown to carry one of three *BRCA-1* mutations: 185delAG, 188del11 or 5382insC[42,43]. Furthermore, 1% carry 6174delT in *BRCA-2*[44]. This is a population that perhaps warrants a separate screening protocol.

DIFFERENT TYPES OF GENETIC SCREENING

Medical screening can loosely be categorized into three groups: screening to provide reproductive choice, postnatal screening and population screening of adults. Reproductive choice is most commonly sought in rare familial conditions in which there is no available disease management. Larger screening programmes that offer limited reproductive choice have already been discussed (Down's syndrome and neural tube defects).

Postnatal screening is now established in most developed countries and in the UK is typically presented in the form of blood droplets applied to a card and then allowed to dry. This is administered to every newborn after milk feeds have begun in the first week of life. The screening tests are essentially biochemical and are primarily aimed at picking up phenylketonuria (Guthrie test) and hypothyroidism, but other conditions such as galactosaemia, maple syrup urine disease and homocystinuria may also be identified. The success of this screening programme lies in its simplicity and cheapness and, furthermore, each disorder fulfils the criteria set out above.

There are many examples of adult population screening programmes, most of which are non-genetic. However, a large proportion do have a genetic component: diabetes, coronary heart disease and cancer. Moreover, the current testing of these conditions is based on measurement of a biochemical or physical marker, and is largely diagnostic rather than predictive.

Predictive testing is not always beneficial. Since the cloning in 1993 of the Huntington's disease gene and the subsequent development of a definitive test, relatively few at-risk individuals have taken it up[4]. This is because a positive result gives information about the inevitable decline in health at a time when the individual may still be in perfect health.

Greenberg distinguishes 'necessary' genes from 'susceptibility' genes[45]. The presence of susceptibility genes increases one's risk of developing disease but is not necessary for disease expression. Such examples include HLA genes in autoimmune-based disease, which influence disease development but are not always present. The main determining factor may not even be genetic, but environmental (e.g. chemical/viral).

The unravelling of the genetics of type 1 and type 2 diabetes has been slow, but the potential to screen a population for genetic susceptibility to diabetes will soon become reality. It is recognized that the major histocompatibility complex contains multiple susceptibility loci (referred to collectively as *IDDM1*), including the class II antigen receptor genes. However, the MHC genes, and a second locus, the insulin gene minisatellite on chromosome 11p15 (*IDDM2*), cannot account for all of the observed clustering of disease in families. There are four additional loci; *IDDM4* (FGF3/11q13), *IDDM5* (ESR/6q22), *IDDM8* (D6S281/6q27) and *IDDM12* (CTLA-4/2q33). Seven other named loci remain to be investigated more thoroughly[46]

ETHICAL ISSUES IN SCREENING FOR GENETIC SUSCEPTIBILITY

It has been suggested that the elucidation of polygenes in multifactorial disorders may lead to a shift in health care, allowing people at risk of disease to be identified. Health benefits will then arise out of the subsequent change in lifestyle in those at risk, providing they are sufficiently motivated[47]. This is an optimistic view and quite possibly the converse may take place with at-risk persons adopting high-risk lifestyles in view of the inevitability of disease. Lipmann has coined the term 'geneticization' to describe the focus on genetic differences between people[48]. Such overemphasis on genetic factors in the aetiology of disease will not only be expensive but also exaggerate personal responsibility for health at the risk of removing collective social and political responsibility.

There is interest, primarily from the private sector, in developing individualized testing systems to identify those at high risk of polygenic disease. There is a great danger that commercial pressures will lead to their hasty introduction before a thorough evaluation has been carried out. Furthermore, these tests may not be available to those who cannot pay, leading to gross inequalities in health access. Conversely, those who cannot pay may actually be better off if the tests are poorly evaluated or offered without counselling. Previous screening programmes for hyperlipidaemia and hypertension have indicated that knowledge of one's own susceptibility can lead to serious psychological problems[49,50]. It is unlikely that rescue counselling and support will be provided by private endeavours. It has been shown that some of these problems can be alleviated or minimized by pre-counselling (as in Huntington's disease), but who will provide this expensive service?

For many common diseases, there may be no public health benefit in screening the general population for genetic susceptibility to them. It is more likely that at-risk families will be targeted based on history, but, nevertheless, screening can be justified only after careful evaluation and demonstration of clear benefits[51]. In addition, there must be an acceptable treatment or preventive management strategy available. If the latter preventive measures involve a general alteration in lifestyle, then this is also likely to apply to everyone in the population, so individualized screening will be expensive and pointless[52-55]. Evaluation research must be carried out to determine the outcome of being labelled low-risk, because detrimental changes in lifestyle may also arise from this knowledge[56].

Additional research needs to be conducted into the psychological, social and behavioural consequences of the screening programme once implemented.

CONSENT AND CONFIDENTIALITY

Those being screened are entitled to receive clear information about the tests involved; they must be made aware of the associated risks, and they must give sufficient time to decide whether to take part and be made aware that they are free to withdraw at any time. The kinds of information required for genetic screening include a knowledge of the condition and its seriousness, the way it is transmitted, reliability of the tests, the procedure for informing about the results and the implications of a positive result. There are special safeguards to cover cases where informed consent is not possible (minors and mentally ill). The issues of confidentiality and disclosure need to be addressed closely, because the individuals being screened may not wish other members of their own families to know of their involvement or outcome even though the result may have a direct bearing on other family members. The main concern lies in situations where non-disclosure may be potentially harmful to other family members. The importance of confidentiality and privacy is set down in Article 8(1) of the European Convention on Human Rights and, in addition to the common law duty not to disclose information, there is also statutory protection (in the UK) in the Data Protection Act 1984, which applies to genetic information stored on computer. Furthermore, professional codes of conduct also serve to protect individuals. Although it is agreed that these accepted standards should be followed as far as possible, there may be exceptional circumstances warranting disclosure (for example, rare cases of malice). The courts recognize that this may also be necessary if disclosure is in the public's interest. Primary responsibility for communicating significant information to other family members should lie with the individual tested and not with the doctor[57]. There is no duty acknowledged by law in the UK that requires health care professionals to disclose information against an individual's wishes. Not uncommonly, evidence of non-paternity can arise out of genetic testing and this in itself poses further ethnical dilemmas for which there is no easy answer.

OWNERSHIP OF DNA

There is a potentially explosive minefield surrounding the issue of exactly who owns a person's DNA once consent has been given for extraction and testing of a sample (usually in the research setting). Once meaningful results have been obtained, the individual then has a right to know (and not to know) the results. Who is responsible for handling this information and imparting it? What arrangements should be made to cope with the aftermath? Storage of DNA for further anonymous testing in genetic research to improve our understanding of disease needs to have consent given at the time of sampling. Assurances on security should also be given.

GENETIC DISCRIMINATION AND MISUSE OF GENETIC INFORMATION

In the UK, the control of genetic/medical information has to a limited extent been legislated for, or guidelines have been drawn up to protect individuals. Nevertheless, the onus to disclose personal information has been placed on many individuals by employers or insurance companies. The potential for abuse of genetic information, especially knowledge of susceptibility to a common disease, is open to the creation of a 'genetic underclass'. Such practice is to be discouraged and in the USA some states have legislated against use of genetic information in setting insurance premiums. In Britain, in 1995, the House of Commons Science and Technology Committee (Human Genetics: the Science and its Consequences) recommended that the insurance industry propose an acceptable (to Parliament) solution to this issue. In 1997, the Association of British Insurers published a policy statement under the section 'Seeking and Use of Genetic Test Results; and stated that:

> In the insurance context, a genetic test is one which is regarded as predictive in an asymptomatic individual

> They go on to say

> The life insurance members (of the ABI) will not ask people to take genetic tests when applying for life insurance.

They also go on to stipulate that for life insurance linked to a new mortgage up to a value of £100 000, the results of any genetic tests already conducted will not be taken into account if it is to the 'detriment of the applicant'. For new applications for other life insurance policies, individual companies will decide for themselves whether to utilize genetic information. New applicants will still be required to report the results of any genetic tests undertaken. With the advent of susceptibility screening programmes for multifactorial diseases, there will undoubtedly be a pressure to alter this voluntary code to take account of the perceived larger-risk population.

Despite theoretically sound arguments that individuals seeking employment in which they may have a genetic susceptibility to develop a work-related illness should be tested, in practice there is no employer in the UK, except for the armed forces, that makes this a requirement. The armed forces require sickle-cell testing for those applying in areas involving exposure to low-oxygen tensions.

STIGMATIZATION AS A RESULT OF GENETIC SCREENING

One example of stigmatization as a consequence of genetic testing was seen at the introduction of sickle-cell screening in the USA during the 1970s. Some carriers experienced discrimination at work and from insurance companies. We must be aware of such possibilities in implementing new screening programmes. To reduce these dangers, education of the test and general population should be a prerequisite.

TESTING OF CHILDREN

Predictive genetic testing of children is clearly appropriate where onset of the condition regularly occurs in childhood or there are useful medical interventions to be offered (Report of Working Party of CGS 1994). Predictive testing for an adult-onset disorder should not be undertaken if the child is healthy and there are no medical interventions that can be offered in the event of a positive test result. It is preferable for the ground to be laid in adolescence and the 'child' given the opportunity to seek testing for him- or herself on reaching an age suitable for making an autonomous decision, and when the social and emotional conditions are right.

The labelling of children at a young age has potential psychological repercussions on subsequent parental interactions[58].

A more delicate issue is the testing of children for carrier status for either a recessive disorder or balanced chromosomal rearrangements. Again testing should be deferred if the only outcome will be to determine any reproductive significance. Wherever testing is being contemplated in childhood, the circumstances should be fully discussed by parents, geneticists and other relevant professionals. For childhood-onset cancers, such as retinoblastoma and Li–Fraumeni syndrome, testing of at-risk children might be appropriate to prevent or increase surveillance for cancer.

CONCLUDING REMARKS

The pace at which molecular and cellular biology is moving is clearly shifting the emphasis from monogenic disorders to polygenic and multifactorial disease research. However, the complexity of inheritance in multifactorial disease hinders the ability to calculate risks and recurrence risks of disease. Based on empirical data, we are able to make estimates of risk in most common disorders, but these are still quite crude. The careful characterization of many diseases such as diabetes and coronary artery disease has resulted in their genetic and environmental dissection. Such reductionism helps to determine the relative contribution of each component, thereby building up a picture of relative risks. Soon, we shall be able to screen at-risk individuals for their susceptibility to a given disease by performing a set of tests and combining the results to aid in genetic counselling.

Who we should test and when are questions currently without answers for many diseases. As more diseases are unravelled, new ethical issues arise over whether it is of benefit to screen for them. Is it cost-effective? Are there any acceptable interventions available? Is it harmful to know of one's own high risk? How will society treat high-risk individuals? How will low-risk individuals behave? Should children be included in screening? There are many more questions than there are answers at present, and it is of paramount importance that we avoid the commercial pressure to implement screening tests before they are fully evaluated. In the same way as drug development in the pharmaceutical industry is subject to rigorous evaluation, it has been proposed that a central body oversee the development of screening tests[57].

ACKNOWLEDGEMENTS

I am grateful to Frances Flinter and Elizabeth Manners for their valuable comments on the manuscript.

FURTHER READING

Report of the Genetics Research Advisory Group: A second report to the NHS central research and development committee on the new genetics. Department of Health 1995.

REFERENCES

1. Kelly T. *Clinical Genetics and Genetic Counselling*. Chicago: Year Book, 1986.
2. World Health Organization. *Control of Hereditary Diseases: report of a WHO Scientific Group*. Geneva: WHO, 1996.
3. Fletcher J, Berg K, Tranoy K. Ethical Aspects of Medical Genetics. A proposal for guidelines in genetic counselling, prenatal diagnosis and screening. *Clin Genet* 1985; **27**:199–205.
4. Craufurd D, Dodge A, Kerzin-Storrar L, Harris R. Uptake of presymptomatic predictive testing for Huntington's disease. *Lancet* 1989; **ii**(8663):603–5.
5. Young ID. *Introduction to Risk Calculation in Genetic Counselling*. Oxford: Oxford University Press, 1991.
6. Harper PS. *Practical Genetic Counselling*. 4th edn 1993. Oxford: Butterworth-Heinemann, 1993.
7. Tattersall RB. Mild familial diabetes with dominant inheritance. *Q J Med*, 1974; **43**:339–57.
8. Vadheim CM, Rimoin DL, Rotter J. Diabetes mellitus. In: Emery AEH, Rimoin DL, eds, *Principles and Practice of Medical Genetics* 1990, Edinburgh: Churchill Livingstone, 1990: 1521–58.
9. Karlsson K, Kjellmer I. The outcome of diabetic pregnancies in relation to the mother's blood sugar level. *Am J Obstet Gynecol* 1972; **112**:213–20.
10. Mills JL, Baker L, Goldman AS. Malformations in infants of diabetic mothers occur before the seventh gestational week. *Diabetes* 1979; **28** 292–3.
11. Mills JL. Malformations in infants of diabetic mothers. *Teratology* 1982; **25**: 385–94.
12. Neave C. Congenital malformations in offspring of diabetics. *Perspect Pediatr Pathol* 1984; **8**:213–22.
13. Hansen U, Persson B, Thunell S. Relationship between hemoglobin A_{1C} in early type 1 (insulin dependent) diabetic pregnancy and the occurrence of spontaneous abortion and fetal malformation in Sweden. *Diabetologia* 1990; **33**:100–4.
14. Reece AE, Davis N, Mahoney NJ, Baumgasten A. Maternal serum alpha-fetoprotein in diabetic pregnancy: correlation with blood glucose control. *Lancet* 1987; **ii**:275.
15. Osler W. *Lectures on Angina Pectoris and Allied States*. New York: D Appleton & Co., 1897.
16. Fogge CH. General xanthelasma and vitilogoidea. *Trans Pathol Soc Lond* 1972; **24**:242.
17. Slack J, Evans KA. The increased risk of death in first degree relatives of 121 men and 96 women with ischaemic heart disease. *J Med Genet* 1966; **3**:239–57.
18. Rissanen AM, Nikkila EA. Coronary heart disease and its risk factors in families of young men with angina pectoris and in controls. *Br Heart J* 1977; **39**:875–83.
19. Rissanen AM. Familial occurrence of coronary heart disease: effect of age at diagnosis. *Am J Cardiol* 1979; **44**:60–6.
20. Rissanen AM. Familial aggregation of coronary heart disease in a high incidence area (North Karelia, Finland). *Br Heart J* 1979; **42**:294–303.
21. Nora JJ, Lortscer RH, Spangler RD, Nora AH, Kimberlig WJ. Genetic–epidemiologic study of early-onset ischemic heart disease. *Circulation* 1980; **61**:603–8.
22. Berg K. *Genetics of coronary heart disease*. In: *Progress in Medical Genetics* (Philadelphia: WB Saunders) 1983: 35–90.
23. Rotter J, Vadheim CM, Rimoin DL. Diabetes mellitus. In: *The Genetic Basis of Common Diseases*, R. A. King, J. Rotter, and A.G. Motulsky (Eds.) Oxford University Press: Oxford, 1992; 413–481.

24. Slack J. Risks of ischaemic heart disease in familial hyperlipoproteinaemic states. *Lancet* 1969; **i**:1380–2.
25. Goldstein JL, Brown MS. Familial hypercholesterolemia: In: *Metabolic Basis of Inherited Diseases*. New York: McGraw-Hill. 1989; 1215–45.
26. Hobbs HH, Brown MS, Goldstein JL. Molecular genetics of the LDL receptor gene in familial hypercholesterolemia. *Hum Mutat* 1992; **1**:445–66.
27. Murphy PD, Bray W. How cancer gene testing can benefit patients. *Mol Med Today* 1997; **3**:147–52.
28. Gayther SA, Ponder BA. Mutations of the BRCA1 and BRCA2 genes and the possibilities for predictive testing. *Mol Med Today* 1997; **3**:168–74.
29. Easton DF, Bishop DT, Ford D, Crockford GP. Genetic linkage analysis in familial breast and ovarian cancer: results from 214 families. The Breast Cancer Linkage Consortium. *Am J Hum Genet* 1993; **52**:678–701.
30. Wooster R, Neuhausen SL, Mangion et al. Localization of a breast cancer susceptibility gene, BRCA2, to chromosome 13q12-13. *Science* 1994; **265**(5181): 2088–90.
31. Couch FJ, Farid LM, Deshano et al. BRCA2 germline mutations in male breast cancer cases and breast cancer families. *Nature Genet* 1996; **13**:123–5.
32. Robledo M, Osorio A, Sentis C, Alberto J, Estevez L, Benitez J. The 12-base-pair duplication/insertion alteration could be a regulatory mutation. *J Med Genet* 1997; **34**:592–3.
33. Jarrett JR. Prophylactic mastectomy. In March JL, ed. *Current Therapy in Plastic and Reconstructive Surgery*. 1989; Toronto: BC Decker. 1989: 64.
34. Fisher J, Maxwell GP, Woods J. Surgical alternatives in subcutaneous mastectomy reconstruction. *Clin Plastic Surg*, 1988; **15**:667–76.
35. Pennisi VR, Capozzi A. Subcutaneous mastectomy data: a final statistical analysis of 1500 patients. *Aesthetic Plastic Surg*, 1989; **13**:15–21.
36. Mant D, Fowler G. Mass screening: theory and ethics. *BMJ* 1990; **300**(6729): 916–8.
37. Nicolaides KH, Brizot ML, Snijders RJ. Fetal muchal translucency: ultrasound screening for fetal trisomy in the first trimester of pregnancy [see comments.] *B J Obstet Gynaecol* 1994; **1001**:782–6.
38. Pandya PP, Brizot ML, Kuhn P, Snijders RT, Nicolaides KH. First-trimester fetal nuchal translucency thickness and risk for trisomies. *Obstet Gynecol* 1994; **84**:420–3.
39. Angastimotos M, Hadjiminas M. Prevention of thalassaemia in Cyprus. *Lancet* 1981; **i**:369–70.
40. Kaback M, Nathan T, Greenwald S. Tay–Sachs disease: heterozygote screening and prenatal diagnosis – US experience and world perspective. In Kaback M, ed, *Tay–Sachs Disease: Screening and Prevention*. 1977: New York: Alan Liss, 13–36.
41. WHO. *Community Approaches to the Control of Hereditary Disease*. Geneva: WHO, 1985.
42. Struewing JP, Abelovich D, Peretz T et al. The carrier frequency of the BRCA 1 185delAG mutation is approximately 1 percent in Ashkenazi Jewish individuals. *Nature Genet* 1995; **11**(2): 198–200.
43. FitzGerald MG, MacDonald DJ, Krainer M. Germ-line BRCA1 mutations in Jewish and non-Jewish women with early-onset breast cancer. *N Engl J Med* 1996; **334**:143–9.
44. Oddoux C, Streiewing JS, Clayton CM. The carrier frequency of the BRCA2 617delT mutation among Ashkenazi Jewish individuals is approximately 1%. *Nature Genet* 1996; **14**:188–90.

45. Greenberg DA. Linkage analysis of 'necessary' disease loci versus 'susceptibility' loci. *Am J Human Genet* 1993; **52**:135–43.
46. Todd JA, Farrall M. Panning for gold: genome-wide scanning for linkage in type 1 diabetes. *Hum Mol Genet* 1996; **5**(Spec No): 1443–8.
47. Baird PA. Genetics and health care: a paradigm shift. *Perspect Biol Med* 1990; **33**:203–13.
48. Lipmann A. *Worrying – and worrying about – the geneticization of reproduction and health*. In Basen G, Eichler M, Lipmann A, eds, *Misconceptions*. Quebec: Voyageur), 1993: 39–65.
49. Lefebvre RC, Hursey KG, Carleton RA. Labeling of participants in high blood pressure screening programs. Implications for blood cholesterol screenings. *Arch Intern Med* 1988, **48**:1993–7.
50. Brett AS. Psychologic effects of the diagnosis and treatment of hypercholesterolemia: lessons from case studies. *Am J Med* 1991; **91**:642–7.
51. Clarke A. Population screening for genetic susceptibility to disease. *BMJ* 1995; **311**:(6996): 35–8.
52. Law MR, Wald NJ, Thompson SG. By how much and how quickly does reduction in serum cholesterol concentration lower risk of ischaemic heart disease? *BMJ* 1994; **308**(6925): 367–72.
53. Chen Z et al. Serum cholesterol concentration and coronary heart disease in population with low cholesterol concentrations. *BMJ* 1991; **303**(6797): 276–82.
54. Law MR, Thompson SG, Wald NJ. Assessing possible hazards of reducing serum cholesterol. *BMJ* 1994; **308**(6925): 373–9.
55. Wald NJ, Law M, Watt HC. Apolipoproteins and ischaemic heart disease: implications for screening. *Lancet* 1994; **343**(8889): 75–9.
56. Kinlay S, Heller RF. Effectiveness and hazards of case finding for a high cholesterol concentration. *BMJ* 1990; **300**(6739): 1545–7.
57. Nuffield Council on Bioethics. *Genetic Screening: Ethnical Issues*. London: Nuffield Council; 1993.
58. Bergman AB, Stamm SJ. The morbidity of cardiac non-disease in school children. *N Engl J Med* 1967; **276**:1008.
59. Smith C. Recurrence risks for multifactorial inheritance. *Am J Hum Genet* 1971; **23**:578–88.
60. Vadheim CM, Rimoin DL, Rotter J. Diabetes mellitus. In: Emery AEH, Rimoin DL, eds. *Principles and Practice of Medical Genetics*. Edinburgh: Churchill Livingstone; 1990: 521–58.

20

Gene Therapy for Type 2 Diabetes: Will it have a Role?

J.A.M. SHAW AND K. DOCHERTY

Department of Molecular and Cell Biology, University of Aberdeen, Institute of Medical Sciences, Foresterhill, Aberdeen AB25 2ZD, UK

In recent years, the need for new therapeutic options in diabetes has become increasingly apparent. The landmark Diabetes Control and Complications Trial (DCCT) has clearly demonstrated that restoration of near-physiological glycaemic control with an intensified insulin injection regimen reduces both the appearance and progression of early microvascular complications in type 1 diabetes mellitus[1]. This was, however, counterbalanced by a significant increase in hypoglycaemia and required considerable on-going patient motivation, in addition to costly health services input.

Insulin analogues with a faster onset of action than unmodified subcutaneously injected insulin have been developed in an attempt to alleviate postprandial hyperglycaemia and reduce later hypoglycaemia, but attainment of a steady-basal insulin level has proved more elusive with currently available forms of insulin[2]. Continuous subcutaneous insulin infusion pumps have thus been employed, but it seems unlikely that these will become suitable for wide-scale application.

Pancreatic transplantation is becoming increasingly viable, although this has largely been restricted to those requiring concomitant renal transplantation given the requirement for life-long immunosuppression[3]. Whole organ transplantation is also dependent on the availability of cadaveric tissue. It had been hoped that these difficulties might be circumvented by transplantation of isolated islet cells but, despite encouraging animal studies, success in patients has been limited[4]. Current immunosuppressive regimens, and in particular the use of cyclosporin A, may inhibit islet function and attempts to

Type 2 Diabetes: Prediction and Prevention. Edited by Graham A. Hitman

avoid the need for immunosuppression by immunobarrier encapsulation techniques have failed to fulfil initial promise. Optimal site for transplantation remains uncertain and purification while maintaining adequate glucose responsivity is technically demanding.

Limited availability of human islet tissue will impose major restrictions on the development of islet cell transplantation and the possible application of porcine islets has thus been examined. Pig pancreases are readily available: use of porcine insulin, differing from human insulin by only a single amino acid, is well validated in patients, and the secretory dynamics of porcine islet insulin are comparable to those of human islets. The isolation of porcine islets has, however, proved particularly challenging, although promising results have been obtained with encapsulated islets in dogs[5] and monkeys[6]. There is also considerable anxiety surrounding the potential for transmission of porcine viral or other infectious agents to human xenograft recipients[7].

GENE THERAPY IN DIABETES

It is hoped that, by utilizing gene therapy or cellular engineering, it may be possible to overcome the problems associated with islet cell transplantation and, in particular, the limits imposed by cadaveric tissue availability[8–12]. As they are terminally differentiated, islet cells cannot readily be induced to propagate in culture. Considerable effort has thus been devoted to the development of islet cell lines that can be grown and replicated in culture, but retain an appropriate level of insulin secretion in response to changes in glucose concentrations within the physiological range of 5–10 mmol/l. Approaches have included cell line derivation from insulinoma explant cultures or via oncogenic viral transformation of isolated human islets. A number of rodent islet cell lines have been generated and, although invaluable resources for research purposes, these cell lines have proved unsuitable for transplantation because of rapid growth and dedifferentiation resulting in loss of glucose-stimulated insulin secretion within the physiological range. Genetic manipulation techniques have been used to improve the phenotype of such cell lines and there have been attempts to engineer insulin expression in non-islet cells, as described below.

Gene therapy may also have a role in the prevention of allograft rejection, as there are a number of ways in which transplanted cells could be genetically modified to resist immune attack. These include expression of immunomodulatory cytokines, such as interleukins 4, 10 or 12[13], protection against host cytokines by interleukin-1-receptor antagonist expression[14], and modification of cellular antigens to reduce recognition by the immune system[15].

GENE THERAPY IN TYPE 2 DIABETES

Until recently, progress towards diabetic gene therapy has largely been considered in terms of potential applications in type 1 diabetes mellitus. There are, however, persuasive reasons for considering that its pertinence to type 2 diabetes may be even greater. Type 2 diabetes accounts for 80% of all diabetes in the UK and around 90% of that in the Western World[16]. Prevalence is rising steadily and it has been estimated that 110 million people worldwide are currently affected, with costs of treating its complications, in the UK alone of at least £2 billion per annum[17,18].

Type 2 diabetes mellitus is a heterogeneous metabolic disorder characterized by defects in both insulin secretion and action[19]. Indeed, regardless of the primary defect, hyperglycaemia itself may lead to insulin deficiency through impaired β-cell function and to insulin resistance through disruption of insulin/receptor interactions. Although there is a strong genetic component, evidenced by concordance in identical twins[20,21], inheritance is clearly polygenic, with identification of specific causative genes remaining elusive[22]. Attempts at identifying potential targets for gene therapy aimed at prevention or cure are thus unlikely to be successful in this multifactorial disease.

The relationship between worsening glycaemic control and the development of complications is clearly established in type 2 diabetes and, although evidence of the calibre of DCCT in type 1 diabetes is still awaited, similar glycaemic targets have been adopted[23,24]. These have proved difficult to attain through conventional therapy with diet, exercise and oral hypoglycaemic agents, and 50% of individuals go on to need insulin[25]. Indeed, the only trial that convincingly demonstrates prevention of progression of microvascular complications with improved glycaemic control in type 2 diabetes involved intensive insulin therapy[27]. Insulin delivery by gene therapy would thus seem equally appropriate, with potentially greater benefit and fewer pitfalls than in type 1 diabetes. Loss of β-cell function as a result of islet cell destruction in type 1 diabetes is irreversible, whereas in type 2 diabetes implantation of engineered cells may protect and prolong the viability of host islets by reducing progressive β-cell exhaustion[27]. Moreover, in type 1 diabetes, implanted β cells are susceptible to recurrence of the autoimmune destructive process in addition to straightforward graft rejection, and there is strong evidence for cytokine-mediated β-cell death in this type of diabetes[28]. Immunobarrier micro- or macroencapsulation devices would therefore need to exclude molecules over a wide range of sizes from immunoglobulins (10^5–10^6 Da) through cytokines (10^4–10^5 Da) to free radicals (10–10^2 Da), while permitting influx of nutrients and oxygen together with efflux of insulin and metabolic waste (lactate, CO_2 and H^+)[29]. This may not be an attainable goal whereas, in type 2 diabetes, it could be sufficient to permit the passage of small molecules ($<10^4$ Da), while protecting the graft from antibody-mediated attack.

The remainder of this chapter examines in greater detail approaches to insulin delivery by gene therapy that have a potential role in type 2 diabetes.

ENGINEERING β CELLS

Insulin-secreting cell lines have been generated from a radiation-induced NEDH (New England Deaconess Hospital) rat insulinoma (RinM5F cells)[30], by transformation of isolated hamster islets with the simian virus SV40 (HIT-T15)[31], and from β-cell tumours that were produced by expression of SV40 large T antigen in β cells of transgenic mice (βTC[32] and MIN6[33]). These cell lines, however, differ in several important respects from normal β cells. RinM5F and HIT-T15 cells have low insulin content and reduced threshold for glucose-stimulated insulin secretion, and do not respond to the normal potentiators of insulin release. MIN6 and βTC have a higher insulin content and better glucose response, but they tend to dedifferentiate with time in culture. Attempts have been made to improve these cells lines by electrofusion with isolated rat islets (BRIN-BD11)[34], or by cloning sublines under different culture conditions (INS-1)[35]. In addition, an understanding of the key role of the glucose-phosphorylating enzyme glucokinase and the glucose transporter GLUT2 in glucose-stimulated insulin secretion[36,37], together with the realization that those cells unresponsive to glucose express hexokinase and GLUT1, has led to a more directed approach to genetic manipulation of these cells.

In a clone of RIN cells (RIN1046-38), which has lost glucose responsiveness in addition to GLUT2 and glucokinase expression over time in culture, Newgard and colleagues[38] have demonstrated reinstatement of glucose-stimulated insulin secretion on stable transfection with GLUT2[38]. The effect was, however, transient and RIN cells remained unsuitable for therapeutic purposes, expressing rat rather than human insulin with an insulin content that was only 10% of that seen in the physiological human β cell. These problems were to some extent overcome by iterative engineering, i.e. the introduction of several genes, including those encoding human insulin, GLUT2 and glucokinase, in a step-wise fashion[39,40]. It is envisaged that further refinement may be possible by ablation of the endogenous genes for hexokinase and GLUT1[39].

Efrat and colleagues[41] have explored an alternative approach to the generation of stable glucose-responsive β-cell lines. Transgenic mice have been engineered in which the SV40 large T antigen is expressed in β cells under the control of a tetracycline-inducible promoter (Figure 20.1). When cultured in the absence of tetracycline, these βTCtet cells replicated well. In the presence of tetracycline, however, expression of large T antigen was

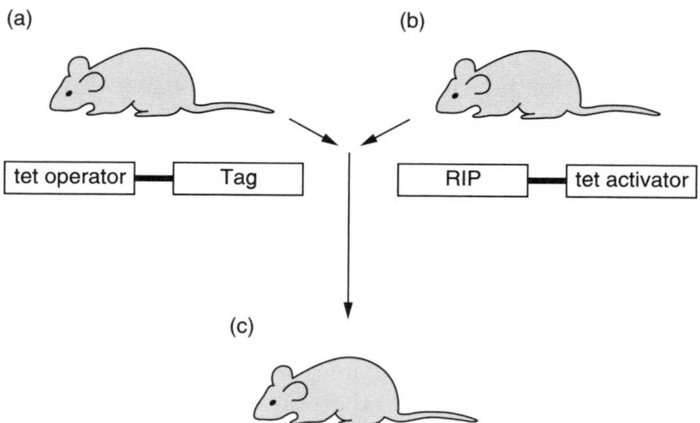

Figure 20.1. Generation of transgenic mice with a genetic switch controlling proliferation and differentiation. One transgenic line contains a tet activator protein (fusion protein combining the tet repressor with the activator domain of VP16) under the control of the insulin promoter (RIP) (b). The tet activator is expressed in β cells. A second transgenic line contains the large T antigen (Tag) downstream of a minimal promoter and repeat sequences from the tet operator (a). This DNA is present in all cells but, because it has a minimal promoter, it is not expressed. Mice are mated so that, in the resultant offspring, the tet activator protein binds to the tet operator sequences in the β cells and switches on expression of Tag (c). When the β cells are treated with a tetracycline analogue, expression of Tag is switched off.

attenuated with no further cell division. Implantation in mice with streptozotocin-induced diabetes resulted in normalization of blood glucose within 2 weeks. Thereafter, continued proliferation of cells in vivo led to increased insulin secretion with eventual fatal hypoglycaemia. When the cells were implanted along with a slow-release tetracycline pellet, proliferation ceased and euglycaemia was maintained for up to 4 months. This approach therefore shows great promise, although it is more likely that cells derived from transgenic pigs, rather than from mice, would be suitable for therapeutic application.

ENGINEERING NON-β CELLS

As alluded to previously, approaches to engineering β cells for the treatment of type 1 diabetes are complicated by the specifications incumbent on any immunobarrier encapsulation device to prevent allograft rejection and cytokine-mediated destruction of the implant[42]. To circumvent autoimmune destruction, attempts have been made to engineer non-β cells that secrete insulin for therapeutic purposes. These cells may also have applications in the treatment of type 2 diabetes.

The ultimate goal of physiological glucose-responsive insulin secretion may not be attainable by genetic manipulation of non-β cells, given the highly specialized mechanism by which insulin gene transcription and secretion of fully processed insulin are regulated by glucose uptake and metabolism in the normal pancreatic β cell. The primary aim of non-β-cell-targeted gene therapy is thus constitutive secretion of insulin at a constant 'trickle', mimicking physiological basal insulin secretion (5–15 μU/ml). This limits hepatic gluconeogenesis that occurs between meals and overnight and which determines the fasting glucose, the most significant factor in overall glycaemic control[43]. None of the available insulin preparations or genetically modified insulin analogues is able to reproduce this stable basal insulin level after subcutaneous injection, and constitutive insulin delivery by genetically manipulated cells would therefore have considerable therapeutic potential.

Such an approach is supported by evidence from the use of continuous subcutaneous insulin infusion in individuals with type 1 diabetes, which suggests that basal insulin supplemented by preprandial insulin boluses results in overall control equal to that obtained with intensive conventional therapy, although with significantly less hypoglycaemia[44]. Earlier studies show that glycaemic control in type 2 diabetes may be attained by fixed rate insulin delivery alone[45]. Constitutive insulin delivery by gene therapy may thus be applicable in combination with preprandial subcutaneous injection of soluble insulin, possibly a fast-acting insulin analogue[46], in type 1 diabetes and with or without adjunctive hypoglycaemic agents in type 2 diabetes. Ultimately, it may be possible to introduce a degree of control at the level of gene transcription by employing either promoters that can be regulated, such as the tetracycline-responsive system[47] or nutrient-responsive elements from the L-type pyruvate kinase gene or the insulin gene itself[48].

There are two potential approaches to the use of engineered non-β cells for gene therapy: transfection of a non-β-cell line grown in culture with encapsulation in a matrix gel or hollow fibres prior to implantation and transduction, with the insulin gene of cells derived from the diabetic individual *in situ* or after harvesting with subsequent reimplantation to circumvent immune rejection.

NEUROENDOCRINE CELL LINES

Early experiments involved neuroendocrine cells that express the regulated secretory pathway with the specific endoproteases (PC2 and PC3) necessary for cleavage of proinsulin to bioactive insulin. Transfection of the mouse pituitary corticotrophic cell line (AtT20) with an insulin gene construct resulted in secretion of fully processed insulin via the regulated secretory pathway, i.e. it was induced by membrane depolarization in the presence of calcium[49]. Insulin release was not, however, affected by changes in glucose concentration and attempts to engineer AtT20 cells with glucose responsivity have met with only partial success.

This cell line expresses an endogenous glucokinase gene and co-transfection with the insulin gene and a cDNA encoding the GLUT2 glucose transporter resulted in insulin secretion in response to glucose, although this was in the subphysiological range with maximum stimulation occurring at glucose concentrations of 10 μmol/l[50]. Glucose responsivity was not seen in cells tranfected with the GLUT1 high-affinity glucose transporter[51].

AtT20 cells stably transfected with an insulin gene construct under the control of a metallothionein promoter and implanted intraperitoneally in nude mice delayed onset of streptozotocin-induced hyperglycaemia by 2 weeks[52,53]. Subsequent hyperglycaemia may have been the result of insulin resistance caused by co-secretion of ACTH. The potential role of neuroendocrine cells in gene therapy is thus limited unless secretion of diabetogenic hormones can be prevented perhaps by gene knockout.

NON-NEUROENDOCRINE CELL LINES

Non-neuroendocrine cells secrete via the constitutive pathway, they do not express the regulated secretory pathway or the enzymes necessary for processing of proinsulin to insulin. Glucose disposal induced by intravenous administration of human proinsulin is only 5–10% of that seen with insulin, although proinsulin has a more prolonged hypoglycaemic effect due to decreased hepatic clearance; it also appears to exert a proportionally greater effect on hepatic gluconeogenesis than on peripheral glucose uptake[54]. Constitutive secretion of proinsulin may therefore have a therapeutic role in type 1 and type 2 diabetes, lowering the fasting glucose level with a lesser risk of hypoglycaemia resulting from peripheral uptake of glucose. Clinical trials of proinsulin have, however, been suspended at present as a result of association with adverse cardiovascular events in one study, although epidemiological data suggest that high levels of proinsulin-like peptides may not be causative, but reflect intrauterine undernutrition and low birthweight, which are known to be associated with increased cardiovascular disease[55].

The mouse LtK^- fibroblast cell line has been stably transfected with a human pre-proinsulin gene driven by the mouse metallothionein promoter; this results in constitutive secretion of proinsulin at a high rate (91 ng/10^6 cells per 24 h)[56]. Proinsulin release was increased in vitro by cadmium administration, presumably because of activation of the metallothionein promoter. Intraperitoneal implantation of 2×10^6 transfected cells in immunocompetent, streptozotocin induced, diabetic C3H mice resulted in a decrease in glucose from about 24 mmol/l to less than 10 mmol/l within 4 days, with subsequent death from hypoglycaemia at 29–46 days. Proinsulin concentration rose from 1 nmol/l at day 14 to 6.1 nmol/l at day 28, presumably as a result of fibroblast multiplication, tumour-like aggregations being present within the peritoneal cavity and liver *post mortem*. Implantation of proinsulin-secreting Ltk^- cells, which had been transfected with a second plasmid that encoded the BALB/c mouse T-cell-differentiation antigen, resulted in an initial decrease in blood glucose concentration, and permanent recurrence of hyperglycaemia after administration of a specific monoclonal antibody to the antigen with no evidence of tumour formation *post mortem*.

Site-directed mutagenesis of the PC2/PC3 cleavage sites to a furin consensus cleavage site has produced a mutant insulin minigene, which allows full insulin processing by furin – a ubiquitously expressed trans-Golgi network protease[57]. Transfection of non-neuroendocrine cell lines, such as NIH3T3 (fibroblast), HepG2 (liver), COS (kidney epithelial) and CHO (ovary epithelial), with this construct results in secretion of fully processed insulin; the extent of insulin processing correlates with the level of endogenous furin expression in each cell line (Table 20.1). Complete conversion can be attained in cells with a low level of endogenous furin by co-transfection with a furin cDNA[58].

The use of engineered myogenic cells for constitutive insulin secretion has certain advantages, because myoblasts, which can be grown, transfected and characterized in culture, fuse to form stable myotubes with no further proliferation in vivo and thus no exponential rise in gene product in an unregulated system. Transient transfection of the C2C12 and L6 mouse myogenic cell lines with the mutant insulin minigene construct results in secretion of fully processed bioactive insulin in vitro, although attempts to select stably transfected clones producing sufficient insulin for in vivo studies have so far proved unsuccessful (A. Hart, J.A.M. Shaw and K. Docherty, unpublished results).

Further progress towards clinical trials with engineered non-syngeneic cell lines is currently hampered by inadequacies in immunobarrier encapsulation

Table 20.1. Insulin processing in non-neuroendocrine cells.

Cell line	Tissue of origin	Processing (%)	Reference
NIH3T3	Mouse fibroblast	85	58
C2C12	Mouse myoblast	75	*
L6	Rat myoblast	75	*
HepG2	Human hepatocyte	70	58
COS	Monkey kidney epithelium	60	58
CHO	Hamster ovary epithelium	50	58
Primary myoblast	Rat myoblast	50	61

Cells were transfected with an insulin gene construct in which PC2 and PC3 cleavage sites had been mutated to allow processing of proinsulin to insulin by endogenous furin.
*A Hart, unpublished data.

techniques, complications of which include pericapsular inflammation, capsule rupture and continuing requirement for adjunctive immunosuppressive therapy[59].

HOST CELL TRANSDUCTION

Muscle-targeted gene therapy, involving primary myoblast derivation and reimplantation after genetic manipulation, may prove to be an elegant method of insulin delivery at a constant rate. Cells are accessible and can be established in culture after a muscle biopsy. Intramuscular injection of genetically engineered myoblasts is straightforward and has been shown to result in long-term stable secretion of gene product at high concentrations into the systemic circulation of rodents[60]. Immunosuppression or encapsulation would be avoided, and surgical removal would remain viable if necessary since both cells and gene expression remain localized after the injection. Recently, primary muscle cells of rat origin have been successfully transfected with wild-type and mutant insulin gene constructs, with in vitro secretion of proinsulin and insulin, respectively[61]. Animal studies with this model are awaited, although ultimately it may become necessary to consider viral transfection techniques to increase efficiency of gene transfer.

An alternative approach to gene delivery, which avoids the need for immunosuppression, is in vivo transfection by direct plasmid injection or utilizing liposomes/viral vectors. Hepatic uptake and short-term expression of insulin gene constructs is seen in rats after intravenous administration of DNA–liposome complexes, resulting in an approximately 30% reduction in plasma glucose[62,63]. Intraportal injection of an insulin cDNA, in a retroviral vector under the control of a long terminal repeat region, results in more stable hepatic cell transduction in rats[64]. After induction of diabetes by streptozotocin, ectopic insulin expression prevented ketoacidosis and death, and normoglycaemia was reinstated during a 24-hour fast, with no adverse effects for up to 20 days. There are, however, concerns about in vivo gene delivery after systemic injection, because the site of incorporation is, to some degree, uncontrolled, with at least a theoretical risk of germline transduction. Unpredictable uptake may result in unacceptable variability in constitutive insulin secretion, and the inability to resect transfected cells easily may render this approach untenable.

CONCLUSIONS

Although progress has at times seemed slow, with new challenges presenting themselves as each obstacle is overcome, this is an exciting time in the development of diabetic gene therapy and there are several diverse techniques that are tantalizingly close to assessment in the first clinical trials. Contrary to previous opinions one or more of these approaches may assume particular relevance in the future therapy of type 2 diabetes.

REFERENCES

1. The Diabetes Control and Complications Trial Research Group. The effect of intensive treatment of diabetes on the development and progression of long-term complications in insulin-dependent diabetes mellitus. *N Eng J Med* 1993; **329**:977–86.
2. Galloway JA, Chance RE. Improving insulin therapy: achievements and challenges. *Horm Metab Res* 1994; **26**:591–8.
3. Sutherland DER. Pancreatic transplantation: an update. *Diabetes Rev* 1993; **1**: 152–65.
4. Weir GC, Bonner-Weir S. Scientific and political impediments to successful islet transplantation. *Diabetes* 1997; **48**:1247–56.
5. Maki T, Ichiro M, O'Neil JJ et al. Treatment of diabetes by xenogeneic islets without immunosuppression. *Diabetes* 1996; 45:342–7.
6. Sun Y, Ma X, Zhou D, Vacaek I, Sun AM. Normalisation of diabetes in spontaneously diabetic cynomologous monkeys by xenografts of microencapsulated porcine islets without immunosuppression. *J Clin Invest* 1996; 98:1414–22.
7. Weiss RA. Transgenic pigs and virus adaptation. *Nature* 1998; 391:327–8.
8. Selden RF, Skoskiewicz MJ, Russel PS, Goodman HM. Regulation of insulin-gene expression. *N Eng J Med* 1987; **317**:1067–76.
9. Docherty K. Gene therapy and cellular engineering in diabetes. In: Pickup JC, ed. *Biotechnology of Insulin Therapy*. Oxford: Blackwell Scientific, 1991; 154–82.
10. Newgard CB. Cellular engineering and gene therapy strategies for insulin replacement in diabetes. *Diabetes* 1994; 43:341–50.
11. Bailey CJ, Docherty K. Exploring the feasibility of insulin gene therapy. In: Flatt PR, Lenzen S, eds. *Frontiers of Insulin Secretion and Pancreatic β-Cell Research*. London: Smith-Gordon, 1995; 781–7.
12. Docherty K. Gene therapy for diabetes mellitus. *Clin Sci* 1997; **92**:321–30.
13. Deng S, Ketchum RJ, Kucher T et al. Adenoviral transfection of canine islet xenografts with immunosuppressive cytokine genes abrogates primary non-function and prolongs graft survival. *Transplant Proc* 1997; **29**:770.
14. Welsh N, Bentzen K, Welsh M. Expression of an insulin/interleukin-1 antagonist hybrid gene in insulin-producing cell lines (HIT-T-15 and NIT-1) confers resistance against interleukin-1 induced nitric oxide production. *J Clin Invest* 1995; **95**:1717–22.
15. Efrat S, Fejer G, Brownlee M, Horowitz MS. Prolonged survival of pancreatic islet allografts mediated by adenovirus immunoregulatory transgenes. *Proc Natl Acad Sci USA* 1995; **92**:6947–51.
16. Neil HAW, Gatling W, Mather HM et al. The Oxford Community Diabetes Study: evidence for an increase in the prevalence of known diabetes in Great Britain. *Diabetic Med* 1987; **4**:539–43.
17. Zimmet P, McCarty D. The NIDDM epidemic: global estimates and projections – a look into the crystal ball. *IDF Bull* 1995; **40**:8–16.
18. King's Fund. *Counting the Cost: The real impact of non-insulin dependent diabetes*. London: British Diabetic Association.

19. Kahn SE, Porte D Jr. The pathophysiology of type II (noninsulin-dependent) diabetes mellitus: implications for treatment. In: Porte D Jr, Sherwin RS, eds. *Ellenberg and Rifkin's Diabetes Mellitus*, 5th edn, Stamford, CT: Appleton & Lange, 1997, 487–512.
20. Barnett AH, Eff C, Leslie RDG, Pyke DA. Diabetes in identical twins: a study of 200 pairs. *Diabetologia* 1981; **20**:87–93.
21. Newman B, Selby JV, Knig M-C, Slemenda C, Fabsitz R, Friedman GD. Concordance for type 2 (non-insulin-dependent) diabetes mellitus in male twins. *Diabetologia* 1987; **30**:763–8.
22. Ghosh S, Schork NJ. Genetic analysis of NIDDM: the study of quantitative traits. *Diabetes* 1996; **45**:1–14.
23. Howard Williams J, Hillson RM, Bron A, Awdry P., Mann JI, Hockaday TD. Retinopathy is associated with higher glycaemia in maturity onset diabetes. *Diabetologia* 1984; **27**:198–202.
24. Natham DM. Insulin treatment of noninsulin-dependent diabetes mellitus. In: Porte D Jr, Sherwin RS, eds. *Ellenberg and Rifkins Diabetes Mellitus* 5th edn. Stamford, CT: Appleton & Lange, 1997: 735–743
25. Berger M. To bridge science and patient care in diabetes. *Diabetologia* 1996; **39**:749–57.
26. Ohkubo Y, Kishikawa H, Araki E et al. Intensive insulin therapy prevents the progression of diabetic microvascular complications in Japanese patients with non-insulin-dependent diabetes mellitus: a randomised prospective six year study. *Diabetes Res Clin Pract* 1995; **28**:103–17.
27. Gray H, O'Rahilly S. β cell dysfunction in non-insulin dependent diabetes mellitus. *Transplant Proc* 1994; **26**:366–70.
28. Gill RG, Coulombe M, Lafferty KJ. Pancreatic islet allograft immunity and tolerance: the two-signal hypothesis revisited. *Immunol Rev* 1996:; 149:75–96.
29. Rabinovitch A, Suarez-pinzon WL, Strynadka K, Lakey JR, Rajotte RV. Human pancreatic islet Beta-cell destruction by cytokines involves oxygen free radicals and aldehyde production. *J Clin Endocrinol Metab* 1996; **81**:3197–202.
30. Gazdar AF, Chick WL, Oie HK et al. Continuous, clonal, insulin- and somatostatin-secreting cell lines established from a transplantable rat islet cell tumour. *Proc Natl Acad Sci USA* 1980; **77**:3519–23.
31. Santerre RF, Cook RA, Cristel RMD et al. Insulin synthesis in a clonal cell line of simian virus 40-transformed hamster pancreatic β-cells. *Proc Natl Acad Sci USA* 1981; **78**:4339–43.
32. Efrat S, Linde S, Kofod H et al. Beta-cell lines derived from transgenic mice expressing a hybrid insulin gene-oncogene. *Proc Natl Acad Sci USA* 1988; **8**:9037–41.
33. Miyazaki J-I, Araki K, Yamamoto E et al. Establishment of a pancreatic β-cell line that retains glucose-inducible insulin secretion: special reference to expression of glucose transporter isoforms. *Endocrinology* 1990; **127**:126–32.
34. McClenaghan NH, Barnett CR, Ah-Singh E et al. Characterization of a novel glucose-responsive insulin-secreting cell line, BRIN-BD11, produced by electrofusion. *Diabetes* 1996; **45**:1132–40.
35. Asfari M, Janjic D, Meda P, Li G, Halban PA, Wollheim CB. Establishment of a 2-mercaptoethanol-dependent differentiated insulin-secreting cell lines. *Endocrinology* 1992; **130**:167–78.
36. Ashcroft FM, Ashcroft SJH. Mechanisms of insulin secretion. In: Ashcroft FM, Ashcroft SJH, eds. *Insulin, Molecular Biology to Pathology*. Oxford: Oxford University Press, 1992: 97–150.

37. Newgard CB. Regulatory role of glucose transport and phosphorylation in pancreatic β-cells. *Diabetes Rev* 1996; **4**:191–206.
38. Ferber S, Beltrande H, Johnson JH et al. GLUT-2 gene transfer into insulinoma cells confers both low and high affinity glucose-stimulated insulin release. *J Biol Chem* 1994; **269**:11523–9.
39. Clark SA, Quaade C, Constandy H et al. Novel insulinoma cell lines produced by iterative engineering of GLUT2, glucokinase and human insulin expression. *Diabetes* 1997; **49**:958–67.
40. Hohmeier HE, BeltrandelRio H, Clark SA, Henkel-Rieger R, Normington K, Newgard CB. Regulation of insulin secretion from novel engineered insulinoma cell lines. *Diabetes* 1997; **46**:968–77.
41. Efrat S, Fusco-Demane D, Lemberg H, Emran OA, Wang X. Conditional transformation of a pancreatic β-cell line derived from transgenic mice expressing a tetracycline-regulated oncogene. *Proc Natl Acad Sci USA* 1995; **92**:3576–80.
42. Tyden G, Reinholt FP, Sundkvist G, Bolinder J. Recurrence of autoimmune diabetes mellitus in recipients of cadaveric pancreatic grafts. *N Engl J Med* 1996; **335**:860–3.
43. Galloway JA, Chance RE. Insulin agonist therapy: a challenge for the 1990's. *Clin Ther* 1990; **12**:460–72.
44. Bode BW, Steed RD, Davidson PC. Reduction in severe hypoglycemia with long-term continuous subcutaneous insulin infusion in type 1 diabetes. *Diabetes Care* 1996; **19**:324–7.
45. Buchwald H, Barbosa J, Varco RL et al. Treatment of a type II diabetic by a totally implantable insulin infusion device. *Lancet* 1981; **i**:1233–5.
46. Gale EAM. Insulin lispro: the first insulin analogue to reach the market. *Pract Diab Int* 1996; **13**:122–4.
47. Gossen M, Bujard H. Tight controls of gene expression in mammalian cells by tetracycline-responsive promoters. *Proc Natl Acad Sci USA* 1992; **89**:5547–51.
48. Mitanchez D, Doiron B, Chen R, Kahn A. Glucose-stimulated genes and prospects of gene therapy for type 1 diabetes. *Endocrine Rev* 1997; **18**:520–40.
49. Moore HP, Walker MD, Lee F, Kelly RB. Expressing a human proinsulin cDNA in a mouse ACTH-secreting cell: intracellular storage, proteolytic processing and secretion on stimulation. *Cell* 1983; **35**:531–8.
50. Hughes SD, Johnson JH, Quaade C, Newgard CB. Engineering of glucose-stimulated insulin secretion and biosynthesis in non-islet cells. *Proc Natl Acad Sci USA* 1992; **89**:688–92.
51. Hughes SD, Quaade C, Johnson JH, Ferber S, Newgard CB. Transfection of AtT20ins cells with GLUT-2 but not GLUT-1 confirms glucose-stimulated insulin secretion. *J Biol Chem* 1993; **11**:335–41.
52. Stewart C, Taylor NA, Docherty K, Bailey CJ. Insulin delivery by somatic gene therapy. *J Mol Endocrinol* 1993; **11**:335–41.
53. Stewart C, Taylor NA, Green IC, Docherty K, Bailey CJ. Insulin-releasing pituitary cells as a model for somatic gene therapy in diabetes mellitus. *J Endocrinol* 1994; **142**:339–43.
54. Robbins DC, Tager HS, Rubenstein AH. Biological and clinical importance of proinsulin. *N Engl J Med* 1984; **310**:1165–75.
55. Yudkin JS. Circulating proinsulin-like molecules. *J Diab Comp* 1993; **7**:113–23.
56. Kawakami Y, Yamaoka T, Hirochika R, Yamashita K, Itakura M, Nakauchi H. Somatic gene therapy for diabetes with an immunological safety system for complete removal of transplanted cells. *Diabetes* 1992; **41**:956–61.

57. Groskreutz J, Sliwkowski MX, Gorman CM. Genetically engineered proinsulin constitutively processed and secreted as mature active insulin. *J Biol Chem* 1994; **269**:6241–45.
58. Yanagita M, Hoshino H, Nakayama K, Takeuchi T. Processing of mutated proinsulin with tetrabasic cleavage sites to mature insulin reflects the expression of furin in non-neuroendocrine cell lines. *endocrinology* 1993; **133**:639–44.
59. Maki T, Mullon CJP, Solomon BA, Monaco AP. Novel delivery of pancreatic islet cells to treat insulin dependent diabetes mellitus. *Clin Pharmacokinet* 1995; **28**:471–82.
60. Dai Y, Roman M, Naviaux RK, Verma IM. Gene therapy via primary myoblasts: long-term expression of factor IX protein following transplantation *in vivo. Proc Natl Acad Sci USA* 1992; **89**:10892–5.
61. Simonson GD, Groskreutz DJ, Gorman CM, MacDonald MJ. Synthesis and processing of genetically modified human proinsulin by rat primary myoblast cultures. *Hum Gen The* 1996; **7**:71–8.
62. Nicolau C, Pape AL, Soriano P, Fargette F, Juhel M-F. *In vivo* expression of rat insulin after intravenous administration of the liposome-entrapped gene for rat insulin I. *Proc Natl Acad Sci USA* 1983; **80**:1068–72.
63. Kaneda Y, Iwai K, Uchia T. Introduction and expression of the human insulin gene in adult rat liver. *J Biol Chem* 1989; **264**:12126–9.
64. Koloddka TM, Finegold M, Moss L, Woo SL. Gene therapy for diabetes mellitus in rats by hepatic expression of insulin. *Proc Natl Acad Sci USA* 1995; **92**:3293–97.

21

Costs and Profits of Prevention

K. BORCH-JOHNSEN

Steno Diabetes Center, Niels Steensens Vej 2, 2820 Gentofte, Denmark

Type 2 diabetes (non-insulin-dependent diabetes mellitus) is a syndrome characterized by relative insulin deficiency, reduced insulin sensitivity and an increased risk of development of microvascular (renal/retinal), neurological and macrovascular complications. Patients with type 2 diabetes may well be entirely without symptoms for years, but during this period the clock will be running for the development of complications and, at diabetes onset, the prevalence of retinopathy is 10–20%[1,2], and of microalbuminuria 19–31%[3-10], and diabetes is often found as a silent bystander in patients who have been hospitalized with acute myocardial infarction or stroke. Based on these epidemiological data, Harris et al.[11] estimated that an average onset of type 2 diabetes occurs at least 4–7 years before clinical diagnosis.

Type 2 diabetes is associated not only with complications that lead to disability, but also with a considerable excess mortality, from both all causes and cardiovascular disease. Mortality rates are two to three times higher for patients with type 2 diabetes than for the general population[12,14].

The long period of time with latent/undiagnosed diabetes, the high prevalence of complications and the excess mortality all indicate the need for more aggressive health policies for early diagnosis and treatment with a focus on secondary prevention (i.e. prevention of development or progression of complications). Methods for primary prevention are, however, also urgently needed.

Type 2 diabetes is among the fastest growing diseases in the world. In 1994, McCarty and Zimmet[15] estimated that the number of individuals with type 2 diabetes in the world would increase from 100 million in 1994 to 215 million in 2010. These estimates are supported by recent estimates from the WHO[16]. The rate of increase is likely to be very unevenly distributed. In

---

Type 2 Diabetes: Prediction and Prevention. Edited by Graham A. Hitman.

Europe and North America, the prevalence will increase by 40–60%, whereas in Asia and Africa the prevalence will increase by 100–170%[15,17]. In other words, this rapidly growing health problem will first hit those parts of the world that have the least financial resources to cope with the problem. The almost epidemic pattern of the disease will be one of the major public health challenges by the turn of the millennium, and the relevant question no longer seems to be whether we can afford to prevent type 2 diabetes but, rather, whether we can afford just to let go. Several questions do, however, need to be answered before preventive strategies can be developed and integrated:

- Why is the prevalence increasing?
- What are the most important risk factors?
- Are the risk factors modifiable?
- Does intervention reduce the risk of diabetes?
- Will the population in general and high-risk groups in particular follow advice and change behaviour?
- What are the relevant prevention strategies?
- What is the cost-effectiveness of these intervention programmes and strategies?

RISK FACTORS FOR DEVELOPMENT OF TYPE 2 DIABETES

The following are the most important risk factors for development of type 2 diabetes:

- genetic susceptibility/ethnicity
- age
- obesity
- physical inactivity
- nutritional factors
- modern lifestyle.

NON-MODIFIABLE RISK FACTORS

Genetic Susceptibility and Ethnicity

Family and twin studies show the important role of genetic predisposition[18], but currently identified genes only explain 5–15% of all cases of type 2 diabetes. Ethnicity also plays an important role, with huge variations in the age-adjusted prevalence rates[19]. There is a marked interaction between genes and the environment in the risk of developing type 2 diabetes, which is most clearly demonstrated in Asian and Pacific populations where the prevalence increases with urbanization and Westernized lifestyle[20]. In relation to prevention, genetic susceptibility is important, because it is an important key to identification of high-risk groups (e.g. familial predisposition and ethnic high-risk groups).

Age

The prevalence of diabetes increases with age[19], and life expectancy is increasing in all parts of the world, leading to an increase in the prevalence of all chronic, non-communicable diseases, including diabetes. Preventive strategies should target a reduction in the morbidity and an increase in the quality of life in old and elderly people. This is possible only if modifiable risk factors can be modified.

MODIFIABLE RISK FACTORS

Obesity

Obesity is a major risk for development of diabetes. In a prospective study of almost 115 000 women aged 30–55 years who were followed for 14 years, the relative risk of developing type 2 diabetes was 40 in women with a body mass index (BMI) of 31 kg/m^2 or more compared with lean women with a BMI of less than 22 kg/m^2 [21]. Ohlson et al.[22] followed a cohort of 54-year-old men for 13.5 years, and the relative risk of diabetes in the highest quintile of BMI was 22 kg/m^2 compared with those in the lowest quintile[22]. Subsequently, this has been confirmed by other groups[23,24], and central obesity with abdominal fat deposits is a particularly strong predictor of development of type 2 diabetes[22,23,25]. In the Nurses' Health Study, weight gain in adult life was strongly associated with an increased risk, whereas weight loss was associated with a decreased risk[22], an observation that was found also in older age groups[24]. Together, these studies indicate that obesity is a modifiable risk factor in which effective intervention (i.e. weight loss) is associated with a decreased risk of developing diabetes mellitus. The problem is the well-known difficulties in obtaining and maintaining a significant weight loss.

Physical Activity

Several studies have shown that low physical activity is associated with an increased risk of type 2 diabetes[26-28]. In the study by Helmrich et al.[27] a cohort of 5990 male students at the University of Pennsylvania were followed for a total of almost 100 000 person-years of observation; they demonstrated a stepwise, combined effect of physical activity and being moderately overweight (BMI $> 26\,kg/m^2$); overweight, physically inactive individuals had a greater than four times increased incidence of type 2 diabetes compared with lean (BMI < 24 kg/m^2) physically active individuals. Trials of individuals with impaired glucose tolerance (IGT) from Sweden[29] and from China[30] have shown that exercise reduces the risk of progressing to type 2 diabetes. In the Chinese study[30], physical exercise reduced the progression rate from IGT to diabetes by 42–46%, independent of the level of obesity. These results are encouraging for future intervention trials.

Nutritional Factors and Modernization of Lifestyle

The rapid increase in the prevalence of type 2 diabetes in developing countries is predominantly found in urbanized areas. The increase has been associated with what has been called a Westernized lifestyle. The most prominent features of this development have been industrialization with decreased physical activity and dietary changes with an increase in total energy intake and a decrease in relative contribution of non-refined carbohydrates as a resource for calories. These factors again lead to obesity and increased prevalence of diabetes. Thus, increased energy intake, reduced physical activity and weight gain are the key elements in Westernized lifestyle leading to type 2 diabetes.

DOES INTERVENTION REDUCE THE RISK OF DIABETES?

As already discussed, weight loss as well as increased physical activity can reduce the risk of developing diabetes in high-risk individuals. The question, from a public health point of view is, however, whether these high-risk strategies will work at a population level. Very few studies have examined the effect of preventive strategies for type 2 diabetes, and our present knowledge is largely based on experience from prevention trials in cardiovascular disease[31]; most of these studies have been disappointing in relation to the two major risk factors for type 2 diabetes: obesity and low physical activity.

NEEDS IN PRIMARY PREVENTION OF TYPE 2 DIABETES

Despite the fact that we know the major risk factors for type 2 diabetes, and theoretically know how to prevent it, studies are urgently needed to focus on how the targets (weight reduction, increased physical activity and dietary changes) can be obtained. Information campaigns do not automatically lead to behaviour modification, and future studies should be organized by teams with expertise not only in medicine and public health, but also in communication and behaviour psychology. Future studies should carefully evaluate the following:

- Whether our message is received by the target population.
- Whether the message is understood.
- Who has and who has not changed behaviour.
- The determinant for compliance/non-compliance with these programmes.

The impact of socioeconomic status, age, sex, social network and level of education on the compliance with different programmes and information campaigns should also be evaluated, with the aim of designing more focused and targeted campaigns that are adjusted specifically to each target population. While waiting for the result of these trials we will have to focus on secondary and tertiary prevention strategies.

SECONDARY AND TERTIARY PREVENTION STRATEGIES

SCREENING FOR AND EARLY TREATMENT OF DIABETES

In 1997, the American Diabetes Association (ADA) revised the diagnostic criteria for diabetes, focusing more on the fasting blood glucose and lowering the fasting plasma glucose level diagnostic for diabetes from 7.8 to 7.0 mmol/l. At the same time, the ADA also recommended screening for diabetes from the age of 45 years[32], because of the high prevalence of complications at diagnosis of diabetes; the hope is that early diagnosis and intensified treatment would reduce the risk of progression of complications to disability and early mortality.

In 1994, a WHO Study Group on Prevention of Diabetes Mellitus[32] stated that 'the question of mass community screening for NIDDM remains controversial', and this statement is still valid 4 years later. The most important considerations in designing a screening programme include:

- sensitivity, specificity and predictive value of the screening test
- identification of the target population
- provision of relevant and effective follow-up care
- cost and benefits to the patient of being diagnosed.

The WHO Study Group also clearly stated that any screening programme should be evaluated in terms of:

- numbers of new cases detected
- cost per new case detected
- action taken for individuals with positive results
- long-term benefits of early detection.

So far, no studies have met all these criteria and, at present, we are seeing more mathematical models on prevention and screening programmes[34–36] than real screening studies.

SCREENING FOR AND EARLY TREATMENT OF COMPLICATIONS

Retinopathy

Early detection of diabetic retinopathy opens the possibility of treatment with laser therapy. Based on clinical and epidemiological data in 1995, Javitt[37] published an analysis of the cost-effectiveness of screening and intervention programmes for diabetic eye disease (retinopathy and macular oedema). The risk of diabetic eye disease was estimated on the basis of the Wisconsin study[38]. Javitt concludes that screening and treatment for eye disease generates US$ 300 million in annual savings and 100 000 person-years of sight even at the current suboptimal level of care (60%). Thus, screening programmes for retinopathy should be developed and integrated in the care of patients with type 2 diabetes to the benefit of both health care providers and patients[37].

Nephropathy

In patients with type 1 diabetes, screening for microalbuminuria and intervention with angiotension-converting enzyme (ACE) inhibitors have been shown to be effective in clinical trials[39,40] and cost-beneficial in health economical analyses[41,42]. In patients with type 1 diabetes, microalbuminuria is a strong predictor of endstage renal failure and death[43], and ACE inhibitor treatment prevents progression to overt nephropathy and endstage renal failure[39,40]. In patients with type 2 diabetes, microalbuminuria is, first of all, a marker of increased mortality, predominantly from cardiovascular disease[44,45], it is still unknown whether treatment will prevent progression of the macrovascular disease.

Neuropathy

One of the most devastating consequences of diabetic neuropathy is the development of foot ulcers, which leads to immobilization and all too often to amputations. Screening for neuropathy, prevention of foot ulcers and early treatment at specialized foot clinics can markedly reduce the risk of amputations by 40–50%[46,47], and the activity is also likely to be cost-beneficial because of costs related to rehabilitation after an amputation.

Macrovascular disease

Cardiovascular and cerebrovascular diseases are the most common causes of death in patients with type 2 diabetes, and age- and sex-adjusted hospitalization rates for vascular diseases of these patients were: stroke eight times, myocardial infarction eight times and peripheral vascular disease 15 times higher than for the general population[48].

Prevention of cardiovascular disease in patients with type 2 diabetes follows the same line as for non-diabetic patients, with smoking cessation, normalization of blood pressure and lipid lowering as the key features. Intervention studies of lipid lowering indicate that the absolute effect of lipid lowering is higher in patients with type 2 diabetes than in non-diabetic individuals[48]. The data from the US study reflected a subgroup analysis with all its limitations. Further studies in type 2 diabetes are needed. Meanwhile, studies focusing on modification of risk factors that can be changed through behaviour modification would be appreciated.

HEALTH ECONOMIC EVALUATION

Economic evaluation can help to ensure that health care resources are used effectively. Health economy is often perceived as a discipline that should help administrators and decision-makers to save money on health care. Based on this misunderstanding, cost–benefit analyses are performed that underestimate costs and overestimate benefits in an attempt to 'prove' that a given health care programme will 'save money'. These analyses are rarely reliable and of no or little help to health care providers.

Health care is not out to make a 'profit' for health care providers. Health economy should be seen as the discipline that helps decision-makers to make priorities that can help to identify programmes providing the highest level of care at the lowest possible cost; as a discipline it should carefully monitor the impact (economic, level of health, quality of life) of any decisions related to the organization of health care.

Health economy is a discipline based on data and results from many different disciplines, including:

- Epidemiology: magnitude of health problems, prevalence, incidence, morbidity, mortality, progress.
- Clinical trials: comparison of treatment programmes.
- Economy: pricing of health care services and of disease manifestation (disability, reduced working hours).

There are several levels of economic evaluations relevant to type 2 diabetes. The first level aims at describing the area by cost of illness studies. This gives the magnitude of the problem, but does not give any data that are relevant to choice of treatment strategies, because it does not evaluate whether changes in organization/treatment strategy will improve care.

The second group of designs aims to evaluate the economic efficiency, and the three principal designs include (1) cost-effectiveness analysis; (2) cost–utility analysis; and (3) cost–benefit analysis.

COST OF ILLNESS STUDIES

The concept of the cost of illness studies was developed in the 1960s[49]; it measures the total costs to society of a disease, by combining direct, indirect and intangible costs. The simple design estimates the annual cost per patient, and uses prevalence data to estimate the total burden of the disease. The direct costs are the most readily accessible data. Direct costs, however, include *all* aspects of medical care, including hospital care, outpatient clinics, general practitioners, nursing, nursing homes, medications, laboratory tests, etc. Also, it includes cost that are 'out of pocket' for the patient. As the distribution of costs between the categories may vary considerably between countries, depending on the organization of the health care system (nationalized, privatized or a mixture of these), it is essential that all costs are included, because comparison between studies and countries will otherwise be impossible.

Indirect costs include the cost to society as a result of disability, premature mortality loss of working capacity, etc. Indirect costs may or may not be included in the cost of illness study, and the major argument against this is that although indirect costs may be relevant to the individual patient and his or her family, it may not be relevant to a society with unemployment, in which a disabled worker will be replaced by another with the same qualifications[50].

Intangible costs relate to anxiety, stress, pain, etc. caused by the disease[51]. As indicated by the word, it is difficult or even impossible to assign monetary costs to intangible costs.

Using the cost of illness design, Laing and Williams[52] estimated that diabetes uses 4–5% of the entire British health care budget, although a more recent Finnish analysis[53] estimated that diabetes consumes 7% of the entire health care budget. Studies from different regions of the world[54-56] have demonstrated considerable variability in cost per patient with type 2 diabetes per year ranging from US$ 330[54] in Argentina to US$ 3500 in Denmark[56]. This difference results partly from differences in general costs between the two countries, but first of all it illustrates the problems related to estimation of costs.

Cost of illness studies provide a baseline for decision-making. Does this health problem have a magnitude or does the cost increase to a level that makes it relevant as a 'high priority area' for development and evaluation? If the answer to this question is yes then the next question is 'which strategy should we use to prevent type 2 diabetes?', or 'when do we screen for type 2 diabetes' or 'when do we try to prevent endstage complications and premature mortality?'. The methods used here are: cost-benefit, cost-effectiveness and cost–utility. All three methods measure costs in monetary terms (normally direct costs only), but differ in outcome measurement:

- Cost–benefit: monetary units (costs saved by programme intervention).
- Cost–effectiveness: physical units (lives saved, deaths avoided, eyes saved from blindness, amputations avoided, etc.).
- Cost–utility: quality adjusted life-years saved [multiplying physical unit (years of life gained) by a quality of life parameter].

These designs may well be combined in the same analysis[41,42]. Cost-benefit and cost-effectiveness analyses have been performed in analyses of prevention strategies for diabetic nephropathy[41,42] and diabetic retinopathy[57–60]. Most of these analyses have been based on data in patients with type 1 diabetes or in mixed cohorts of patients with type 1 and type 2 diabetes.

In 1997, the ADA recommended screening for diabetes in middle-aged and elderly people[32]. Similar recommendations are on their way in other countries. Recent publications are also supporting implementation of primary prevention programmes[61,62]. Before jumping to conclusions, there are reasons to recommend strict evaluation of all future programmes. Screening for disease may do harm by inducing fear, anxiety and stress and, if screening and intervention does not change the prognosis, we may do more harm than good. The next ten years should focus on:

- Trials of primary prevention of type 2 diabetes with a focus not only on outcome (± diabetes mellitus) but also on costs, compliance and intangible costs.
- Trials using different information campaigns and screening strategies in high-risk populations, focusing not only on immediate outcome (prevalence, false-positive, false-negative, etc.), but also on impact on prognosis, costs, compliance and intangible costs.
- Tertiary prevention trials specifically in patients with type 2 diabetes, with the aim of evaluating different screening and intervention strategies for late diabetic complications in previously diagnosed patients.

CONCLUSION

Prevention of type 2 diabetes through behaviour modification is a theoretical possibility that also has support in clinical trials. Further large-scale, primary prevention trials, in high-risk groups with normal and impaired glucose tolerance, should be performed and carefully evaluated. This is an area that calls for true multidisciplinary collaboration in planning, implementation and evaluation of research programmes.

While waiting for these results, secondary prevention and intervention programmes, which focus on early detection of (1) type 2 diabetes and (2) micro- and macrovascular complications, should be implemented and carefully evaluated, with the aim of optimizing these programmes outside the highly specialized diabetes clinics.

REFERENCES

1. Klein R, Klein BEK, Moss SE, Davis MD, DeMets DL. The Wisconsin Epidemiologic Study of Diabetic Retinopathy. III. Prevalence and risk of diabetic retinopathy when age at diagnosis is 30 or more years. *Arch Ophthalmol* 1984; **102**:527–32.
2. Knuiman MW, Welborn TA, McCann VJ, Stanton KG, Constable IJ. Prevalence of diabetic complications in relation to risk factors. *Diabetes* 1986; **35**:1332–9.
3. Ballard DJ, Humphrey LL, Melton III J et al. Epidemiology of persistent proteinuria in Type II diabetes mellitus. *Diabetes* 1988; **37**:405-12.
4. Fabre J, Balant LP, Dayer PG, Fox HM, Vernet AT. The kidney in maturity onset diabetes mellitus: A clinical study of 510 patients. *Kidney Int* 1982; **21**:730–8.
5. Humphrey LL, Ballard DJ, Frohnert PP, Chu C-P, O'Fallon M, Palumbo PJ. Chronic renal failure in non-insulin-dependent diabetes mellitus. A population-based study in Rochester, Minnesota. *Ann Intern Med* 1989; **111**:788–96.
6. Stadl E, Stiegler H. Microalbuminuria in a random cohort of recently diagnosed Type 2 (non-insulin-dependent) diabetic patients living in the Greater Munich Area. *Diabetologia* 1993; **36**:1017–20.
7. Wingard DL, Barrett-Connor EL, Scheidt-Nave C, McPhillips JB. Prevalence of cardiovascular and renal complications in older adults with normal or impaired glucose tolerance or NIDDM. *Diabetes Care* 1993; **16**:1022–5.
8. Damsgaard EM, Mogensen CE. Microalbuminuria in elderly hyperglycaemic patients and controls. *Diabetic Med* 1986; **3**:430–5.
9. Olivarius N de F, Andreasen AH, Keiding N, Mogensen CE. Epidemiology of renal involvement in newly-diagnosed middle-aged and elderly diabetic patients. Cross-sectional data from the population-based study 'Diabetes care in general practice'. *Diabetologia* 1993; **36**:1007–16.
10. Wirta O, Pasternack A, Mustonen J, Oksa H, Koivula T, Helin H. Albumin excretion rate and its relation to kidney disease in non-insulin-dependent diabetes mellitus. *J Intern Med* 1995; **237**:367–73.
11. Harris MI, Klein R, Welborn TA, Knuiman MW. Onset of NIDDM occurs at least 4–7 yr before clinical diagnosis. *Diabetes Care* 1992; **15**:815–19.
12. Garcia MJ, McNamara PM, Gordon T et al. Morbidity and mortality in diabetics in the Framingham population. *Diabetes* 1974; **23**:105–11.
13. Dowse GK, Zimmet PZ, Gareeboo H et al. Abdominal obesity and physical inactivity as risk factors for NIDDM and impaired glucose tolerance in Indian, Creole, and Chinese Mauritians. *Diabetes Care* 1991; **14**:271–82.
14. Whittal DE, Glatthaar C, Knuiman MW et al. Deaths from diabetes are underreported in national mortality statistics. *Med J Aust* 1990; **152**:598–600.
15. McCarty, D, Zimmet P. *Diabetes 1994 to 2010: Global Estimates and Projections.* Melbourne: International Diabetes Institute, 1994.

16. World Health Organization. *The World Health Report*. Geneva: WHO, 1997.
17. Amos AF, McCarty DJ, Zimmet P. The rising global burden of diabetes and its complications: estimates and projections to the year 2010. *Diabetic Med* 1997; **14**:S7–85.
18. Hamman RF. Genetic and environmental determinants of non-insulin dependent diabetes mellitus (NIDDM). *Diabetes Metab Rev* 1993; **8**:287–338.
19. King H, Rewers M. WHO Ad Hoc Diabetes Reporting Group. Global estimates for prevalence of diabetes mellitus and impaired glucose tolerance in adults. *Diabetes Care* 1993; **16**:157–77.
20. Zimmet P, Dowse G, Serjeantson S, Finch C, King H. The epidemiology and natural history of NIDDM – Lessons from the South Pacific. *Diabetes Metab Rev* 1990; **6**:91–124.
21. Colditz GA, Willett WC, Rotnitzky A, Manson JE. Weight gain as a risk factor for clinical diabetes mellitus in women. *Ann Intern Med* 1995; **122**:481–6.
22. Ohlson LO, Larsson B, Björntorp P et al. Risk factors for type 2 (non-insulin dependent) diabetes mellitus: thirteen and one-half years of follow-up of the participants in a study of Swedish born men in 1913. *Diabetologia* 1988; **31**: 798–805.
23. Chan JM, Rimm EB, Colditz GA, Stampfer MJ, Willett WC. Obesity, fat distribution, and weight gain as risk factors for clinical diabetes in men. *Diabetes Care* 1994; **17**:961-9.
24. Holbrook TL, Barrett-Connor E, Wingard TL. The association of lifetime weight and weight control patterns with diabetes among men and women in an adult community. *Int J Obesity* 1989; **13**:723–9.
25. Hartz AJ, Rupley DC, Kalkhoff RD, Rimm AA. Relationship of obesity to diabetes: influence of obesity level and body fat distribution. *Prev Med* 1983; **12**: 351–7.
26. Schranz A, Tuomilehto J, Marti B, Jarrett JR, Grabauskas V, Vassalo A. Low physical activity and worsening of glucose tolerance: results from a 2-year follow-up of a population sample in Malta. *Diabetes Res Clin Pract* 1991; **11**:127–36.
27. Helmrich SP, Ragland DR, Ieung RW, Paffenberger RS Jr. Physical activity and reduced occurrence of non-insulin-dependent diabetes mellitus. *N Engl J Med* 1991; **325**:147–52.
28. Manson JE, Rimm EB, Stampfer MJ et al. Physical activity and incidence of non-insulin-dependent diabetes mellitus in women. *Lancet* 1991; **338**:774–8.
29. Eriksson KF, Lindgärde F. Prevention of type 2 (non-insulin-dependent) diabetes mellitus by diet and physical exercise: the six-year Malmö feasibility study. *Diabetologia* 1991; **34**:891–8.
30. Pan XR, Li GW, Hu YH et al. Effects of diet and exercise in preventing NIDDM in people with impaired glucose tolerance. The Da Qing IGT and Diabetes Study. *Diabetes Care* 1997; **20**:537–44.
31. WHO. *Prevention of Coronary Heart Disease. Report of a WHO Expert Committee.* WHO Technical Report Series, No. 678. Geneva: World Health Organization, 1982.
32. The Expert Committee on the Diagnosis and Classification of Diabetes Mellitus. Report of the Expert Committee on the diagnosis and classification of diabetes mellitus. *Diabetes Care* 1997; *20*:1183–97.
33. Prevention of Diabetes Mellitus. Report of WHO Study Group. Geneva: WHO Technical Report Series, No. 844. World Health Organization, 1994.
34. Eastman RC, Javitt JC, Herman VH et al. Model of complications of NIDDM. *Diabetes Care* 1997; **20**:725–34.

35. Segal L, Dalton A, Richardson J. *The Cost-effectiveness of Primary Prevention for Non-insulin Dependent Diabetes Mellitus*. Centre for Health Program Evaluation, 1996.
36. Engelgau MM, Aubert RE, Thompson TJ, Herman WH. Screening for NIDDM in Nonpregnant Adults. A review of principles, screening tests, and recommendations. *Diabetes Care* 1995; **18**:1006–18.
37. Javitt JC. Cost savings associated with detection and treatment of diabetic eye disease. *PharmacoEconomics* 1995; **8**(suppl 1): 33–9.
38. Klein R, Klein BEK, Moss SE et al. The Wisconsin epidemiology study of diabetic retinopathy. II. Prevalence and risk of diabetic retinopathy when age at diagnosis is less than 30 years. *Arch Ophthalmol* 1984; **102**:520–6.
39. Mathiesen ER, Borch-Johnsen K, Jensen DV et al. Improved survival in patients with diabetic nephropathy. *Diabetologia* 1989; **32**:884–6.
40. Viberti G, Mogensen CE, Groop LC et al. Effect of captopril on progression to clinical proteinuria in patients with insulin-dependent diabetes mellitus and microalbuminuria. *JAMA* 1994; **271**:275–9.
41. Siegel JE, Krolewski AS, Warram JH et al. Cost-effectiveness of screening and early treatment of nephropathy in patients with insulin-dependent diabetes mellitus. *J Am Soc Nephrol* 1992; **3**:3111–19.
42. Borch-Johnsen K, Wentzel H, Viberti GC et al. Is screening and intervention for microalbuminuria worthwhile in patients with insulin dependent diabetes? *BMJ* 1993; **306**:1722–5.
43. Andersen AR, Christiansen JS, Andersen JK et al. Diabetic nephropathy in type 1 (insulin-dependent) diabetes: an epidemiological study. *Diabetologia* 1983; **25**:496–501.
44. Mogensen CE. Microalbuminuria predicts clinical proteinuria and early mortality in maturity-onset diabetes. *N Engl J Med* 1984; **310**:356–60.
45. Jarret RJ, Viberti GC, Argyropoulos A, Hill RD, Mahmud U, Murrels TJ. Microalbuminuria predicts mortality in non-insulin-dependent diabetes. *Diabetic Med* 1984; **1**:17–19.
46. Edmunds ME, Blundell MP, Morris HE et al. Improved survival of the diabetic foot: the role of the specialised foot clinic. *Q J Med* 1986; **60**:763–71.
47. Cethia KK, Berry AR, Morrison JD et al. Changing pattern of lower limb amputation for vascular disease. *Br J Surg* 1986; **73**:701–3.
48. Jacobs J, Sena M, Fox N. The cost of hospitalization for the late complications of diabetes in the United States. *Diabetic Med* 1991; **8** Spec No: S23–9.
49. Rice DP. *Estimating the Costs of Illness. Health Economic Series*, PHS Publication no. 947–6. Washington: Government Printing Office, 1966.
50. Drummond M. Cost of illness studies. A major headache? *PharmacoEconomics* 1992; **2**:1–4.
51. Leese B. The cost of diabetes and its complications. *Soc Sci Med* 1992; **35**:1303–10.
52. Laing W, Williams R. *Diabetes. A Model for Health Care Management*. London: Office of Health Economics, 1989.
53. Kangas T. *The Finndiab Report. Health of People with Diabetes in Finland*. Helsinki, 1995.
54. Gagliardino JJ, Olivera EM, Barragan H et al. A simple economic evaluation model for selecting diabetes health care strategies. *Diabetic Med* 1993; **10**:351–4.
55. Triomphe A, Flori Y-A, Costagliola D et al. The cost of diabetes in France. *Health Policy* 1988; **9**:39–48.
56. Damsgaard EMS. Known diabetes and fasting hyperglycaemia in the elderly. *Dan Med Bull* 1990; **37**:530–46.

57. Javitt JC, Aiello LP, Bassi LJ et al. Detecting and treating retinopathy in patients with type I diabetes mellitus: savings associated with improved implementation of current guidelines. *Ophthalmology* 1991; **98**:1565–74.
58. Canner JK, Chiang YP, Javitt JC. PROPHET: A Monte Carlo based simulation network model for a chronic progressive disease: the case of diabetic retinopathy. *Proceedings of the Winter Simulation Conference* 1992; **25**:1041–9.
59. Dasbach E, Fryback D, Newcomb PN et al. Cost-effectiveness of strategies for detecting diabetic retinopathy. *Med Care* 1991; **29**:20–39.
60. Fendrick AM, Javitt JC, Chiang YP. Cost-effectiveness of the screening and treatment of diabetic retinopathy: what are the costs of underutilization? *Int J Technol Assess Health Care* 1992; **8**:694–707.
61. Bennett PH. Primary prevention of NIDDM: A practical reality. *Diabetes/Metab Rev* 1997; **13**:105–11.
62. Assal J-P. Primary Prevention of NIDDM: A future dream. *Diabetes/Metab Rev* 1997; **13**:113–17.

Index

Index compiled by Keyword Publishing Services Ltd